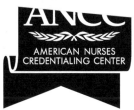

AMERICAN NURSES
CREDENTIALING CENTER

NURSING REVIEW AND RESOURCE MANUAL

Medical-Surgical Nursing, 3rd Edition

Published by American Nurses Credentialing Center

Authors: Nancy Henne Batchelor, MSN, RN-BC, CNS, Paula Gillman, MSN, RN-C, ANP-BC, GNP-BC, Jeanine Goodin, MSN, RN-BC, CNRN, Deborah Jane Schwytzer, MSN, RN-BC, CEN, Jo Nell Wells, PhD, RN-BC, OCN, and Eileen Werdman, MSN, RN-BC, CNS

CONTINUING EDUCATION SOURCE

NURSING CERTIFICATION REVIEW MANUAL

CLINICAL PRACTICE RESOURCE

Library of Congress Cataloging-in-Publication Data

Medical-surgical nursing : review and resource manual / by Nancy Henne Batchelor ... [et al.].
— 3rd ed.
    p. ;   cm.
  Rev. ed. of: Medical-surgical nursing review and resource manual. 2nd ed. c2007.
  Includes bibliographical references and index.
  ISBN 978–1-935213–21-5
  I. Batchelor, Nancy Henne. II. American Nurses Credentialing Center. III. Medical-surgical
nursing review and resource manual.
    [DNLM: 1. Education, Nursing, Continuing. 2. Perioperative Nursing—methods. WY 18.5]
    617'.0231076—dc23

The American Nurses Credentialing Center (ANCC), a subsidiary of the American Nurses
Association (ANA), provides individuals and organizations throughout the nursing profession
with the resources they need to achieve practice excellence. ANCC's internationally renowned
credentialing programs certify nurses in specialty practice areas; recognize healthcare organizations
for promoting safe, positive work environments through the Magnet Recognition Program® and
the Pathway to Excellence® Program; and accredit providers of continuing nursing education. In
addition, ANCC's Institute for Credentialing Innovation provides leading-edge information and
education services and products to support its core credentialing programs.

ISBN 13: 978-1-935213-21-5

© 2011 American Nurses Credentialing Center.
8515 Georgia Ave., Suite 400
Silver Spring, MD 20910

Medical-Surgical Nursing Review and Resource Manual, 3rd Edition

October 2011

Please direct your comments and/or queries to: revmanuals@ana.org

The healthcare services delivery system is a volatile marketplace demanding superior knowledge, clinical skills, and competencies from all registered nurses. Nursing autonomy of practice and nurse career marketability and mobility in the new century hinge on affirming the profession's formative philosophy, which places a priority on a lifelong commitment to the principles of education and professional development. The knowledge base of nursing theory and practice is expanding, and while care has been taken to ensure the accuracy and timeliness of the information presented in the **Medical-Surgical Nursing Review and Resource Manual, 3rd Edition,** clinicians are advised to always verify the most current national guidelines and recommendations and to practice in accordance with professional standards of care used with regard to the unique circumstances that apply in each practice situation. In addition, the editors wish to note that provision of information in this text does not imply an endorsement of any particular products, procedures or services.

Therefore, the authors, editors, American Nurses Association (ANA), American Nurses Association's Publishing (ANP), American Nurses Credentialing Center (ANCC), and the Institute for Credentialing Innovation cannot accept responsibility for errors or omissions, or for any consequences or liability, injury, and/or damages to persons or property from application of the information in this manual and make no warranty, express or implied, with respect to the contents of the **Medical-Surgical Nursing Review and Resource Manual, 3rd Edition.** Completion of this manual does not guarantee that the reader will pass the certification exam. The practice examination questions are not a requirement to take a certification examination. The practice examination questions cannot be used as an indicator of results on the actual certification.

Published by:

American Nurses Credentialing Center
The Institute for Credentialing Innovation
8515 Georgia Avenue, Suite 400
Silver Spring, MD 20910–3402
www.nursecredentialing.org

Introduction to the Continuing Education (CE) Contact Hour Application Process for *Medical-Surgical Nursing Review and Resource Manual, 3rd Edition*

The Institute for Credentialing Innovation now offers the continuing education contact hours for this manual online at www.NursingWorld.org, the American Nurses Association's Web site. This process involves answering approximately 25–30 questions that test knowledge of the information contained within this manual. The continuing education contact hours can be completed at any time and a certificate can be printed from the Web site immediately upon successful completion of the test. After studying the manual and given an online multiple-choice test, the exam candidate will be able to:

1. Pass the posttest with at least 75% of the answers correct.
2. Select responses to test questions based on key principles, standards of practice, and theoretical basis of nursing practice.
3. Choose accepted therapeutic interventions in answering questions related to quality nursing practice.
4. Utilize direct and indirect professional role responsibilities and applications regarding nursing practice in answering test questions.

Upon completion of this manual *and* the online CE test, a nurse can receive a total of 34 continuing education contact hours at a price of $68, only $2 per CE. (ANA members receive a discount on CEs.) **The entire process—online test and evaluation form—must be completed by December 31, 2013, in order to receive credit.** To begin the process, please e-mail **revmanuals@ana.org**. Your patience with this process is greatly appreciated.

Inquiries or Comments
If you have any questions about the CE contact hours, please e-mail The Institute at revmanuals@ana.org. You may also mail any comments to Editor/Project Manager at the address listed below.

Duplicate CE Certificates
Once you have successfully passed the CE test, you may go back and re-print your certificate as often as you wish.

Conflicts of Interest

A conflict of interest occurs when an individual has an opportunity to affect educational content about healthcare products or services of a commercial company with which she or he has a financial relationship.

The planners and presenters of this CNE activity have disclosed no relevant financial relationships with any commercial companies pertaining to this activity.

The Institute for Credentialing Innovation
American Nurses Credentialing Center
Attn: Editor/Project Manager
8515 Georgia Avenue, Suite 400
Silver Spring, MD 20910-3492
Fax: (301) 628-5342

A maximum of 34 contact hours may be earned by learners who successfully complete this continuing nursing education activity.

The American Nurses Association Center for Continuing Education and Professional Development is accredited as a provider of continuing nursing education by the American Nurses Credentialing Center's Commission on Accreditation.

ANCC Provider Number 0023

ANA is approved by the California Board of Registered Nursing, Provider Number 6178.

The ANA Center for Continuing Education and Professional Development includes ANCC's Institute for Credentialing Innovation.

Contents

MEDICAL-SURGICAL
NURSING REVIEW AND RESOURCE
MANUAL, 3RD EDITION

Taking the Certification Examination

When you sign up to take a national certification exam, you will be instructed to go online and review the testing and review handbook (www.nursecredentialing.org/documents/certification/application/generaltestingandrenewalhandbook.aspx). Review it carefully and be sure to bookmark the site so you can refer to it frequently. It contains information on test content and sample questions. This is critical information; it will give you insight into the nature of the test. The agency will send you information about the test site; keep this in a safe place until needed.

GENERAL SUGGESTIONS FOR PREPARING FOR THE EXAM

Step One: Control Your Anxiety
Everyone experiences anxiety when faced with taking the certification exam.
- Remember, your program was designed to prepare you to take this exam.
- Your instructors took a similar exam, and probably have talked to students who took exams more recently, so they know how to help you prepare.
- Taking a review course or setting up your own study plan will help you feel more confident about taking the exam.

Step Two: Do Not Listen to Gossip About the Exam
A large volume of information exists about the tests based on reports from people who have taken the exams in the past. Because information from the testing facilities is limited, it is hard to ignore this gossip.
- Remember that gossip about the exam that you hear from others is not verifiable.
- Because this gossip is based on the imperfect memory of people in a stressful situation, it may not be very accurate.

- People tend to remember those items testing content with which they are less comfortable; for instance, those with a limited background in women's health may say that the exam was "all women's health." In fact, the exam blueprint ensures that the exam covers multiple content areas without overemphasizing any one.

Step Three: Set Reasonable Expectations for Yourself
- Do not expect to know everything.
- Do not try to know everything in great detail.
- You do not need a perfect score to pass the exam.
- The exam is designed for a beginner level—it is testing readiness for *entry-level* practice.
- Learn the general rules, not the exceptions.
- The most likely diagnoses will be on the exam, not questions on rare diseases or atypical cases.
- Think about the most likely presentation and most common therapy.

Step Four: Prepare Mentally and Physically
- While you are getting ready to take the exam, take good physical care of yourself.
- Get plenty of sleep and exercise, and eat well while preparing for the exam.
- These things are especially important while you are studying and immediately before you take the exam.

Step Five: Access Current Knowledge

General Content
You will be given a list of general topics that will be on the exam when you register to take the exam. In addition, examine the table of contents of this book and the test content outline, available at www.nursecredentialing.org/cert/TCOs.html.
- What content do you need to know?
- How well do you know these subjects?

Take a Review Course
- Taking a review course is an excellent way to assess your knowledge of the content that will be included in the exam.
- If you plan to take a review course, take it well before the exam so you will have plenty of time to master any areas of weakness the course uncovers.
- If you are prepared for the exam, you will not hear anything new in the course. You will be familiar with everything that is taught.
- If some topics in the review course are new to you, concentrate on these in your studies.
- People have a tendency to study what they know; it is rewarding to study something and feel a mastery of it! Unfortunately, this will not help you master unfamiliar content. Be sure to use a review course to identify your areas of strength and weakness, then concentrate on the weaknesses.

Depth of Knowledge
How much do you need to know about a subject?
- You cannot know everything about a topic.
- Remember that the depth of knowledge required to pass the exam is for entry-level performance.

- Study the information sent to you from the testing agency, what you were taught in school, what is covered in this text, and the general guidelines given in this chapter.
- Look at practice tests designed for the exam. Practice tests for other exams will not be helpful.
- Consult your class notes or clinical diagnosis and management textbook for the major points about a disease. Additional reference books can be found online at www .nursecredentialing.org/cert/refs.html.
- For example, with regard to medications, know the drug categories and the major medications in each. Assume all drugs in a category are generally alike, and then focus on the differences among common drugs. Know the most important indications, contraindications, and side effects. Emphasize safety. The questions usually do not require you to know the exact dosage of a drug.

Step Six: Institute a Systematic Study Plan

Develop Your Study Plan

- Write up a formal plan of study.
  - Include topics for study, timetable, resources, and methods of study that work for you.
  - Decide whether you want to organize a study group or work alone.
  - Schedule regular times to study.
  - Avoid cramming; it is counterproductive. Try to schedule your study periods in 1-hour increments.
- Identify resources to use for studying. To prepare for the examination, you should have the following materials on your shelf:
  - A good pathophysiology text.
  - This review book.
  - A physical assessment text.
  - Your class notes.
  - Other important sources, including: information from the testing facility, a clinical diagnosis textbook, favorite journal articles, notes from a review course, and practice tests.
  - Know the important national standards of care for major illnesses.
  - Consult the bibliography on the test blueprint. When studying less familiar material, it is helpful to study using the same references that the testing center uses.
- Study the body systems from head to toe.
- The exams emphasize health promotion, assessment, differential diagnosis, and plan of care for common problems.
- You will need to know facts and be able to interpret and analyze this information utilizing critical thinking.

Personalize Your Study Plan

- How do you learn best?
  - If you learn best by listening or talking, attend a review course or discuss topics with a colleague.
  - Read everything the test facility sends you as soon as you receive it and several times during your preparation period. It will give you valuable information to help guide your study.
  - Have a specific place with good lighting set aside for studying. Find a quiet place with no distractions. Assemble your study materials.

Implement Your Study Plan

You must have basic content knowledge. In addition, you must be able to use this information to think critically and make decisions based on facts.

- Refer to your study plan regularly.
- Stick to your schedule.
- Take breaks when you get tired.
- If you start procrastinating, get help from a friend or reorganize your study plan.
- It is not necessary to follow your plan rigidly. Adjust as you learn where you need to spend more time.
- Memorize the basics of the content areas you will be required to know.

Focus on General Material

- Most of what you need to know is basic material that does not require constant updating.
- You do not need to worry about the latest information being published as you are studying for the exam. Remember, it can take 6 to 12 months for new information to be incorporated into test questions.

Pace Your Studying

- Stop studying for the examination when you are starting to feel overwhelmed and look at what is bothering you. Then make changes.
- Break overwhelming tasks into smaller tasks that you know you can do.
- Stop and take breaks while studying.

Work With Others

- Talk with classmates about your preparation for the exam.
- Keep in touch with classmates, and help each other stick to your study plans.
- If your classmates become anxious, do not let their anxiety affect you. Walk away if you need to.
- Do not believe bad stories you hear about other people's experiences with previous exams.
- Remember, you know as much as anyone about what will be on the next exam!

Consider a Study Group

- Study groups can provide practice in analyzing cases, interpreting questions, and critical thinking.
  - You can discuss a topic and take turns presenting cases for the group to analyze.
  - Study groups also can provide moral support and help you continue studying.

Step Seven: Strategies Immediately Before the Exam

Final Preparation Suggestions

- Use practice exams when studying to get accustomed to the exam format and time restrictions.
  - Many books that are labeled as review books are simply a collection of examination questions.
  - If you have test anxiety, such practice tests may help alleviate the anxiety.
  - Practice tests can help you learn to judge the time it should take you to complete the exam.

- Practice tests are useful for gaining experience in analyzing questions.
- Books of questions may not uncover the gaps in your knowledge that a more systematic content review text will reveal.
- If you feel that you don't know enough about a topic, refer to a text to learn more. After you feel that you have learned the topic, practice questions are a wonderful tool to help improve your test-taking skill.
- Know your test-taking style.
  - Do you rush through the exam without reading the questions thoroughly?
  - Do you get stuck and dwell on a question for a long time?
  - You should spend about 45 to 60 seconds per question and finish with time to review the questions you were not sure about.
  - Be sure to read the question completely, including all four answer choices. Choice "a" may be good, but "d" may be best.

The Night Before the Exam
- Be prepared to get to the exam on time.
  - Know the test site location and how long it takes to get there.
  - Take a "dry run" beforehand to make sure you know how to get to the testing site, if necessary.
  - Get a good night's sleep.
  - Eat sensibly.
  - Avoid alcohol the night before.
  - Assemble the required material—two forms of identification, admission card, pencil, and watch. Both IDs must match the name on the application, and one photo ID is preferred.
  - Know the exam room rules.
  - You will be given scratch paper, which will be collected at the end of the exam.
  - Nothing else is allowed in the exam room.
  - You will be required to put papers, backpacks, etc., in a corner of the room or in a locker.
  - No water or food will be allowed.
  - You will be allowed to walk to a water fountain and go to the bathroom one at a time.

The Day of the Exam
- Get there early. You must arrive at the test center at least 15 minutes before your scheduled appointment time. If you are late, you may not be admitted.
- Think positively. You have studied hard and are well-prepared.
- Remember your anxiety-reduction strategies.

Specific Tips for Dealing With Anxiety
Test anxiety is a specific type of anxiety. Symptoms include upset stomach, sweaty palms, tachycardia, trouble concentrating, and a feeling of dread. But there are ways to cope with test anxiety.
- There is no substitute for being well-prepared.
- Practice relaxation techniques.
- Avoid alcohol, excess coffee, caffeine, and any new medications that might sedate you, dull your senses, or make you feel agitated.
- Take a few deep breaths and concentrate on the task at hand.

Focus on Specific Test-Taking Skills
To do well on the exam, you need good test-taking skills in addition to knowledge of the content and ability to use critical thinking.

All Certification Exams Are Multiple Choice
- Multiple-choice tests have specific rules for test construction.
- A multiple-choice question consists of three parts: the information (or stem), the question, and the four possible answers (one correct and three distracters).
- Careful analysis of each part is necessary. Read the entire question before answering.
- Practice your test-taking skills by analyzing the practice questions in this book and on the ANCC Web site.

Analyze the Information Given
- Do not assume you have more information than is given.
- Do not overanalyze.
- Remember, the writer of the question assumes this is all of the information needed to answer the question.
- If information is not given, it is not relevant and will not affect the answer.
- Do not make the question more complicated than it is.

What Kind of Question Is Asked?
- Are you supposed to recall a fact, apply facts to a situation, or understand and differentiate between options?
  - Read the question thinking about what the writer is asking.
  - Look for key words or phrases that lead you (see Figure 1–1). These help determine what kind of answer the question requires.

Figure 1–1. Examples of Key Words and Phrases

avoid	initial	most
best	first	significant
except	contributing to	likely
not	appropriate	of the following
		most consistent with

Read All of the Answers
- If you are absolutely certain that answer "a" is correct as you read it, mark it, but read the rest of the question so you do not trick yourself into missing a better answer.
- If you are absolutely sure answer "a" is wrong, cross it off or make a note on your scratch paper and continue reading the question.
- After reading the entire question, go back, analyze the question, and select the best answer.
- Do not jump ahead.
- If the question asks you for an assessment, the best answer will be an assessment. Do not be distracted by an intervention that sounds appropriate.
- If the question asks you for an intervention, do not answer with an assessment.

- When two answer choices sound very good, the best one is usually the least expensive, least invasive way to achieve the goal. For example, if your answer choices include a physical exam maneuver or imaging, the physical exam maneuver is probably the better choice provided it will give the information needed.
- If the answers include two options that are the opposite of each other, one of the two is probably the correct answer.
- When numeric answers cover a wide range, a number in the middle is more likely to be correct.
- Watch out for distracters that are correct but do not answer the question, combine true and false information, or contain a word or phrase that is similar to the correct answer.
- Err on the side of caution.

Only One Answer Can Be Correct
- When more than one suggested answer is correct, you must identify the one that best answers the question asked.
- If you cannot choose between two answers, you have a 50% chance of getting it right if you guess.

Avoid Changing Answers
- Change an answer only if you have a compelling reason, such as you remembered something additional, or you understand the question better after rereading it.
- People change to a wrong answer more often than to a right answer.

Time Yourself to Complete the Whole Exam
- Do not spend a large amount of time on one question.
- If you cannot answer a question quickly, mark it and continue the exam.
- If time is left at the end, return to the difficult questions.
- Make educated guesses by eliminating the obviously wrong answers and choosing a likely answer even if you are not certain.
- Trust your instinct.
- Answer every question. There is no penalty for a wrong answer.
- Occasionally a question will remind you of something that helps you with a question earlier in the test. Look back at that question to see if what you are remembering affects how you would answer that question.

ABOUT THE CERTIFICATION EXAMS

The American Nurses Credentialing Center Computerized Exam
The ANCC examination is given only as a computer exam, and each exam is different. The order of the questions is scrambled for every test, so even if two people are taking the same exam, the questions will be in a different order. The exam consists of 175 multiple-choice questions.
- 150 of the 175 questions are part of the test and how you answer will count toward your score; 25 are included to refine questions and will not be scored. You will not know which ones count, so treat all questions the same.
- You will need to know how to use a mouse, scroll by either clicking arrows on the scroll bar or using the up and down arrow keys, and perform other basic computer tasks.
- The exam does not require computer expertise.

- However, if you are not comfortable with using a computer, you should practice using a mouse and computer beforehand so you do not waste time on the mechanics of using the computer.
- Know what to expect during the test.
- Each ANCC test question is independent of the other questions.
- For each case study, there is only one question. This means that a correct answer on any question does not depend on the correct answer to any other question.
- Each question has four possible answers. There are no questions asking for combinations of correct answers (such as "a and c") or multiple-multiples.
- You can skip a question and go back to it at the end of the exam.
- You cannot mark key words in the question or right or wrong answers. If you want to do this, use the scratch paper.
- You will get your results immediately, and a grade report will be provided upon leaving the testing site.

INTERNET RESOURCES

- ANCC Web site: www.nursecredentialing.org
- ANA Bookstore: www.nursesbooks.org. Catalog of ANA nursing scope and standards publications and other titles that may be listed on your test content outline
- National Guideline Clearinghouse: www.ngc.gov

2

Development

Nancy Henne Batchelor, MSN, RN-BC, CNS

INTRODUCTION

- Theories attempt to explain aspects of human development.
- Theories provide a scientific basis for practice.
- Theories conceptualize a framework to address practice situations.
- Theories provide a perspective in which to view practice situations.

PSYCHOLOGICAL THEORIES

- Assumption: Aging is a dynamic developmental process.
  - Incorporate beliefs of biological and sociological theories.
    - Weave adaptive coping mechanisms into how a person behaves.
    - Memory, learning, emotions, motivation are part of psychological coping.
    - Mechanisms are challenged as one ages.

Maslow's Hierarchy of Needs
- Physiologic: Air, food, water, elimination, and shelter
  - Safety and security: Feeling emotionally and physically safe and secure
  - Love and belonging: Feeling good about oneself, respect for others, and personal and professional success
- Self-actualization: Reaching one's full potential
  - Some needs are perceived as more prevailing than others.
  - Higher needs are met only after lower needs have been satisfied.

Piaget's Stages of Cognitive Development

- Sensorimotor: Birth to 1½ years
  - Learning through sensory input
- Preoperational: 1½ to 7 years
  - Egocentric or one-dimensional thinking
  - Incomplete understanding of cause and effect
- Concrete Operational: 7 to 11 years
  - Able to understand cause and effect
  - Able to classify information
- Formal Operational: 11 years and older
  - Able to think abstractly
  - Able to reason about hypothetical situations
  - Egocentric

Erickson's Theory

- Trust vs Mistrust: Infancy to 1 year
  - Require consistency and nurturing
  - Security attained through having needs met
- Autonomy vs Shame and Doubt: 1 to 2 years
  - Assert independence
  - Overprotection and punishment lead to shame and doubt
- Initiative vs Guilt: 3 to 5 years (early childhood)
  - Engage in purposeful, active behavior
  - Increase responsibility
- Industry vs Inferiority: 6 to 10 years (middle childhood)
  - Master knowledge and intellectual skills
  - Expansive imagination
- Identity vs Identity Confusion: 10 to 20 years (adolescence)
  - Explore roles
  - Ask who, what, and where
  - Preteens and teens model behaviors of young adults
  - Safety concerns: Seat belt usage, abstinence from underage drinking, increased awareness of legal consequences of behavior
- Intimacy vs Isolation: 20s to 30s (early adulthood)
  - Form close relationships, maintain friendships
  - Find and manage career, children, home
- Generativity vs Stagnation: 40s to 60s (middle adulthood)
  - Continue tasks of early adulthood: friendships, family, career
  - Transmit positive things to next generation
  - Parent, teach, social activism
  - Leave a legacy
  - Assist grown children
  - Find areas of new satisfaction
  - Care for aging parents
  - Safety concerns: drinking and driving, safety belt use
  - Awareness of cognitive changes and drug interactions
  - Evaluate role overload
- Integrity vs Despair: 60s and older (late adulthood)
  - Life review, reflection, and evaluation
  - Adapt to physical changes of aging

- Redirect energies and talents to new direction
- Develop personal view of death
- Safety concerns: seat belt use, drinking and driving
- Check for cognitive changes and drug interactions
- Because of increased life expectancy, this stage can be subdivided
  - Psychologist Robert Peck identifies three subdivisions:
    - Body Transcendence vs Body Preoccupation
      - Adjust to changes and decline caused by physical aging
      - Find satisfying interpersonal and social activities
    - Ego Differentiation vs Role Preoccupation
      - Achieve feelings of worth and self-significance from areas other than work
    - Ego Transcendence vs Ego Preoccupation
      - Accept that death is inevitable without dwelling on it

PHYSICAL AND COGNITIVE THEORIES

Early Adulthood
- Physical functioning
  - Peak of strength, energy, and endurance
  - Fully developed body function by mid-40s
  - Senses are sharpest
- Health
  - Most without chronic conditions
  - Most medical interventions due to injury or pregnancy
- Cognitive development
  - Postformal thought
    - Problem-solving by relativistic thinking rather than pure logic
    - Draw upon previous experiences to problem-solve
    - Rely on intuition and logic

Middle Adulthood
- Physical functioning
  - Declines are small and gradual, noticeable in mid-forties
  - Hearing: perception of high-pitched sounds declines (presbycusis)
  - Vision: focus and visual acuity declines
  - Strength and coordination decline due to loss of muscle mass secondary to sedentary lifestyle
  - Endurance maintained
  - Decline in reproductive capacity
- Health
  - Middle-aged are typically healthy
  - Hypertension increases from midlife forward
  - Leading causes of death: heart disease, cancer, accidents
  - Stress causes physiological response and weakens immune system
  - Positive lifestyle factors are associated with less stress
- Cognitive
  - Crystallized intelligence improves through middle age
  - Remember and use information acquired over a lifetime

- Postformal thought
  - Relies on subjective feelings and intuition as well as logic
  - Interprets meaning
  - Reconciles or chooses among conflicting views

Older Adulthood

- Physical functioning
  - Changes are highly variable.
  - Declines may be effects of disease rather than causes.
  - Healthier lifestyles may maintain higher physical function.
  - Changes in brain result in slower response time.
- Health
  - Many have two or more chronic diseases.
  - Depression is underdiagnosed in older adults.
  - Dementia increases and may be due to disease:
    - Hypertension
    - Stroke
    - Parkinson's disease
- Cognitive
  - Crystallized intelligence is maintained.
  - Problem-solving intact, but slower processing time.
  - Deterioration may be related to disuse.

DR. K. WARNER SCHAIE'S STAGES OF ADULT DEVELOPMENT
- Acquisitive (childhood/adolescence)
- Achieving (early adulthood)
  - Attain long-term goals: career, family, society
- Responsible (middle adulthood)
  - Protect and nourish spouses, families, careers
- Executive (middle adulthood)
  - Take broader perspective, concerned about world
- Reintegrative (late adulthood)
  - Focus on tasks of personal meaning

SOCIOLOGICAL THEORIES OF AGING

- The theories of Elaine Cumming and William Henry, sociologists, deal with roles and relationships assumed by people as they age.

Disengagement

- As individuals age, they disengage and become self-centered.
- Internalization and withdrawal from society.
- Separation is desired by society and older adults.
- Serves to maintain social equilibrium.

Activity

- Robert Havighurst and Ruth Albrecht promoted the idea that activity is necessary to promote life satisfaction and positive self-concept.

- Activity can delay the negative effects of old age.
- Three assumptions:
  - It is better to be active than nonactive.
  - It is better to be happy than unhappy.
  - The individual is the best judge of his/her happiness.

Continuity

- Bernice Neugarten, Robert Havighurst, and Sheldon Tobin promoted the theory that character and personality is consistent with earlier stages and continues through the rest of life.
  - Previous habits, preferences, values, and beliefs do not change with age.

Age Stratification

- The aging person and society are interdependent and interact dynamically.
- Each person's place in society is based on a cohort: psychological, social, or biological.
- New cohorts experience society differently than others.
- Society can be divided according to age and roles.
- People, roles, and society continually change.
- Interactions between older persons and society are ever-changing.

Person–Environment Fit

- Lawton's theory that a person's competencies change throughout life and play a role in helping the person deal with changing environments.
  - Competencies
    - Ego strength
    - Motor skills
    - Biological health
    - Cognitive capacities
    - Sensory-perceptual capacities
    - As competencies are altered in old age, so is the ability to interact with environment.

BIOLOGICAL THEORIES OF AGING

Error Theory

- Errors occur during DNA transcription, leading to aging or death of cells.
- If left unchecked, errors produce cells unlike the original cells.

Free Radical Theory

- Molecular reactions within cell membranes interfere with RNA–DNA transcription.
  - Molecular particles break off and attach to other molecules, causing altered cell structure.

Cross-Link Theory

- Proteins become cross-linked or entwined, causing altered metabolic processes.
  - Nutrients and wastes between cellular compartments interfere with cellular transport, causing organ and body system failure.

Wear and Tear Theory
- Tissues have a preprogrammed amount of available energy and eventually wear out when energy is depleted.

Programmed Aging/Hayflick Limit Theory
- Cells have limited ability to replicate.
- Life expectancy/aging phenomenon is a preprogrammed, species-specific biological clock.

Immunity Theory
- Immune function decreases with age.
  - T and B cells respond differently to invading organisms.
  - Aging increases cancer risk due to decreased resistance to tumor cells.
  - Aging increases production of autoantigens, leading to autoimmune disease.

Emerging Biological Theories

NEUROENDOCRINE CONTROL
- Complex interactions governing hormone production decline over time.
- Identifies roles of hypothalamus, DHEA, and melatonin in longevity immune function and aging process.

METABOLIC/CALORIC RESTRICTION
- All organisms have a finite amount of metabolic lifetime.
- Those with higher metabolic rates have shorter life spans.

DNA-RELATED RESEARCH
- Cells have limited capacity to divide.

GENETIC THEORY
- Life span is largely determined by the genes one inherits.
  - Genes explain 35% of life span.
  - Remaining determinants: behaviors, exposures, and luck.

CHANGES ACROSS THE LIFE SPAN/LIFE TRANSITIONS

Developmental Transitions
- Processes that occur over time and that require changes in identities, roles, relationships, abilities, and patterns of behavior (Schumacher & Meleis, 1994).
- A person moves through socially prescribed norms into new categories, roles, and statuses (Ebersole & Hess, 1998).
- Involve a disruption in usual life patterns—considered to be periods of instability.

Box 2-1. Common Life Transitions

Marriage	Travel
Birth	Home ownership
Retirement	Divorce
Death	School graduation
Disabling accident	Moving
New jobs	

Box 2-2. Conditions Influencing the Outcome of Transitions

Meaning
Expectations
Level of knowledge
Planning
Emotional reserves
Physical reserves
Level of support

Nursing Measures That Positively Influence Outcome of Transition
- State of readiness, preparedness, and sufficient anticipatory guidance
- Education: includes knowledge and practice of new skills
- Environmental exposure and support

Role Transitions for the Older Adult
- Parent to grandparent
- Primary caregiver to care recipient
- Health to illness
- Work to retirement
- Paid worker to volunteer
- Widowhood
- Role reversal: independence to dependence
- Relocation

Nursing Role for Patients Experiencing Transition
- Provide an environment that encourages independence, exploration, and recognition of uncertainty resulting from transition.
- Help patients locate available resources for specific needs.
- Facilitate adjustment to widowhood through recognition and referral to social networks.
- Evaluate attitudes about retirement.
- Provide referrals for assistance with health-related financial planning and income management.
- Educate patients regarding common changes associated with aging.
- Promote optimum functioning, prevention and early treatment of health problems, and stress management techniques.

Interventions to Assist Older Adults in Responding to Life Transitions

LIFE REVIEW AND LIFE STORY
- Assess one's life in totality.
- Reflect on past experience to resolve troublesome and traumatic events.

SELF-REFLECTION
- Awareness of self and one's place in the world; expression of feelings
  - Journaling
  - Writing letters and e-mail
  - Art

STRENGTHEN INNER RESOURCES
- Physical, emotional, and spiritual

EMPOWERMENT
- Include in care planning and caregiving activities
- Provide options and freedom to choose
- Equip for self-care and self-direction through education, sharing, and support

ADVOCATE
- Provide support, feedback, and reinforcement

REFERENCES

Ebersole, P., & Hess, P. (2006). *Toward healthy aging: Human needs and nursing response* (7th ed.). St. Louis, MO: Mosby.

Eliopolous, C. (2010). *Gerontological nursing* (7th ed.). Philadelphia: Lippincott Williams & Wilkins.

Miller, C. A. (2008). *Nursing for wellness in older adults: Theory and practice (5th ed.)*. Philadelphia: Lippincott Williams & Wilkins.

Osborn, K. S., Wraa, C. E., & Watson, A. B. (2010). *Medical surgical nursing: Preparation for practice*. Saddle River, NJ: Pearson.

3

Communication

Jeanine Goodin, MSN, RN-BC, CNRN,
& Jo Nell Wells, PhD, RN-BC, OCN

Therapeutic & Interviewing Skills

COMMUNICATION OVERVIEW

- Open lines of communication between nurse and patient are essential so the patient is able to express any emergent needs or problems. The patient remains the focus of therapeutic communication.
- When you plan to have lengthy interactions with a patient, it is important to address physical care priorities so the discussion is not interrupted. Make the patient comfortable by ensuring that any symptoms are under control and that any elimination needs have been met.
- Effective verbal communication requires appropriate intonation, clear and concise phrasing, proper pacing of statements, and proper timing and relevance of a message.
- Nurses strengthen helping relationships by establishing trust, empathy, autonomy, confidentiality, and professional competence.

THERAPEUTIC COMMUNICATION TECHNIQUES

- Therapeutic communication techniques are specific responses that encourage the expression of feelings and ideas and convey acceptance and respect. Therapeutic relationships and achievement of desired patient outcomes are facilitated by the following skills.

Active Listening

- Be attentive to what the patient is saying both verbally and nonverbally. Some effective communicators suggest it is important to remember that we have two ears and one mouth and we should use them in that 2:1 ratio. Several nonverbal skills facilitate attentive listening. Townsend (2003) suggests the following guidelines for therapeutic listening:
  - S: Sit facing the patient.
  - O: Open posture: keep arms and legs uncrossed.
  - L: Lean toward the patient to convey that you are involved and interested in the interaction.
  - E: Establish and maintain eye contact to convey involvement and willingness to listen.
  - R: Relax. This conveys a feeling of interest in and comfort with the patient.

Sharing Observations

- Avoid making assumptions and drawing unnecessary conclusions about the other person without validating them. Do comment on how the other person looks, sounds, or acts. Avoid stating observations that will embarrass or anger the patient because this can lead to resentment. Therapeutic examples include: "You look sad...," "You seem different today...," or "I see you haven't eaten your breakfast."

Sharing Empathy

- Empathy is the ability to understand and accept another person's reality, to accurately perceive feeling, and to communicate this understanding to the other. Statements reflecting empathy are highly effective because they tell the patient that the nurse hears the feeling content, as well as factual content, of the communication. Example: The nurse says to an angry patient who has low mobility after a motor vehicle accident, "It must be very frustrating to want to be more active and not be able to do so."

Sharing Hope

- Appropriate encouragement and positive feedback are important in fostering hope and self-confidence and for helping people achieve their potential and reach their goals. You can reassure patients that there are many kinds of hope and that meaning and personal growth can come from the illness experience. Example: The nurse says to a patient discouraged about a poor prognosis, "I believe you will find a way to face your situation, because I have seen your courage and creativity in the past."

Sharing Humor

- Humor is an important but underused resource in nursing interactions that can improve the patient's self-esteem and make the nurse seem more approachable. The nurse's goal in using humor is to bring hope and joy to the situation and enhance the patient's well-being and the therapeutic relationship. Humor must be used carefully when communicating with patients of another culture or within earshot of patients or their loved ones who have been given distressing healthcare news or experienced unsuccessful health care (McCabe, 2004).

Sharing Feelings

- Feelings are not right, wrong, good, or bad, although they are pleasant or unpleasant. If people do not express feelings, stress may increase and illness will worsen. It is appropriate to share feelings of caring, or even cry with others, as long as the nurse is in control of the expression of those feelings and does so in a way that does not burden the patient or break confidentiality. A social support system of colleagues is helpful. Employee assistance programs, peer group meetings, and the use of interdisciplinary teams including social work and pastoral care can provide means for nurses to safely express feelings away from patients.

Using Touch

- Touch can bring the sense of caring and human connection to the patient. Comfort touch, such as holding a hand, is especially important for vulnerable patients who are experiencing severe illness with its accompanying physical and emotional losses. In older persons, touch increases a sense of safety, increases self-confidence, and decreases anxiety (Gleeson & Timmins, 2004). Nurses need to be sensitive to others' reactions to touch and use it wisely. Touch should be as gentle or as firm as needed and delivered in a comforting, nonthreatening manner. There are times when you withhold touch; for example, with highly suspicious and angry persons who might respond negatively or even violently to the nurse's touch.

Using Silence

- Silence allows the patient to think and gain insight. In general, allow the patient to break the silence, particularly when the patient has initiated it (Stuart & Laraia, 2005). Silence is especially therapeutic during times of profound sadness or grief. It also allows the nurse to observe nonverbal messages and demonstrates the nurse's patience and willingness to wait for a response when the other person is unable to reply quickly.

Providing Information

- It is usually not helpful to hide information from patients, particularly when they seek it. If a physician withholds information, the nurse needs to clarify the reason with the physician. Patients have a right to know about their health status and what is happening in their environment. Distressing information needs to be communicated with sensitivity, at a pace appropriate to what the patient can absorb, and in general terms at first. Example: "Mrs. Burgess, your heart sounds have changed from earlier today, and so has your blood pressure. I'll let your doctor know."

Clarifying

- During a conversation, either party may need to assess accurate understanding of a statement or restate an unclear or ambiguous message to make the meaning clear. For example, the nurse asks the patient to rephrase what he or she just said, explain further, or give an example of what the patient means. Sometimes you will not understand the patient's message and need to let the patient know this is the case. Example: "I'm not sure I understand what you mean by 'having a bad day.' What is different now?"

Focusing

- The nurse uses focusing to guide the direction of conversation to important areas. This is a useful technique when the conversation is vague or rambling or a patient begins to repeat himself or herself. Example: "We've talked a lot about your dizzy spells, but let's look more closely at the timeline for the last two dizzy episodes."

Paraphrasing

- Restate the patient's message more briefly, using your own words, to let the patient know that you are actively involved in the search for understanding. For example, a patient says, "I've been a smoker all my life and never had any problems. I can't understand why I need to stop now." Example: "You're not convinced you need to stop smoking because you've stayed healthy?"

Asking Relevant Questions

- Focused questions are used when you need more specific information for decision-making. Remember to ask only one question at a time and fully explore one topic before moving to another. Use open-ended questions to allow the patient to take the lead and introduce pertinent information about a topic. Examples: "What's your biggest problem at the moment?" "How has your pain affected your life at home?" A useful exercise is to try conversing without asking the other person a single question, instead use general leads such as "Tell me about it...," making observations, paraphrasing, focusing, and providing information.

Summarizing

- A concise review of key aspects of a conversation aids recall, brings a sense of satisfaction and closure to an individual conversation, and is especially helpful during the termination phase of a nurse–patient relationship. It clarifies expectation and shows the patient that the nurse has analyzed communication. Example: "You've told me a lot of things about why you don't like this town and how unhappy you've been. We've also come up with some possible ways to make things better, and you've agreed to try some and let me know if any of them help."

Self-Disclosure

- Self-disclosure needs to be relevant and appropriate and made to benefit the patient rather than the nurse. Use it sparingly, so the patient is the focus of the interaction. Example: "I stopped smoking with the help of a counselor, and it was still very difficult. What are your thoughts about seeing a counselor?"

Confrontation

- This approach is used when the patient's words differ from what his or her body language is saying. Share your observations only after you have established trust, and do it gently, with sensitivity, to help the patient become more aware of inconsistencies in their feelings, attitudes, beliefs, and behaviors (Stuart & Laraia, 2005).

Nontherapeutic Communication Techniques

- Try to avoid the following communication techniques to allow for therapeutic communication. Achievement of desired patient outcomes is hindered or blocked by these forms of communication.

Asking Personal Questions

- Avoid nosy, invasive, and unnecessary questions that are not relevant to the situation but simply serve to satisfy the nurse's curiosity. Remember to ask open-ended questions rather than "Why?" questions.

Giving Personal Opinions

- At times, patients need suggestions and help to make choices; however, the patient, not the nurse, must make the decision. Offer your suggestions as options, and remember that the problem and its solution belong to the patient, not the nurse.

Changing the Subject

- This approach tends to block further communication so the patient withholds important information or fails to openly express feelings. In some instances, changing the subject serves as a face-saving maneuver. If the nurse or patient changes the subject, reassure the patient that you will return to his or her concerns at a more private time.

Automatic Responses

- Making stereotyped remarks about others reflects poor nursing judgment and threatens nurse–patient and team relationships. Avoid clichés (stereotyped comments) such as "You can't win them all," "Older adults are often confused," or "Administration does not care about staff." Remember to focus on the patient's comments to appear approachable and caring.

False Reassurance

- Although the nurse who uses this communication technique is trying to be kind, offering reassurance not supported by facts or based in reality will do more harm than good. False reassurance tends to block conversation and discourage further expression of feelings.

Sympathy

- The nurse's own emotional issues can prevent effective problem-solving and impair good judgment when the nurse over-identifies with the patient. Nurse objectivity is lost and the nurse is not able to help the patient work through the situation (Arnold & Boggs, 2003). Use empathy rather than sympathy. Example of sympathy: "I'm so sorry about...." A more empathic approach: "The loss of...is a major change. How do you think it will affect your life?"

Asking for Explanations

- Avoid the use of "Why?" questions. Patients tend to see this technique as a way to accuse or test them when the nurse already knows the answer. This approach can foster resentment, insecurity, and mistrust. In the place of "why" questions, use therapeutic techniques such as asking open-ended questions or sharing observations.

Approval or Disapproval

- Judgmental responses by the nurse often contain terms such as *should, ought, good, bad, right,* or *wrong.* Agreeing or disagreeing sends the subtle message you have the right to make value judgments about patient decisions.

Defensive Responses

- The patient's concerns are ignored when the nurse focuses on the need for self-defense or the defense of others. Attempt to listen uncritically and avoid defensiveness, to defuse anger, and to uncover deeper concerns.

Passive or Aggressive Responses

- Passive responses serve to avoid conflict or sidestep issues. Aggressive responses provoke confrontation at the other person's expense and reflect feelings of anger, frustration, resentment, and stress. Avoid triangulation, which is complaining to a third party rather than confronting the problem or expressing concerns directly to the source. Assertive communication is a far more professional approach for the nurse to take.

Arguing

- Challenging or arguing against perceptions denies that they are real and valid to the patient. The therapeutic nurse gives information or presents reality in a way that avoids argument.

INTERVIEWING SKILLS

- A helping relationship between nurse and patient does not just happen; the nurse creates it with care, skill, and trust. A natural progression of four goal-directed phases characterizes the nurse–patient relationship. Those phases are:

Preinteraction Phase

- In this phase, the nurse prepares for the first face-to-face meeting with the patient. The nurse reviews the medical and nursing history and talks to other caregivers who have information about the patient, which allows the nurse to anticipate health concerns or issues that may arise.

Orientation Phase

- This phase occurs when the nurse and patient meet and get to know one another and sets the tone for the relationship. The nurse and patient observe one another. The nurse assesses the patient's health status, prioritizes the patient's problems, and identifies the patient's goals. The nurse forms contracts with the patient that specify who will do what and lets the patient know when to expect the relationship to be terminated.

Working Phase

- In this phase, the nurse and patient work together to solve problems and accomplish goals. The nurse and patient take actions to meet the set goals. The nurse encourages and helps the patient to express feelings about his or her health, provides information the patient needs to understand and change behavior, and uses appropriate self-disclosure and confrontation.

Termination Phase

- This is the ending of the relationship and occurs most therapeutically by reminding the patient that termination is near. Evaluate goal achievement with the patient and separate from the patient by relinquishing responsibility for his or her care. Achieve a smooth transition to other caregivers for the patient as needed.

PROFESSIONAL COMMUNICATION AND BARRIERS TO COMMUNICATION

- In the healthcare setting, communication is necessary and integral to the delivery of safe patient care. Professional communication involves multiple interfaces and patient handoffs among numerous healthcare practitioners at varying levels of educational preparation. Safe and effective clinical practice involves many situations in which vital information must be communicated accurately. Effective communication can lead to these positive outcomes: better information flow, more effective interventions, enhanced safety, improved employee morale, increased patient and family satisfaction, adherence to treatment, improved treatment outcomes, and decreased lengths of stay. Nurses must collaborate with other disciplines in the provision of care. A common barrier to effective communication between healthcare providers is hierarchies. When healthcare professionals do not communicate effectively, patient safety may be compromised.
- Barriers to interprofessional communication between healthcare providers:
  - Complexity of care
  - Concerns about clinical responsibilities
  - Concerns of diluted professional identity
  - Culture
  - Differences in accountability, payment, and rewards
  - Differences in personality
  - Disruptive behavior
  - Emphasis on rapid decision-making
  - Gender
  - Generational differences
  - Hierarchy
  - Historical interprofessional and intraprofessional rivalries
  - Language and jargon differences
  - Personal expectations and values
  - Differences in schedule and professional routine
  - Varying levels of educational preparation, qualifications, and status
  - Differences in requirements, regulations, and norms of professional education and licensure
- Communication barriers between the patient and healthcare provider
  - Physical barriers
    - Space between participants
    - Characteristics of the room
      - Acoustics
      - Arrangement of the furniture
      - Audiovisual equipment
      - Lighting
      - Temperature
    - Noise level
    - Sensory impairments
      - Hearing, speech, or vision deficits
        - Accents or dialects
      - Effects of medications, disease, or treatment

- Language and vocabulary
  - Fluency in the same language
  - Medical terminology
- Psychosocial barriers
  - Developmental age or stage
    - Regression may occur with stress or illness.
  - Low literacy levels or difficulty reading healthcare information
    - Healthcare provider must recognize the sensory input level of the patient.
    - Risk factor for the patient not comprehending information and resuming poor health patterns.
      - Patients with low health literacy are more likely to have increased hospitalizations, higher healthcare costs, medication noncompliance, depression, and diabetes complications.
    - Provide the patient with nonmedical terminology, pictures, and diagrams.
  - Personal state
    - Emotional state
    - Preconceived ideas
      - About role of caregiver
      - Related to disease or diagnosis
    - Previous experiences
      - Within the healthcare system
      - With persons with similar diagnosis or needs
    - Personal or societal beliefs
      - Impact of values, morals, or judgments
    - Body language, eye contact, facial expressions, touch, tone of voice, and nods of the head
- Communication with other healthcare team members
  - Healthcare jargon is appropriate to convey precise meanings.
  - Both oral and written; important elements of oral exchanges must be documented in the medical record.
- Transfer of care
  - Communication must occur between healthcare providers, whether the transfer of care is temporary or permanent.
  - Information shared should be concise but complete.
  - SBAR method provides a standardized structure for concise, factual communication.
    - S: Situation
    - B: Background
    - A: Assessment
    - R: Recommendations
      - Include any issues, tests, and results that are in process or pending.
  - Information may be oral or written.
    - The opportunity to clarify information and ask or answer questions is essential to this process.
    - SBAR should be used for any situation where patient information is communicated between members of the healthcare team.
- Encountering difficult people or situations
  - Address the behavior in private.
    - Away from patients and families
    - Away from patient care areas

- May be beneficial to have a neutral third party present.
- Describe the issue, conflict, or behavior.
  - Remain calm.
  - Use "I" statements.
  - Describe the effects of words or actions.
- If the issue remains unresolved, use appropriate chain of command to address concerns.
  - Nursing chain of command
  - Family services chain of command
  - Medical staff office chain of command
  - State nurses' association

REFERENCES

Arnold, E. (2009). Communication and the nurse-patient relationship. In E. Arnold & K. Kverno, *Psychiatric-mental health nursing review and resource manual* (3rd ed., pp. 29–46). Silver Spring, MD: American Nurses Credentialing Center.

Arnold, E., & Boggs, K. U. (2003). *Interpersonal relationships: Professional communication skills for nurses* (4th ed.). St. Louis, MO: Saunders.

Corlett, K. (2010). Communication. In P. K. Y. Chiplis, K. Corlett, M. J. Gilmer, & C. J. Richardson, *Pediatric nursing review and resource manual* (2nd ed., pp. 19–26). Silver Spring, MD: American Nurses Credentialing Center.

Gleeson, M., & Timmins, F. (2004). Touch: A fundamental aspect of communication with older people experiencing dementia. *Nursing Older People, 16*(2), 18.

Institute for Healthcare Improvement. (n.d.). *SBAR technique for communication: A situational briefing model.* Retrieved from http://www.ihi.org/IHI/Topics/PatientSafety/SafetyGeneral/Tools/SBARTechniqueforCommunicationASituationalBriefingModel.htm

McCabe, C. (2004) Nurse–patient communication: An exploration of patients' experiences. *Journal of Clinical Nursing, 13*(1), 41.

O'Daniel, M., & Rosenstein, A. H. (n.d.). *Professional communication and team collaboration.* Retrieved from http://www.ahrq.gov/qual/nurseshdbk/docs/O'DanielM_TWC.pdf

Potter, P. A., & Perry, A. G. (2009). *Fundamentals of nursing* (7th ed.). St. Louis, MO: Mosby Elsevier.

Stuart, G. W., & Laraia, M. T. (2005). *Principles and practice of psychiatric nursing* (8th ed.). St. Louis, MO: Mosby.

Townsend, M. (2003). *Psychiatric mental health nursing: Concepts of care.* Philadelphia: F.A. Davis.

Williams, E. *Healthcare communication.* (n.d.). Retrieved from http://www.associatedcontent.com/article/470318/healthcare_communication-pg2.html

4

Basic and Applied Sciences

*Deborah Jane Schwytzer, MSN, RN-BC, CEN,
Jeanine Goodin, MSN, RN-BC, CNRN,
& Jo Nell Wells, PhD, RN-BC, OCN*

Fluid and Electrolyte Balance

GENERAL APPROACH

Homeostasis Overview
- *Homeostasis* is the delicate balance within the internal environment of the body that maintains an optimal and healthy condition for functioning of all body systems despite alterations in the external environment.
- It is the balance of such systems as intracellular and extracellular cellular structure, body temperature, serum electrolyte values, pH, fluid and blood volumes, nutrition, and elimination. Any changes at the cellular or organ level can affect the entire body and its functioning.
- The body attempts to maintain homeostasis through many mechanisms, including release of hormones into the bloodstream affected by a negative feedback mechanism or regulatory processes that rely on simple diffusion. If these processes are not fully functional, death can occur.
- The liver, lungs, kidneys, and brain help maintain homeostasis through metabolism, detoxification, hormone release, and exchange of materials.

Fluid and Electrolyte Balance

- An important mechanism of homeostasis is the maintenance of the body's fluid and electrolyte balance. This mechanism primarily involves the kidneys, which regulate water fluid volume (solvent) and composition (solutes). The skin and lungs also contribute to this balance to a lesser degree.
- The fluid compartments of the body include the intracellular fluid (ICF; approximately 65% of total body weight [TBW]) and the extracellular fluids (approximately 35% of TBW). The extracellular fluid (ECF) consists of the interstitial fluid (ISF), the plasma (IVF), and the transcellular fluids, which include the cerebrospinal fluid (CSF), intraocular fluids, and fluids in the serous membranes, GI tract, respiratory tract, and urinary tissues. Variance of composition occurs with age, body mass, and gender. Men generally have a slightly higher TBW than women due to lean body mass. Because elderly people tend to have a smaller TBW of water (approximately 45% to 55%) and infants generally will have larger TBW of water (70% to 80%), these groups are more susceptible to fluid-related problems.
- Water is the main component of body fluids and serves many functions in normal cellular function and maintenance of homeostasis. It provides a medium for chemical reactions in the cells; the transport of nutrients, electrolytes, and oxygen to the cells; and transport of waste products away from the cells. Water is also essential for temperature control, serves as an insulator, and acts as a lubricant.

Red Flags

- Electrolytes are essential for the functioning of the various processes of homeostasis. They assist in the maintenance of water, acid, and base balance, and mediate enzyme reactions. The normal serum electrolyte values needed for fluid and electrolyte balance and potential causes of an elevation or decrease are listed in Table 4–1 below.

Table 4–1. Serum Levels Important to Fluid and Electrolyte Balance

Test	Normal Values	Function	Potential Causes of Elevation	Potential Causes of Decrease
Carbon dioxide	23–30 mEq/L	Maintains metabolic acid–base balance	Respiratory acidosis Compensated metabolic acidosis Emphysema Severe vomiting	Respiratory alkalosis Diabetic ketoacidosis (DKA) Starvation Lactic acidosis Renal failure Dehydration
Calcium	9.0–10.5 mg/dL	Maintains muscle contractility, cardiac function, neural transmission, and cofactor in blood clotting Adds strength to bones and teeth	Hypothyroidism Hyperparathyroidism Metastatic bone tumor Addison disease Prolonged immobilization	Hypoparathyroidism Renal failure Hyperphosphatemia Hypoalbuminemia Malabsorption Pancreatitis Alkalosis

Chloride	99–107 mEq/L	Maintains electrical neutrality Major role in fluid balance and renal function	Diarrhea Hyperalimentation	DKA Vomiting
Magnesium	1.3–2.1 mEq/L	Facilitate metabolic activities and electrical conductivity Essential for cardiac, skeletal, and smooth muscle contraction Cofactor in clotting cascade	Renal insufficiency Addison's disease Excessive ingestion of magnesium-containing antacids Hypothyroidism	Malnutrition Malabsorption Hypoparathyroidism Alcoholism Chronic renal tubular disease DKA
Phosphorus	3.0–4.5 mg/dL	Contributes to electrical activity of the body and acid-base homeostasis Cofactor in metabolism Important in body energy stores	Hypoparathyroidism Renal failure Bone metastasis Hypocalcemia Acidosis Hemolytic anemia	Inadequate dietary intake Chronic antacid ingestion Hyperparathyroidism Hypercalcemia Chronic alcoholism
Potassium Most prevalent cation (+) in intracellular fluid	3.4–5.3 mEq/L	Protein synthesis, glucose storage, and electrical activity of heart muscles and others Regulates intracellular osmolarity	Acute renal failure Metabolic acidosis Anuria Oliguria	Dehydration Vomiting/diarrhea Starvation Stress DKA
Protein, total	6.4–8.3 g/dL	Maintains colloid osmotic pressure, supplies amino acids	Dehydration Nausea Vomiting Excessive exercise	Malnutrition Starvation Malabsorption syndrome Burns Chronic renal failure
Sodium Most prevalent cation (+) in extracellular fluid	137–147 mEq/L	Maintains extra-cellular volume, cardiac and skeletal muscle contraction through sodium/potassium pump	Diabetes insipidus Congestive heart failure (CHF) Hepatic failure Severe vomiting	Vomiting Diarrhea SIADH Burn injury Renal failure

- Electrolyte location is essential for neuromuscular activities. Transfer of electrolytes across compartment membranes is essential to the delicate homeostatic balance of the body and its functioning. The composition of electrolytes within the various fluid compartments varies as shown in Table 4–2.

Table 4-2. Electrolyte Composition

Fluid Compartment	Intravascular (Plasma) mEq/L	Interstitial mEq/L	Intracellular mEq/L
Cations			
Sodium ion	142	145	10
Potassium ion	4	4	160
Calcium ion	5	3	
Magnesium ion	3	2	35
Anions			
Chloride ion	103	115	2
Bicarbonate ion	27	30	8
Phosphate ion	2	2	140
Sulfate ion	1	1	
Organic acids	5	5	
Protein	16	1	55

- Water and electrolyte movement between the ICF and ECF compartments are controlled by several processes. Water movement is driven by hydrostatic pressure and osmotic pressures that exist in the compartments. Hydrostatic pressure is the force within a fluid compartment that pushes water out of the vasculature into the tissues in areas of higher vascular pressure and from tissues into the vasculature in areas of higher interstitial hydrostatic pressure. Also referred to as filtration, this process requires the use of a biologic membrane between the compartments. Osmotic pressure allows for movement of water across a semipermeable membrane from an area of lower solute (more dilute) concentration to an area of higher solute (less dilute) concentration. Osmosis will stop when the concentration is equal on both sides of the membrane or when the hydrostatic pressure has equalized.
- Electrolyte movement is based on the concentration of the electrolyte, moving towards the area of lower concentration, and the electrical charge gradient, moving to maintain an intracellular and extracellular equilibrium of electrolytes and charge. This movement involves diffusion, facilitated diffusion, or active transport. The diffusion of electrolyte or molecules occurs as an attempt is made to equalize concentrations on both sides of a semipermeable membrane without energy requirement. Solutes diffuse from an area of higher concentration to an area of lower concentration of that solute. Facilitated diffusion moves solutes from areas of higher concentration to areas of lower concentration to equalize concentration but requires the use of carrier molecules to facilitate the movement of the molecule. Active transport requires the use of energy to move a solute against the concentration gradient to maintain a higher concentration of one molecule electrolyte on one side of a membrane. The sodium-potassium pump is an example of this type of transport.

- Normal fluid balance in the adult is the result of a balance of the intake of approximately 2,500 mL fluid and output of approximately 2,500 mL. The regulation of water balance involves the presence of hormones regulated by osmoreceptors in various areas of the body as well as the functioning of the renal and gastrointestinal systems. A sensed state of fluid volume deficit or high serum osmolarity stimulates the release of antidiuretic hormone (ADH) from the posterior pituitary gland and the sense of thirst. In response, the patient will drink water and the presence of ADH will enhance renal reabsorption of water in the distal and collecting tubules. If receptor sites in the kidneys do not respond appropriately to the presence of ADH, excessive water loss will occur as experienced with the disease processes of diabetes insipidus. Similarly, if excessive ADH is released, water retention will occur as experienced with the syndrome of inappropriate antidiuretic hormone hypersecretion (SIADH). Aldosterone, a mineralocorticoid secreted by the adrenal cortex, increases sodium retention in the kidneys and with these levels, water will be drawn in. If the body's fluid volume increases, the increased sodium levels and increased volume will stimulate the cardiomyocytes to release atrial natriuretic peptides (ANP) and B-type natriuretic peptides (BNP). ANP and BNP block the release of ADH and aldosterone and cause diuresis, resulting in the excretion of sodium and water. The renal system regulates fluid and electrolyte balance through adjustments in the concentration of electrolytes and the volume of water as it is filtered in the tubules. The gastrointestinal system also facilitates a balance of water and electrolytes in the body. Oral intake, secretion, and reabsorption of gastric fluids and the production and elimination of feces are a component of fluid and electrolyte balance. The insensible water loss of approximately 900 mL/day through the lungs and skin contributes to this balance as well.
- Fluid volume and electrolyte replacement and balance between the intracellular space (ICS) and extracellular space (ECS) can be accomplished through oral replacement or through the use of intravenous (IV) fluids. Commonly used crystalloids can be classified as three types:
  - Isotonic solutions are solutions that contain electrolyte concentrations similar to the ICF and expand only ECF volume.
  - Hypotonic solutions contain a lower concentration of electrolytes than the intracellular fluids and a higher concentration of water. These solutions typically will be utilized to increase intracellular fluids in dehydration.
  - Hypertonic solutions contain a higher electrolyte concentration than the intracellular fluids and will "pull" fluids from the tissues and cells into the extracellular space. This type of solution can be used to increase circulating volume, increase cardiac output, and decrease cellular edema.
- The composition of common crystalloid solutions is shown in Table 4–3 below.

Table 4–3. Composition of Common Crystalloid Solutions (per 1,000 mL)

Type	Sodium (mmol)	Potassium (mmol)	Calcium (mmol)	Bicarb	Chloride (mmol)	Glucose (mmol)	Lactate (mmol)	pH	Tonicity
0.9% Saline	154				154			5.0	Isotonic
0.9% with 20 mEq KCl	154	20			174			6.0	Hypertonic
0.45% Saline	77				77			5.0	Hypotonic
5% Dextrose in Water (D5W)						277		3.5 to 6.5	Isotonic

cont.

Table 4–3. Composition of Common Crystalloid Solutions (per 1,000 mL) (cont.)

5% Dextrose in 0.9% Saline (D5NS)	154				154	277		3.5 to 6.5	Hypertonic
5% Dextrose in 0.45% Saline (D5/.45NS)	77				77	277		4	Hypertonic
Ringer's Lactate	130	4	3		109		28	6.5	Isotonic
5% Dextrose in Ringer's Lactate (D5LR)	130	4	3	109	277	28	4 to	6.5	Hypertonic
Plasma	140	4.5	2.3	26	100			7.4	Isotonic

ECF and Electrolyte Imbalances

HYPOVOLEMIA (EXTRACELLULAR FLUID DEFICIT)

Description
- Decreased circulating fluid volume due to fluid or blood loss from the extracellular space
- Presentation:
  - Increased heart rate with thready pulse
  - Decreased blood pressure and postural hypotension
  - Increased respiratory rate and depth
  - Lethargy
  - Thirst
  - Decreased renal output and increased specific gravity
  - Dry, scaly skin with poor skin turgor
  - Dry mucous membranes and tongue
  - Decreased GI motility, constipation
  - Obvious bleeding

Etiology
- Inadequate fluid intake
- Increased insensible fluid loss such as in fever or excessive perspiration
- GI loss such as found in diarrhea, vomiting, N/G suctioning, colostomy, or fistula drainage
- eHHeHemorrhage
- Diabetes insipidus
- Osmotic diuresis
- Excessive diuretic use: Fluids that have leaked from the intravascular space to the interstitial space as seen in peripheral edema, burns, and ascites, which causes a relative hypovolemia
- Trauma

- Clotting disorders
- Blood loss from internal sources such as bleeding GI ulcers, esophageal varicosities, hemorrhoids, and ruptured vascular sources

Prevention and Screening
- Discuss importance of maintaining adequate hydration, particularly during periods of exercise, fever, or hot weather.
- Encourage use of sports or electrolyte-balanced drinks to replace water and electrolytes lost.
- Encourage oral fluid intake in elderly because sensation of thirst decreases with aging.
- Maintain adequate hydration in patients who cannot care for themselves such as those with altered level of consciousness or debilitated.
- Assure adequate hydration in patients with severe vomiting, diarrhea, presence of nasogastric suctioning, open wounds, or excessive urine output.

Laboratory Findings
- Increased BUN and creatinine
- Increased Hgb
- Increased Hct
- Increased urine specific gravity

Nursing Management

NONPHARMACOLOGIC TREATMENT
- Increase oral intake if possible.
- Monitor IV infusion of fluids and blood products.
- Treat cause.
- Maintain mucous membrane integrity.
- Prevent complications of possible dysrhythmias, altered level of consciousness, and poor skin turgor.
- Monitor intake and output and daily weights.
- Increase accessibility of oral fluids, especially in the elderly and debilitated.

PHARMACOLOGIC TREATMENT
- IV infusion of fluids and blood products as ordered

Special Considerations
- Close monitoring of IV infusion of large quantities of fluids and blood products in patients with comorbidities affecting the cardiac, neurological, or renal systems is essential to avoid complications of pulmonary edema and sudden increase in cardiac workload.

Follow-up

EXPECTED OUTCOMES
- Fluid volume status will be returned to normal without disturbance of electrolyte balance.
- Underlying cause has been addressed and resolved.

COMPLICATIONS
- Decreased cardiac output and poor perfusion of tissues
- Hypovolemic shock

HYPERVOLEMIA (EXTRACELLULAR FLUID DEFICIT)

Description
- Increased circulating fluid volume due to fluid shifts into the extracellular spaces
- Presentation:
  - Bounding pulse
  - Increased blood pressure and central venous pressure (CVP)
  - Distended neck veins
  - Dyspnea, crackles, rales
  - Headache, confusion
  - Lethargy
  - Muscle spasms
  - Pitting edema
  - Periorbital edema
  - Weight gain
  - Seizures or coma

Etiology
- Excessive fluid intake
- Excessive hypotonic or isotonic IV fluids
- Heart failure
- Renal failure
- Primary polydipsia
- Cushing's syndrome
- SIADH
- Corticosteroid use
- Excessive ADH and aldosterone release
- Excessive intake of sodium-containing foods
- Elevated serum sodium — "water follows sodium"

Prevention and Screening
- Monitor for risk factors such as cardiac, renal, or liver disease history.
- Assessing early signs and symptoms of fluid volume excess can prevent complications.
- Monitor patient compliance when prescribed diuretics and low-sodium diet for existing disease processes.
- Monitor electrolytes for changes in serum sodium levels. Elevated sodium levels can lead to fluid retention and excessive fluid volume complications.

Laboratory Findings
- Decreased BUN
- Decreased Hgb
- Decreased Hct
- Decreased Serum osmolality
- Decreased urine specific gravity

Nursing Management

NONPHARMACOLOGIC TREATMENT
- Treat cause

- Fluid management through monitoring of intake and output
- Controlled IV infusion rates
- Monitor daily rate to assure weight loss as appropriate
- Sodium-restricted diet
- Monitor K+ with diuretic therapy

PHARMACOLOGIC TREATMENT
- Use of diuretics

Special Considerations
- Close monitoring of the cardiac, renal, and pulmonary systems is necessary because of the increased workload of these systems due to the excess fluid present.

Follow-up

EXPECTED OUTCOMES
- Fluid volume status will return to normal without disturbance of electrolyte balance.
- Underlying cause has been addressed and resolved.
- Skin integrity will remain intact.

COMPLICATIONS
- Increased circulating volume can increase cardiac workload and cardiac failure.
- Pulmonary edema and impaired gas exchange.
- Peripheral edema and ascites can precipitate skin breakdown.

HYPERNATREMIA

Description
- Abnormally high serum sodium level (serum sodium > 145 mEq/L)
- Presentation:
  - Restlessness, agitation, seizures, or coma
  - Dry mucous membranes
  - Excessive thirst
  - Oliguria
  - Muscle weakness and sluggishness
  - Weight loss
  - Peripheral edema
  - Elevated blood pressure

Etiology
- Excessive sodium intake from hypertonic IV saline solutions, IV solutions with sodium bicarbonate, or isotonic solutions
- Tube feedings with high sodium content without water supplements
- Inadequate water intake is seen in patients with altered level of consciousness, cognitively impaired, or NPO
- Dehydration
- Excessive water loss due to fever, perspiration, heat stroke, hyperventilation, diarrhea
- Polyuria commonly found in diabetes insipidus, uncontrolled diabetes, Cushing's syndrome

- Excessive corticosteroid usage
- Hyperaldosteronism
- Alterations in hypothalamus thirst-response centers
- Medications such as lithium, demeclocycline, colchicine, amphotericin B, gentamicin, vinblastine, which affect renal response to ADH

Prevention and Screening
- Discuss importance of adequate fluid intake to prevent dehydration.
- Discuss compliance with medications and medical follow-up for preexisting disease processes.
- Discuss use of oral rehydration solutions, which should be used only at times of potential dehydration because they contain high sodium content.

Nursing Management

NONPHARMACOLOGIC TREATMENT
- Treat cause
- Possible dialysis
- Fluid management through monitoring of intake and output, controlled IV infusion rates
- Monitor daily weight to ensure weight loss as appropriate
- Sodium-restricted diet

PHARMACOLOGIC TREATMENT
- Use of diuretics
- IV fluids of D5W or hypotonic saline solutions

Special Considerations
- If hypernatremia has occurred over a period of time, slow reduction of sodium level occurs to prevent rapid shifting of fluids into the cells and potential for the development of cerebral edema, herniation, and permanent neurological losses.
- Hypernatremia can occur in the adult population due to the lack of administration of water to hospitalized patients, particularly those who are critically ill or intubated.

Follow-up

EXPECTED OUTCOMES
- Underlying cause has been treated.
- Normal neurological function is maintained.
- Normal hydration status is maintained as shown by good skin turgor, weight stabilized, and alert and oriented mentation.

COMPLICATIONS
- Seizures and coma

HYPONATREMIA

Description
- Abnormally low serum sodium level (serum sodium < 136 mEq/L)

- Presentation:
  - Irritability, restlessness, agitation, seizures, or coma
  - Dry mucous membranes
  - Excessive thirst
  - Postural hypotension
  - Tachycardia, weak and thready pulse
  - Cool and clammy skin
  - Headache
  - Muscle spasms, weakness, and sluggishness
  - Nausea, vomiting, abdominal cramps
  - Oliguria

Etiology
- Excessive diaphoresis
- Use of diuretics
- Wound drainage
- Renal disease
- Low-sodium diet
- Increased aldosterone secretion
- NPO
- Burns
- Freshwater submersion
- Syndrome of inappropriate antidiuretic hormone hypersecretion (SIADH)
- Hyperglycemia
  - Medication usage such as lithium carbonate, vasopressin, and diuretics
  - Nephrotic syndrome
  - Irrigation with hypotonic solutions

Risk Factors
- Presence of above etiology
- Excessive potassium depletion
- Acute water intoxication

Prevention and Screening
- Discuss importance of adequate fluid intake to prevent dehydration.
- Discuss compliance with medications and medical follow-up for preexisting disease processes.

Nursing Management

NONPHARMACOLOGIC TREATMENT
- Treat cause
- Fluid management through monitoring of intake and output and controlled IV infusion rates
- IV fluids of hypertonic solutions if extreme hyponatremia
- Sodium-supplemented diet

PHARMACOLOGIC TREATMENT
- Decrease use of diuretics if possible, particularly loop diuretics and thiazides.

Special Considerations
- Infusion of hypertonic solutions can be irritating to vessels. Monitoring of IV site is needed to prevent infiltration and pain.

Follow-up

EXPECTED OUTCOMES
- Intake and output will approximate themselves.
- Patient will be awake, alert, and oriented.
- Cause has been identified and is being treated.

COMPLICATIONS
- Potential safety needs exist due to weakness and confusion. Supervision and use of side rails may be needed.

HYPERKALEMIA

Description
- Abnormally high serum potassium level (serum potassium > 5.0 mEq/L)
- Presentation:
  - Irritability, anxiety
  - Abdominal cramping
  - Diarrhea and nausea
  - Weakness and paresthesia
  - Irregular pulse and cardiac arrhythmias such as ventricular fibrillation, PVCs, or arrest
  - EKG changes such as tall, peaked T wave; prolonged PR interval; loss of P wave

Etiology
- Excessive or chronic use of potassium-sparing diuretics
- Excessive intake of potassium-rich foods, salt substitute containing potassium, or medication high in potassium
- Excessive or rapid parenteral administration of potassium supplements
- Crush injuries
- Fever
- Burns
- Sepsis
- Acidosis—potassium exits cells and enters the serum in acidotic states
- Renal disease
- Uncontrolled diabetes
- ACE inhibitors
- Multiple blood transfusions (due to preservatives)

Risk Factors
- Presence or history of above etiologies.
- The presence of leukocytosis in leukemia can cause an elevated potassium level.

Prevention and Screening
- Frequent monitoring of serum lab values in patients with disease processes such as renal failure or trauma, which can predispose patient to retention of potassium ion.
- Discuss compliance with medications and medical follow-up for preexisting disease processes.

Nursing Management

NONPHARMACOLOGIC TREATMENT
- Treat cause.
- Fluid management through monitoring of intake and output, control IV infusion rates.
- Stop all potassum supplements.
- Potassium-restricted diet; foods such as bananas, oranges, avocados, broccoli, spinach, dry fruits, coffee, chocolate, and organ and preserved meats should be avoided.
- Dialysis.

PHARMACOLOGIC TREATMENT
- Use of diuretics if possible, such as furosemide (Lasix)
- Administration of sodium polystyrene sulfonate (Kayexalate), a cation exchange resin, either orally or as enema

Special Considerations
- Excessive use of salt substitutes may predispose patient to altered potassium levels
- Some medications can cause an elevation in potassium level, such as potassium preparations of antibiotics, tetracycline, heparin, and aldosterone antagonists.

Follow-up

EXPECTED OUTCOMES
- Patient will show no cardiac arrhythmia.
- Underlying cause treated.
- Normal potassium level will be present.
- Patient and family will understand the dietary restrictions that can prevent hyperkalemia.
- Patient and family will understand the appropriate use of potassium supplements and salt substitutes.

COMPLICATIONS
- Prolonged hyperkalemia can lead to flaccid paralysis and cardiac arrest if untreated.
- Hyperkalemia can precipitate muscle weakness. The safety needs of the patient must be met.

HYPOKALEMIA

Description
- Abnormally low serum potassium level (serum potassium < 3.5 mEq/L)
- Presentation:
  - Fatigue
  - Weak and irregular pulse
  - Muscle weakness and cramps

- Nausea, vomiting, and ileus
- Paresthesia
- Decreased reflexes
- Polyuria
- Hyperglycemia
- EKG changes such as ST depression, flattened T wave, bradycardias, ventricular dysrhythmias
- Postural hypotension
- Confusion

Etiology
- GI loss through excessive vomiting, diarrhea, use of laxatives
- Cushing's syndrome
- Wound drainage
- Excessive diaphoresis
- NPO
- Alkalosis
- Renal disease that impaired reabsorption
- Excessive laxative use
- Water intoxication
- Total parenteral nutrition

Risk Factors
- Any of above etiology

Prevention and Screening
- Discuss compliance with medications and medical follow-up for preexisting disease processes.
- Use of appropriate IV solutions for rehydration.
- Use of potassium-sparing medications.
- Discuss need for diet rich in potassium, such as bananas, oranges, spinach, broccoli.

Nursing Management

NONPHARMACOLOGIC TREATMENT
- Treat cause
- Dietary intake of foods high in potassium such as bananas, raisins, avocado, mushrooms, spinach and potatoes

PHARMACOLOGIC TREATMENT
- Generally, potassium levels < 3.0 mEq/L require supplementation. KCl is the drug of choice either as an oral supplement or through IV infusion if patient cannot tolerate oral preparations or if severe hypokalemia exists.

Special Considerations
- IV supplementation of potassium can be painful and irritating to veins.
- Rapid infusion of potassium can cause depression of cardiac contractility and death. Potassium should not be administered at a rate more than 20 mEq/hour.

- Some medications, such as insulin, aspirin, prednisone, lithium, laxatives, gentamycin, and aldosterone, can cause decreased potassium levels.
- Diets low in meat and vegetables can cause low potassium levels.

Follow-up

EXPECTED OUTCOMES
- Normal potassium level
- Underlying cause treated
- Patient and family will acknowledge appropriate use of potassium supplements and food rich in potassium for oral intake
- Patient and family will identify signs and symptoms of hypokalemia and need to report to the healthcare provider.

COMPLICATIONS
- Cardiac dysrhymias
- Paralytic ileus
- Shock
- Sudden cardiac death

Hypercalcemia

Description
- Abnormally high serum calcium level (serum calcium > 10.5 mg/L)
- Presentation:
  - Increased heart rate and blood pressure
  - In high levels of calcium, heart rate will slow
  - Blood clots
  - Muscle weakness
  - Decreased deep tendon reflexes
  - Mental confusion and lethargy
  - Decreased peristalsis, constipation, and abdominal pain
  - Hypoactive bowel sounds
  - Flank pain
  - Bone pain and pathological fractures

Etiology
- Excessive oral intake of calcium and calcium-containing products such as nutritional supplements
- Excessive oral intake of vitamin D
- Renal failure
- Use of thiazide diuretics
- Hyperparathyroidism
- Malignancies of breast, lung, prostate, and bone
- Hyperthyroidism
- Immobility
- Dehydration
- Acidosis
- Leukemia

Risk Factors
- Bed rest or extended immobility
- Increased intake of high-calcium foods and fluids
- Thiozide diuretics can cause calcium excretion from the kidneys

Prevention and Screening
- Discuss compliance with medications and medical follow-up for preexisting disease processes.
- Discuss need to avoid over-the-counter medications that contain high levels of calcium or vitamin D.
- Discuss need to restrict calcium intake in foods.

Nursing Management

NONPHARMACOLOGIC TREATMENT
- Treat cause
- Dialysis
- Encourage early ambulation to prevent calcium loss from bone
- Discourage use of high-calcium foods
- Use of normal saline IV infusion to increase renal excretion of calcium
- Monitor and treat dysrhythmias due to elevated calcium levels

PHARMACOLOGIC TREATMENT
- Decrease use of medications containing calcium or vitamin D.
- Medications that increase excretion of calcium and bind with calcium such as Lasix, Mithracin, and Penicillamine.
- Use of medications that inhibit calcium reabsorption from bone are calcitonin, phosphorus, bisphosphonates, and prostaglandin synthesis inhibitors such as NSAIDs and aspirin.

Special Considerations
- Fluid intake of 3–4 liters/day is suggested to increase excretion of excess calcium.

Follow-up

EXPECTED OUTCOMES
- Patient will have a normal calcium level.
- Underlying cause has been diagnosed and is being treated.
- Patient is free from pathological fractures and decreased mobility.

COMPLICATIONS
- Osteoporosis and pathological fracture
- Renal calculi
- Cardiac dysrhymias
- Pancreatitis

HYPOCALCEMIA

Description
- Abnormally low serum calcium level (serum calcium < 8.5 mg/L)
- Presentation:
  - Poor dietary intake of calcium
  - Painful muscle spasms
  - Paresthesia, numbness, and tingling
  - Trousseau's sign: spasms of fingers when blood pressure cuff inflated on upper arm
  - Chvostek's sign: facial twitch one side of face evoked by tapping on face just below and in front of ear
  - Heart rate either slow or fast with weak, thready pulse
  - Hypotension
  - Prolonged ST and QT intervals

Etiology
- Inadequate calcium and vitamin D intake
- Lactose intolerance
- Malabsorption syndromes
- Acute and chronic renal disease
- Diarrhea
- Steatorrhea
- Alkalosis
- Removal or destruction of the parathyroid glands
- Acute pancreatitis
- Immobility
- Alcoholism

Risk Factors
- Presence of any etiologies listed.
- Removal or irradiation of the parathyroid, causing hyposecretion of parathyroid hormone.
- Patients having a small bowel resection, partial gastrectomy, or Crohn's disease can experience a loss of calcium reabsorption from the surface of the intestine.
- Some medications, such as caffeine, achohol, and corticosteroids, decrease calcium absorption.

Prevention and Screening
- Discuss compliance with medications and medical follow-up for preexisting disease processes.
- Discuss need to increase calcium intake in foods.
- Teach methods to decrease strain on bones to prevent fracturing and pain.

Nursing Management
NONPHARMACOLOGIC TREATMENT
- Treat cause.
- Reduce stimuli to prevent excitement of nervous system by darkening room, limiting visitors, using a soft voice, and decreasing noises.
- Injury prevention such as seizure precautions, fall precautions, pathological fractures.

PHARMACOLOGIC TREATMENT
- Calcium replacement either orally or via IV
- Medications that enhance calcium absorption, such as vitamin D

Special Considerations
- Patients with hypocalcemia may experience alterations in nervous impulses and may require safety precautions.
- Decreased calcium levels also can interfere with the normal blood coagulation.

Follow-up

EXPECTED OUTCOMES
- Serum calcium level within normal limits
- No seizure activity
- No cardiac dysrhythmias
- Safety needs are met

COMPLICATIONS
- Osteoporosis and pathological fractures
- Laryngospasm
- Seizures

HYPERMAGNESEMIA

Description
- Abnormally high serum magnesium level (serum magnesium > 2.5 mEq/L)
- Presentation:
  - Peripheral vasodilatation
  - Flushing
  - Bradycardia and hypotension
  - Lethargy
  - Respiratory insufficiency and depression
  - Coma
  - Loss of deep tendon reflexes
  - Cardiac arrest
  - Nausea and vomiting

Etiology
- Excessive magnesium intake such as magnesium-containing antacids, laxatives, and IV supplementation
- Renal insufficiency, which decreases magnesium excretion
- Adrenal insufficiency
- Diuretic abuse
- Burns
- Shock
- Sepsis

Risk Factors
- In patients with renal failure, chronic use of magnesium-containing antacids can cause hypermagnesia.
- Tissue breakdown as seen in extensive burns and shocks can lead to release of magnesium from the intracellular space into the vasculature.

Prevention and Screening
- Education about appropriate use of magnesium-containing medications.
- Monitor for history of adrenal disease processes.

Nursing Management

NONPHARMACOLOGIC TREATMENT
- Treat cause
- Dialysis

PHARMACOLOGIC TREATMENT
- Discontinue all magnesium-containing medications.
- Use of loop diuretics.
- Administer calcium to decrease cardiac effects.

Special Considerations
- Alterations in the ability of blood to clot in hypermagnesia can occur as platelet adhesiveness and thrombin formation times are affected.

Follow-up

EXPECTED OUTCOMES
- Causative etiology has been determined and is being treated.
- Patient and family will identify potential sources of magnesium intake.
- Neurological function such as deep tendon reflexes will return to baseline.
- Muscle strength and function will return to normal with no residual paralysis.

COMPLICATIONS
- Coma
- Cardiac arrest
- Respiratory arrest

HYPOMAGNESEMIA

Description
- Abnormally low serum magnesium level (serum magnesium < 1.3 mEq/L)
- Presentation:
  - Hyperactive deep tendon reflexes
  - Numbness and tingling
  - Tetany
  - Skeletal muscle weakness
  - Depression or confusion
  - Anorexia

- Nausea, constipation, abdominal distension
- Paralytic ileus

Etiology
- Malnutrition and starvation
- Diarrhea
- Malabsorption syndromes
- Chronic diarrhea and steatorrhea
- Crohn's disease
- Acute pancreatitis
- Nephrotic syndrome
- Ethanol ingestion
- Medications such as diuretics, aminoglycoside antibiotics, cyclosporine, insulin

Risk Factors
- Alcoholism can be a risk factor for development of hypomagnesia due to poor dietary intake.
- Patients on long-term parenteral nutrition can develop hypomagnesia due to loss of GI function and absorption in the small intestine.

Prevention and Screening
- Instruct patient in the signs and symptoms of hypomagnesemia to prevent neurological symptoms
- Instruct patient in the proper use of medications and need for appropriate follow-up.

Nursing Management

NONPHARMACOLOGIC TREATMENT
- Treat cause
- Monitor for effectiveness of supplements

PHARMACOLOGIC TREATMENT
- Discontinue medications such as loop diuretics, aminoglycosides antibiotics, and any medications containing phosphorus.
- Replacement of magnesium via IV with magnesium sulfate or orally with an extended release mechanism such as Mag-Ox or Slow-Mag.

Special Considerations
- Patients receiving IV replacement of magnesium should be closely monitored for respiratory arrest or areflexia during infusion.

Follow-up

EXPECTED OUTCOMES
- Cause of hypomagnesia will be found and treated.
- Serum magnesium returns to normal range.
- Patient and family will verbalize magnesium-rich foods that should be included in diet, such as seafoods, nuts, and green vegetables.

COMPLICATIONS
- Seizures
- Parasthesia

HYPERPHOSPHATEMIA

Description
- Abnormally high serum phosphorus level (serum level of > 4.5 mEq/L)
- Presentation
  - Signs and symptoms of hypocalcemia such as tetany
  - Increased RBC count
  - Soft tissue calcification
  - Altered mental status, delirium, coma
  - Muscle cramping
  - Hypotension
  - Cataracts

Etiology
- Chemotherapy
- Tumor lysis syndrome
- Increased phosphorus intake
- Hypothyroidism
- Decreased renal excretion due to renal insufficiency
- Burns or heat-related illnesses
- Renal failure
- Muscle necrosis due to trauma or illness
- Prolonged immobility
- Hypercalcemia

Risk Factors
- Phosphorus levels are primarily controlled through excretion from the kidney. Renal disease can increase a patient's probability of developing hyperphosphotemia.
- Multiple blood transfusions can increase phosphorus levels due to leakage of phosphorus out of the cells

Prevention and Screening
- Instruct patient in appropriate use of medications prescribed to decrease phosphorus levels and enhance calcium levels.
- Maintain adequate hydration.

Nursing Management

NONPHARMACOLOGIC TREATMENT
- Treat cause
- Treat hypocalcemia, which commonly is a comorbidity
- Hemodialysis

PHARMACOLOGIC TREATMENT
- Oral binders of phosphorus such as sevelamer (Renagel)
- Eliminate or substitute medications high in phosphorus

Special Considerations
- Phosphorus maintains acid–base balance in the body.
- Serves in the mineralization of bones, and teeth.

Follow-up

EXPECTED OUTCOMES
- Underlying cause is identified and is being treated.
- Serum phosphorous returning to normal value.
- Patient and family can identify those foods which should be avoided such as red meats, poultry, eggs, hard cheeses, bran, or oatmeal cereals.
- Patient and family understand the importance of choosing over-the-counter medications low in phosphorus.

COMPLICATIONS
- Airway compromised due to laryngospasm
- Tetany

HYPOPHOSPHATEMIA

Description
- Abnormally low serum phosphorus level (serum phosphorus < 2.0 mg/dL)
- Presentation:
  - Muscular weakness such as diplopia, dysphagia, dysarthria
  - Weakness of large muscle groups of trunk or extremities
  - Decreased respiratory rate and tidal volume
  - Hypotension
  - Parasthesia
  - Hyporeflexia
  - Increased irritability, confusion, and coma

Etiology
- Alcohol withdrawal
- DKA—recovery phase
- Chronic ingestion of phosphate-binding antacids
- Malnutrition
- Total parenteral nutrition (TPN) with inadequate phosphorus supplementation
- Malabsorption syndromes
- Hypocalcemia
- Medications such as diamox, insulin, epinephrine
- Aluminum-containing antacids and diuretics

Risk Factors
- Because phosphorus is absorbed in the jejunum, patients with GI dysfunction will be at risk for phosphorus imbalances.
- Aluminum-containing antacids and diuretics bind with phosphorus and promote excretion in the kidney.

Prevention and Screening
- Patient and family should be aware that 1 quart of milk can provide the daily requirement of phosphorus.

- Decrease alcohol intake.
- Control glucose levels within normal ranges.

Nursing Management

NONPHARMACOLOGIC TREATMENT
- Treat cause.
- Encourage improved diet.
- Monitor for airway compromise, hyporeflexia, and signs of alcohol withdrawal.

NONPHARMACOLOGIC TREATMENT
- Replacement of phosphate either orally or IV.
- Replace all other electrolytes to normal serum levels.

Special Considerations
- Airway management is an issue because these patients can develop neurological complications.

Follow-up

EXPECTED OUTCOMES
- Cause will be identified and treated.
- Patient will maintain a patent airway and gag reflex.
- Patient will be free of neurological seizures or hyperactivity.

COMPLICATIONS
- Respiratory distress
- Dysrhythmias
- Heart failure
- Seizures and coma

ACID–BASE BALANCE OVERVIEW

- Homeostasis and the functioning of the cell is dependent on the acid–base balance of the body. This balance is a function of the chemical and physiological components of the body and is reflected in the concentration of hydrogen ions in the body. Hydrogen ions are acidic and must be maintained within a strict limit to allow for optimal functioning of all physiologic systems. The body normally functions at a slightly basic pH of 7.35 to 7.45 (a pH of 7.0 is neutral). Changes in the normal blood pH often interfere with many physiological functions, such as changes in the shape of hormones and enzymes so that they no longer are able to perform their normal functions. The pH also can alter the distribution of electrolytes, alter the fluid and electrolyte balance, and impact the effectiveness of many hormones and drugs.
- Acids are substances or compounds that release hydrogen in solution; basic solutions will accept these hydrogen ions. Even a slight variation in the pH of as little as 0.4 in either direction can be fatal in humans. A pH < 6.9 or > 7.8 is usually believed to be fatal.
- Sources of acids in the body include the normal waste products of carbohydrate, protein, and fat metabolism. Lactic acid formation is a byproduct of anaerobic metabolism as a result of hypoxia, sepsis, and shock.

- Bicarbonate, the most common base in the body, is the result of the breakdown of carbonic acid. Bicarbonate also is absorbed from foods, produced in the pancreas, and reabsorbed from the kidneys.
- In extracellular fluid, a constant ratio of 1 molecule of carbonic acid to 20 bicarbonate ions is necessary for optimal functioning. Both of these substances and their constant ratio are the result of the production and elimination of carbon dioxide and hydrogen ions, through either the lungs or the kidneys.
- Acidosis is present when the body fluid pH is < 7.35. A state of acidosis can produce complications such as myocardial irritability, decreased myocardial contractility, pulmonary vascular constriction, systemic and cerebral vasodilatation, and a depressed cortical function. Carbonic acid (H_2CO_3) is the most common acid in the body.
- An alkalosis state is present when the body fluid pH is < 7.45. A state of alkalosis can cause bronchoconstriction, pulmonary vascular dilatation, myocardial irritability, systemic and cerebral vasoconstriction, and increased neuromuscular irritability. Bicarbonate (HCO_3^-) is the most common base present.
- Oxygenation is another important component to be considered when assessing the total functioning of the body's ability to maintain adequate acid–base balance. Every living cell in the body needs oxygen for aerobic metabolism and the prevention of anaerobic metabolism and lactic acid formation. Normally only 3% of the body's oxygen is dissolved in the plasma and available to the cells for metabolism. The PaO_2 is a measurement of the partial pressure of oxygen in the plasma and not the total oxygen content of the body. Normal PaO_2 is between 80 mm Hg and 100 mm Hg. Results < 80 mm Hg are classified as hypoxia. SaO_2 (oxygen saturation) is the measure of the degree to which the hemoglobin oxygen-binding sites are occupied. Because these sites can be occupied by oxygen or carbon monoxide, it is important to consider what molecules are present and have the potential for binding to these sites. The presence of carbon monoxide in the blood can result in a normal SaO_2 despite a hypoxic state.
- The pH is maintained in the body through three systems:
  - Buffer systems, which include the bicarbonate-carbonic acid buffer system, are the fastest to respond to excess acids in the system. Bicarbonate combines with the excess hydrogen ions of the acid to form carbonic acid, which is then dissociated into carbon dioxide and water. Phosphates, as well as plasma proteins—particularly hemoglobin in the red blood cells—also serve as buffers to maintain the carbonic acid and bicarbonate ratio.
  - The respiratory system regulation of acid–base balance is controlled by the central nervous system. Sensors in the brain are sensitive to changes in the amount of CO_2 in the brain tissue and will initiate increased or decreased respiration depth and rate eliminate or retain CO_2 to maintain appropriate levels.
  - The kidneys work to retain or secrete hydrogen ions and bicarbonate as needed to maintain a constant ratio of 1:20. These compensatory efforts will potentially take hours to days to correct the problem.
  - All of these processes can be considered compensatory efforts and will be considered when interpreting the arterial blood gases.
  - The aging process can cause some alterations to these buffer systems and their responsiveness to pH changes. The aging kidneys can become less responsive to minor changes in hydrogen ions due to disease such as fever, infection, and pneumonia, and some medications such as diuretics and digoxin can cause increased excretion of hydrogen and thus increase pH. Aging of the respiratory system can cause decreased gas exchange due to thickened vessels and less alveolar membrane, causing an increase in CO_2 retention and a decrease in pH.

- Arterial blood gases are laboratory specimens that measure oxygen, carbon dioxide, pH, and bicarbonate in the arterial blood. They are typically utilized to determine the body's acid–base balance. Normal blood gas results and potential causes for deviation from normal are shown in Table 4–4 below.

Table 4–4. Arterial Blood Gas Values

Test	Normal Range	Potential Causes of Elevation	Potential Causes of Decrease
pH (Hydrogen ion concentration)	7.35–7.45	Metabolic alkalosis Loss of gastric fluids Diuretic therapy Hypokalemia Salicylate toxicity	Metabolic acidosis Respiratory acidosis Ketones Renal failure Starvation Diarrhea
pCO_2 (Partial pressure of carbon dioxide in arterial blood)	35–45 mm Hg	Respiratory acidosis Emphysema Pneumonia Respiratory depression	Respiratory alkalosis Hyperventilation Diarrhea
pO_2 (Partial pressure of oxygen in arterial blood)	83–100 mm Hg	Hyperventilation Oxygen therapy Exercise	Respiratory depression High altitude Carbon monoxide poisoning
Bicarbonate (HCO_3^-) (Bicarbonate concentration in the plasma)	19–24 mmol/L	Bicarbonate infusion Metabolic alkalosis	Metabolic acidosis Diarrhea Pancreatitis

INTERPRETING ABGS

- Analyze the pH first. Is the pH value normal, low (acidotic: < 7.4) or high (alkalotic: > 7.4)?
- Analyze the $PaCO_2$ to determine if the primary respiratory value is normal, high (acidotic: > 45 mm Hg), or low (alkalotic: < 35 mm Hg).
- Analyze the HCO_3 to determine if the primary metabolic value is normal, low (acidotic: < 22 mEq/L), or high (alkalotic: > 26 mEq/L).
- Evaluate the pH–$PaCO_2$ relationship. If the pH is acidotic and the $PaCO_2$ is acidotic, the patient is experiencing respiratory acidosis. If the pH is alkalotic and the $PaCO_2$ is alkalotic, the patient is experiencing respiratory alkalosis.
- If the pCO_2 value is the opposite direction of the pH, the imbalance is of respiratory origin.
- Evaluate the pH–HCO_3^- relationship. If the pH is acidotic and the HCO_3^- is acidotic, the patient is experiencing metabolic acidosis. If the pH is alkalotic and the HCO_3^- is alkalotic, the patient is experiencing metabolic alkalosis.
- If the HCO_3^- value is the same direction as the pH, the imbalance is of metabolic origin.

- Look for possible compensation. In general, two imbalances will be demonstrated. In the process of compensation, the body attempts to normalize the pH through the processes of the respiratory system and the kidneys. Both of these systems will assist in the compensation to return to the pH to a normal physiologic state but they respond to changes and begin to compensate at different rates. The lungs can respond more quickly and are more sensitive to changes, but are limited in their efforts over time. The renal system is more powerful in its functions to compensate for an imbalance but its response usually takes hours to days. To determine the primary acid–base imbalance cause, look for the value that is demonstrating the same acidosis/alkalosis indication.
- Renal compensation can be considered if initial respiratory acidosis has been found ($pH < 7.35$ and $PaCO_2 > 45$ mm Hg). The effects of the kidneys attempting to compensate will be seen as $HCO_3^- > 26$ mEq/L and pH moving toward the 7.35 to 7.45 range.
- Renal compensation can be considered if initial respiratory alkalosis has been found ($pH > 7.45$ and $PaCO_2 < 35$ mm Hg). The effects of the kidneys attempting to compensate will be seen as $HCO_3^- < 22$ mEq/L and pH moving toward the 7.35 to 7.45 range.
- Respiratory compensation can be considered if initial metabolic acidosis has been found ($pH < 7.35$ and $HCO_3^- < 22$ mEq/L). The effects of the respiratory system attempting to compensate will be seen as $PCO_2 < 35$ mm Hg and pH moving toward the 7.35 to 7.45 range.
- Respiratory compensation can be considered if initial metabolic alkalosis has been found ($pH > 45$ and $HCO_3^- > 26$ mEq/L). The effects of the respiratory system attempting to compensate will be seen as $PCO_2 > 45$ mm Hg and pH moving toward the 7.35 to 7.45 range.
- Full compensation can be considered when the pH has returned to within the normal range, 7.35 to 7.45.
- Examples of primary cause and compensation mechanisms are shown in Table 4–5 below.

Table 4-5. Acid–Base Disturbances and Compensatory Mechanisms

pH	pCo_2	HCO_3^-	Disturbance	Potential Causes	Compensation Mechanism
↓	↑	Normal	Respiratory acidosis	Respiratory depression, central nervous system (CNS) trauma, acute respiratory distress syndrome (ARDS), pneumonia, chronic obstructive pulmonary disease (COPD), other pulmonary disease	Renal
↑	↓	Normal	Respiratory alkalosis	Hyperventilation, pain, anxiety, sepsis, tetany, fever, pulmonary emboli	Renal
↓	Normal	↓	Metabolic acidosis	Diabetes, shock, renal failure, burns, starvation, malnutrition	Respiratory

↑	Normal	↑	Metabolic alkalosis	Severe vomiting, nasogastric drainage, excessive sodium bicarbonate intake, hepatic failure, Cushing syndrome	Respiratory

ALTERATIONS IN ACID–BASE IMBALANCE

- Respiratory acidosis is caused by under-elimination of hydrogen ions or excess carbon dioxide in the body. It is the result of elevated CO_2 from hypoventilation or a compensatory response to bicarbonate retention by the kidneys. Decreases in chest wall expansion due to skeletal deformities or muscular weakness, airway obstruction, and respiratory depression from drugs and electrolyte imbalances are some factors that can cause this condition. ABG findings typically will reveal pH decreased, $PaCO_2$ elevated, and HCO_3^- normal if uncompensated. The HCO_3^- will be elevated if the body is attempting to compensate for the condition. Increased oxygen intake can assist in the correction of this condition.

- Respiratory alkalosis is caused by over-elimination of hydrogen ions or a level of carbon dioxide below normal in the body. It is the result of a decreased CO_2 level from hyperventilation or a compensatory response to bicarbonate elimination by the kidneys. Fear, anxiety, mechanical ventilation, excessive use of drugs such aspirin or catecholamine, and alcohol intoxication can cause this condition. ABG findings typically will reveal plasma pH elevated, $PaCO_2$ decreased, and HCO_3^- normal if uncompensated. The HCO_3^- will be decreased if the body is attempting to compensate for the condition. Immediate compensation for this condition can be achieved by assisting the patient to retain carbon dioxide through calming down and breathing into a nonrebreather mask or paper bag.

- Metabolic acidosis is caused by production of acid and the presence of excessive hydrogen ions secondary to illness. Diseases such as renal failure, sepsis, and diabetic ketoacidosis, as well as loss of bicarbonate from the lower GI tract through diarrhea or fistula drainage, are some illnesses and conditions that can cause this diagnosis. ABG findings typically will reveal plasma pH decreased, $PaCO_2$ normal if uncompensated, and HCO_3^- decreased. The $PaCO_2$ will decrease if the body is attempting to compensate for the condition. Compensation primarily occurs by increased ventilation, fixing the underlying cause; in extreme situations, sodium bicarbonate can be administered intravenously. The kidney can also work to increase excretion of hydrogen ions in the urine.

- Metabolic alkalosis is caused by the presence of excessive base or loss of hydrogen ions secondary to illness. Severe vomiting, excessive gastric suctioning, diuretics, or excessive intake of bicarbonate products such as antacids can cause this condition. ABG findings typically will reveal plasma pH decreased, $PaCO_2$ normal if uncompensated, HCO_3^- elevated. The $PaCO_2$ will increase if the body is attempting to compensate for this condition. Compensation typically occurs by increasing carbon dioxide retention by the lungs, increasing retention of hydrogen ions by the kidneys, and treating the underlying cause of the condition.

MEDICINAL THERAPIES

- Complementary and alternative medicine (CAM) is defined as treatment practices that are not widely accepted or practiced by mainstream clinicians in a given culture. CAM use is widespread in the United States. Its popularity can be attributed to the perception that herbs are safer and "healthier" than conventional drugs, the desire for a sense of control over one's care, emotional comfort from taking action, cultural influences, limited access to professional care, lack of health insurance, convenience, media hype and aggressive marketing, and recommendations from family and friends.
- Medicinal and herbal therapies often include dietary supplements. Dietary supplements can be defined as vitamins, minerals, herbs or other botanicals, amino acids, and substances such as enzymes, organ tissues, glandular extracts, and metabolites intended to promote health and relieve symptoms of disease.
- Dietary supplements are regulated under the Dietary Supplement Health and Education Act of 1994 (DSHEA) and the Current Good Manufacturing Practices (CGMPS) ruling issued in 2007. Under DSHEA, dietary supplements are presumed safe until proven harmful. Many people think that because herbs are natural plants they will not cause harm or side effects, but this is not always true. Dietary supplements can interact with conventional drugs, sometimes with serious results. It is important for patients to tell their healthcare providers about all therapies they are currently using or thinking of using.
- The nurse's responsibility regarding patient use of herbal medicinal therapies is to apply the Nursing Process within the guidelines of your state Nurse Practice Act. Practice only within the scope of these laws. Some general nursing guidelines structured within the Nursing Process steps follow.

Assess

- Be sure to ask patients if they are using medicinal herbs or other dietary supplements during the drug history and before administering prescribed medications. Use a nonjudgmental attitude when doing this assessment. Discuss with your patient the importance of telling his or her healthcare providers about any complementary or alternative practices they use to ensure coordinated and safe care.

Plan

- Plan the care for the patient using herbal or alternative therapies by communicating information to the physician and encouraging the patient to do likewise. The Office of Dietary Supplements, National Institutes of Health, maintains an online resource (http://ods.od.nih.gov) providing fact sheets on herbals studied in the United States.

Implement

- Teach the patient about possible interactions between herbal therapies and prescribed medications. In general, discourage the use of herbal products in pregnant women, nursing mothers, infants or young children, and older adults with liver or cardiovascular disease.

Evaluate

- Determine patient response to prescribed medications and herbal therapies.
- A number of herbals are safe and effective for a variety of conditions, while some are harmful. For some herbals this information is unknown.

- Patients should be instructed that some herbals are deemed unsafe based on the most recent studies or anecdotal reports. Some unsafe herbals are: borage, calamus, coltsfoot, comfrey life root, kava, pokeweed, and ephedra (ma huang).
- Some commonly used dietary supplements or medicinal herbs are described below. Possible side effects and adverse reactions are included. Additionally, known food–drug and drug–drug interactions are addressed and implications for patient teaching are included.

Table 4-6. Commonly Used Dietary Supplements/Medicinal Herbs

Medicinal Herbals & Dietary Supplements	Uses	Adverse Effects	Drug Interactions
Aloe	Topically for wound healing Orally as a laxative or for diabetes, asthma, epilepsy, and osteoarthritis FDA-approved as a natural food flavoring	Topical use: No significant side effects Oral use: Abdominal cramps and diarrhea	Furosemide and loop diuretics Diarrhea caused by the laxative effect can decrease the absorption of many drugs In patients with diabetes, may lower blood glucose levels
Black Cohosh	Hot flashes and other menopausal symptoms, in the short term (6 months) Arthritis and muscle pain	Headaches and stomach discomfort	No known interactions with prescription meds Do not take with liver disorders
Coenzyme Q-10	Parkinson's disease Heart failure Breast cancer patients undergoing chemotherapy	Mild	Not known Being studied by NIH
Chamomile	Inflammatory diseases of gastrointestinal and upper respiratory tracts Sleeplessness Anxiety	Rare allergic reaction	Likely unsafe taken in medicinal amounts during pregnancy Should be avoided if breastfeeding
Echinacea	Upper respiratory tract infections Stimulate immune system Less commonly for wounds and skin problems such as acne or boils	Rare; sometimes allergic reactions and GI symptoms	There are many drug interactions; always check with physician before taking May increase caffeine effects

cont.

Table 4–6. Commonly Used Dietary Supplements/Medicinal Herbs (cont.)

Feverfew	Migraine headache prevention	Well-tolerated with short-term therapy GI upsets: nausea, digestive problems, and bloating	Warfarin, aspirin, heparin, ibuprofen
Flaxseed and flaxseed oil	Laxative Hot flashes and breast pain High cholesterol	Well-tolerated Can cause GI effects of bloating, flatulence, and abdominal discomfort	Take with plenty of water to avoid increased constipation or, in rare cases, intestinal blockage. May lower the body's ability to absorb p. o. medications; take 1 hour before or 2 hours after other p. o. meds
Garlic	Lower cholesterol and hypertension Platelet aggregate inhibitor Prevent stomach and colon cancers	Well-tolerated Bad breath, unpleasant taste, heartburn	Avoid with warfarin, heparin, and aspirin Avoid with saquinavir and other anti-HIV drugs
Ginger root	Nausea and vomiting; exerts an antiemetic effect	Few; GI discomfort	Avoid with warfarin, heparin, aspirin, other anticoagulants Can lower blood sugar—use cautiously with antidiabetic meds
Gingko biloba	Alzheimer's disease and dementia to improve memory Increase blood flow Leg pain Tinnitus	Headache GI upsets Allergic reactions Increased bleeding	Avoid with aspirin, heparin, warfarin, and other anticoagulants Avoid in patients at risk for seizures
Ginseng	Age-related diseases Increase physical endurance	Well-tolerated Headaches Sleep and GI problems Breast tenderness and menstrual irregularities Hypertension	Avoid with aspirin, heparin, warfarin, and other anticoagulants Avoid with MAO inhibitors May lower blood sugar levels so avoid if taking antidiabetic meds

Licorice root	Stomach ulcers Bronchitis Sore throat Viral infections (hepatitis)	High blood pressure and heart problems due to salt and water retention and low potassium levels	Immunosuppressive drugs, digoxin, and antihypertensive meds Avoid in pregnancy
Saw palmetto	Benign prostatic hyperplasia and urinary problems	Stomach discomfort Tender breasts Decline in sexual desire	Finasteride and anti- androgen drugs Warfarin and other anticoagulants
St. John's wort	Orally for mild to moderate depression Topically for pain and inflammation	Generally well- tolerated Do not take if taking antidepressant medications	Variety of known adverse interactions and is likely to have more that are unknown May cause increased sensitivity to sunlight
Soy	High cholesterol levels and high blood pressure Hot flashes, osteo- porosis, and memory problems Prevention of breast and prostate cancer	Well-tolerated Possibly minor stomach and bowel problems such as nausea, bloating, and constipation Rare allergic reactions	Avoid with tamoxifen and other drugs that can block estrogen receptors Antibiotics may decrease the effects of soy
Valerian	Sleep disorders and anxiety-related restlessness	Generally well- tolerated FDA rates it safe when consumed in amounts commonly used in food for 4–6 weeks Possible effects include daytime drowsiness, dizziness, depression, fatigue, headaches, dyspepsia, and pruritus	Avoid with barbiturates and other sleep medications, alcohol, and antihistamines
Vitamin E supplements	Boosts the immune system Widens blood vessels and keeps blood from clotting within them. Cells use vitamin E to interact with each other and to carry out many important functions	Eating vitamin E in foods is not risky or harmful. In supplement form, high doses of vitamin E might increase the risk of bleeding and hemorrhagic stroke.	Avoid with anti- coagulant or anti- platelet medicines, such as warfarin (Coumadin®). Avoid with other antioxidants (such as vitamin C, selenium, and beta-carotene) when taking statin meds Avoid with chemo- therapy or radiation therapy for cancer

cont.

Table 4–6. Commonly Used Dietary Supplements/Medicinal Herbs (cont.)

| Zinc | Severe diarrhea, malabsorption To decrease the length of time of the common cold (as a lozenge); as a pill or a nose spray, doesn't seem to help prevent colds Acne (ointment form) Age-related macular degeneration (AMD) when taken with other medicines | Routine use of zinc supplements is not recommended Might cause nausea, vomiting, diarrhea, metallic taste, kidney and stomach damage, and other side effects. Using zinc on broken skin may cause burning, stinging, itching, and tingling | Black coffee decreases zinc absorption Avoid with many medications, such as certain antibiotics and chemotherapy |

Nutrition

GENERAL APPROACH

- In the healthcare setting, it can be easy to place a patient's nutritional needs secondary to the diseases, tests, or treatments needed for the care and recovery process. An appropriate diet can improve the short- and long-term outcomes of many disease processes. This section will review important aspects of nutritional assessment, risks for malnourishment, and interventions for the adult.

NUTRITION

- Protein, carbohydrates, and fat are nutrients in food that provide the body with energy. This energy is used to maintain body temperature, cardiac output, respiratory and muscle function, protein synthesis, and the storage and metabolism of food. Proper nutrition is essential in promoting and maintaining health. Nutrition, hydration, and electrolyte balance are interrelated and can have a significant impact on a person's functional status, immune system, and overall state of health.

Nutrition Standards
- In the United States, the U.S. Department of Agriculture (USDA) and the U.S. Department of Health and Human Services (DHHS) revise the *Dietary Guidelines for Americans* every 5 years. The most recent guidelines (2010) emphasize three major goals for Americans: to balance calories with physical activity to manage weight; to consume more of certain foods and nutrients such as fruits, vegetables, whole grains, fat-free and low-fat dairy products, and seafood; and to consume fewer foods with sodium, saturated fats and trans fats, cholesterol, added sugars, and refined grains. Also contained within these guidelines are recommendations for the general population as well as specific population groups. The intention of the recommendations is to help people choose an overall healthy diet.

- In 1992, the USDA developed the Food Guide Pyramid to translate nutrition recommendations into a graphic pyramid format, with the intention to communicate three key nutrition principles: variety, moderation, and proportion. The pyramid was redesigned in 2005 to facilitate understanding of these principles and also to stress the importance of physical activity to promote health. The USDA Web site also provides additional information for people of all ages and with special conditions (such as pregnancy) as well as the opportunity to create individualized meal plans at www.mypyramid.gov.
- Food pyramids also have been developed for people who are adopting specialized diets. The Vegetarian Food Pyramid was developed to assist vegetarians with daily food choices. The Atkins Pyramid was developed to reflect the current trend toward low-carbohydrate diets, and emphasizes building the diet on protein sources and vegetables rather than on grains.

NUTRITION SCREENING

- To identify patients who are malnourished or at risk for malnutrition, the first step is to complete a nutrition screening. The Joint Commission Patient Care Standards require that a nutritional screening be completed within 24 hours of admission to the hospital. This involves collecting a limited amount of health-related information that can identify malnutrition, and generally can be completed within 10 to 15 minutes. This screening may be repeated or followed up with a more comprehensive screening during a patient's hospital stay. The information gathered during a nutrition screening varies according to the patient population, type of care offered by the facility, and the patient's medical problem. Although multiple screening tools are available, there is no single screening method that is universally accepted, and healthcare facilities frequently develop specific techniques that meet their particular needs. Based on the screening results, an in-depth nutritional assessment should be performed. When patients are hospitalized for longer than a week, a nutritional assessment should be part of the daily plan of care. The initial nutritional screening typically includes the following:
  - Inspection
  - Measured height and weight
  - Weight history
  - Usual eating habits
  - Ability to chew and swallow
  - Recent changes in appetite and food intake
- Various methods are available for obtaining current dietary intake information. These include the 24-hour recall, the food frequency questionnaire, and the food diary. When patients are hospitalized, nutritional intake is documented through the use of calorie counts and direct observation. These are further described in Table 4–6.

Table 4–7. Methods for Collecting Current Dietary Intake

Method	Description	Advantages/Disadvantages
24-hour recall	This is the easiest and most popular method for obtaining information about dietary intake. The patient or family member is asked to recall everything consumed within the past 24 hours.	Advantage: • Able to elicit specific information about dietary intake over a specific period of time Disadvantages: • Patient or family member may not be able to recall the type or amount of food eaten • Intake within the past 24 hours may not be reflective of usual intake • The truth may be altered for a variety of reasons • Snack items and the use of gravies, sauces, and condiments may be underreported
Food frequency questionnaire	This tool is used to collect information on how many times per day, week, or month a person eats a particular food.	Disadvantages: • Does not always quantify the amount of intake • Relies on the patient's or family member's memory for how often a food was consumed
Food diary	This tool collects information about what a person has consumed for a certain period of time. Three days, which often includes 2 weekdays and a weekend day, are typically used. This is most complete and accurate if you instruct the patient to record the information immediately after eating.	Disadvantages: • Noncompliance • Inaccurate recording • Atypical intake on the recording days • Conscious altering of diet during the recording period
Direct observation	This process can detect problems not readily identified through the other methods for obtaining dietary intake or nutrition information. With this method, the caregiver observes the feeding techniques used and the type and amount of foods consumed.	Advantage: • Observing the typical feeding techniques by the patient or caregiver and the interaction between the patient and caregiver can be helpful if assessing failure to thrive or unintentional weight loss. This is best used with young children or older adults.

Nutrition Assessment

- A nutrition assessment is more comprehensive than a screening. It is generally completed by a registered dietitian or as a collaborative effort among the nurses, dietitian, or other members of the healthcare team. It involves the collection and analysis of pertinent health information for the purpose of identifying specific nutrition problems or causes of problems. The nutrition assessment should be sensitive enough to detect subtle nutrition problems and specific enough to identify problem areas. The components of a comprehensive nutritional assessment generally include the following:

HISTORY
- *Medical/Health History*
  - Current complaints
  - Past medical conditions
  - Surgical history
  - Family medical history
  - Chronic disease risk
  - Mental and emotional health status
- *Medication History*
  - Prescription drugs
  - Over-the-counter drugs
  - Dietary and herbal supplements and vitamins
- *Personal/Social History*
  - Age
  - Occupation
  - Educational level
  - Socioeconomic status
  - Cultural and ethnic identity and food preferences
  - Alcohol intake
  - Cigarettes and other tobacco use
  - Illegal drug use
  - Religious beliefs
  - Home and family situation
  - Cognitive changes affecting appetite and self-feeding
  - Psychosocial issues such as depression or isolation
- *Food/Nutrition History*
  - Food preferences and eating habits
  - Meal schedule
  - Special diets
  - Food allergies and intolerances
  - Nutrition and health knowledge
  - Food availability
  - Control over food choices and preparation
  - Physical activity and exercise patterns

CLINICAL EVALUATION
- Chronic illnesses
- Physical exam
- Oral health
- Chewing and swallowing

- Cognitive or psychological assessment
- Lab work (e.g., CBC, electrolytes, BUN, creatinine, serum proteins, pre-albumin, albumin, lipids)

ANTHROPOMETRIC ASSESSMENT
- Body mass index (BMI)
- Skinfold measurements
- Waist circumference (fat distribution)
- Weight changes (usual weight)
  - These are noninvasive methods of evaluating nutritional status, and include height, weight, and assessment of body fat. Obtain a current weight and height to provide baseline data and ensure accurate measurements because patients tend to overestimate height and underestimate weight. Subsequent measurements may indicate a change in nutritional status. Patients should be measured and weighed while wearing minimal clothing and no shoes. An unintentional weight loss of 10% over a 6-month period at any time significantly affects nutritional status and should be evaluated.
  - The BMI is a measure of nutritional status that is not dependent on frame size. It indirectly estimates total fat stores within the body based on the relationship of weight to height, and the normal BMI is between 18.5 and 24.9. (*Note.* BMI often overestimates fat stores in muscular athletes and underestimates fat stores in the elderly.) The lowest risk for malnutrition is associated with scores between 18.5 and 25, and scores above and below these values are associated with increased health risks. BMI tables are readily available. A calculation for estimating BMI can be completed using one of these two formulas:

$$BMI = \frac{\text{Weight (lb)}}{\text{Height (in inches)}^2} \times 703$$

$$BMI = \frac{\text{Weight (kg)}}{\text{Height (in meters)}^2}$$

MALNUTRITION

- The term *malnourished* can refer to those who are undernourished or those who are obese. Malnutrition is a multinutrient problem because foods that are positive sources of calories and protein are often high-quality sources of other nutrients. In an undernourished patient, protein catabolism exceeds protein intake and synthesis, and which results in a negative nitrogen balance, weight loss, decreased muscle mass, and weakness. Multiple body systems are impacted by malnutrition: the function of the heart, liver, lungs, gastrointestinal tract, and immune system are decreased. Hypoproteinemia occurs as protein synthesis in the liver decreases. Common complications of severe malnutrition include:
- Leanness and cachexia
- Decreased activity tolerance
- Lethargy
- Intolerance to cold
- Edema
- Dry, flaking skin and various types of dermatitis
- Poor wound healing

- Infection (especially postoperative infection and sepsis)
- Possible death
- Protein-energy malnutrition (PEM) may be present in three forms: marasmus, kwashiorkor, and marasmic-kwashiorkor. They are described in Table 4–8. Unrecognized or untreated PEM often results in dysfunction or disability and leads to increased morbidity or mortality. Acute PEM may develop in patients who were adequately nourished prior to hospitalization but experienced starvation due to a catabolic state resulting from infection, stress, or injury. Chronic PEM may occur in patients who have cancer, end-stage kidney or liver disease, or chronic neurological disease.

Table 4–8. Types of Protein-Energy Malnutrition (PEM)

Type of PEM	Description
Marasmus	Calorie malnutrition in which body fat and protein are wasted. Occurs due to an inadequate intake of calories or prolonged starvation. Serum proteins are generally preserved.
Kwashiorkor	Protein malnutrition caused by inadequate protein quantity and quality despite adequate caloric intake. May also result from long-term use of dextrose-containing IV fluids. Body weight is typically normal and serum proteins are low. Serum albumin is < 3.5 g/dL.
Marasmic Kwashiorkor	Combined protein and energy malnutrition caused by prolonged inadequate intake of protein and calories. Persons with this form of PEM typically present with muscle, fat, and visceral protein wasting. Often presents clinically when metabolic stress is imposed on an individual who is chronically starved. Without nutritional support, this type of PEM is associated with the highest risk of morbidity and mortality.

Psychosocial Factors Affecting Nutrition
- Psychosocial factors play an important role in the desire to eat as well as the attainment of nutritional foods. Multiple psychosocial factors may impact a person's nutritional status and contribute to malnutrition. These include:
  - Lack of education
  - Poverty
  - Substance abuse
  - Decreased appetite
  - Decline in functional ability to eat independently
  - Lack of transportation
  - Culture
  - Social isolation
  - Depression
  - Dementia

Oral, Dental, and Swallowing Conditions Affecting Nutrition
- The following oral and swallowing conditions may affect people of all ages, and may impact a person's ability to eat a well-balanced diet.
  - Tooth decay
  - Periodontal disease

- Missing teeth or ill-fitting dentures
- Xerostomia
- Taste disorders
- Oral infections
- Oral or throat lesions
- Medications causing nausea or dry mouth or affecting taste, appetite, or level of consciousness
- Dysphagia

Nutrition Interventions

- The treatment of malnutrition is initially directed at correcting reversible causes whenever possible. An example would be to replace ill-fitting dentures or treat periodontal disease, which may improve dietary intake without the need for other interventions. Also, avoiding restrictive diets when possible without exacerbating an underlying disease may also improve dietary intake. For example, foods low in fat may be too calorie-restrictive for some persons or not tolerated by others. Foods may also be made more calorie-dense without increasing the volume of food when the patient is only able to tolerate small meals. Calorie density may be increased by using whole milk in place of low-fat milk; adding protein powder or another dietary supplement to cereals, soups, sauces, or beverages; adding butter to hot savory foods; or adding sugar, corn syrup, or honey to sweet foods. Milkshakes may also be made with a variety of calorie-dense dairy products and healthy fruits. Other interventions include:
  - Schedule oral supplements so as to not interfere with meals.
  - Refer patients with dysphagia to a speech therapist.
  - Aid persons with eating problems.
  - Monitor bowel regimens and treat constipation and diarrhea.

Effects of Illness on Nutrition

- The role of nutrition in illness has long been a topic of interest. Although the current focus is on health promotion and disease prevention through healthy eating and exercise, the impact of nutrition in illness is significant. A disease process and its treatments can lead to malnutrition in multiple ways, such as decreasing appetite and food intake, interfering with digestion and absorption of nutrients, or altering nutrient metabolism and excretion. Certain medications may cause gastrointestinal discomfort or anorexia or can interfere with nutrient function or metabolism. Patients who are on bed rest are susceptible to developing pressure ulcers, the presence of which increases metabolic stress as well as protein and energy needs of the body.
- During an acute illness, the dietary changes required are generally temporary and can be adjusted to accommodate a person's lifestyle and individual preferences. However, chronic illnesses may demand long-term dietary and lifestyle modifications, as in the case of diabetes. The challenge for nurses is to aid their patients in appreciating the potential benefits of treatment and to accept the modifications in diet that can improve their health status.

REFERENCES

Ignatavicius, D. D. (2010). Care of patients with malnutrition and obesity. In D. D. Ignatavicius and M. L. Workman (Eds.), *Medical-surgical nursing: Patient-centered collaborative care*. St. Louis, MO: Saunders.

Ignatavicius, D. D., & Workman, M. L. (2010). *Medical-surgical nursing: Patient-centered collaborative practice*. St. Louis, MO: Saunders Elsevier.

Lehne, R. (2009). *Pharmacology for nursing care* (7th ed.). Philadelphia: W.B. Saunders.

Medline Plus. (2011). *Echinacea: Are there interactions with medications?* Retrieved from http://www.nlm.nih.gov/medlineplus/druginfo/natural/981.html#DrugInteractions

Morton, P. G., & Fontaine, D. K. (2009). *Critical care nursing: A holistic approach*. Philadelphia: Wolters Kluwer/Lippincott Williams & Wilkins.

Pagana, K. D., & Pagana, T. J. (2009). *Mosby's diagnostic and laboratory test reference* (9th ed.). St. Louis, MO: Mosby Elsevier.

Perrin, K. O. (2009). *Understanding the essentials of critical care nursing*. Upper Saddle River, NJ: Pearson.

Potter, P. A., & Perry, A. G. (2009). *Fundamentals of nursing* (7th ed.). St. Louis, MO: Mosby Elsevier.

Rolfes, R. R., Pinna, K., & Whitney, E. (2009). *Understanding normal and clinical nutrition*. Belmont, CA: Wadsworth Cengage Learning.

U.S. Department of Agriculture. (2011). *Anatomy of MyPyramid*. Retrieved from http://www.mypyramid.gov/downloads/MyPyramid_Anatomy.pdf

U.S. Department of Health & Human Services. (2011). *Dietary guidelines for Americans, 2010*. Retrieved from http://www.health.gov/dietaryguidelines/2010.asp

Wilson, B. A., Shannon, M. T., & Shields, K. M. (2009). *Prentice Hall nurse's drug guide 2009*. Upper Saddle River, NJ: Pearson.

5

Behavioral Sciences

Nancy Henne Batchelor, MSN, RN-BC, CNS,
& Deborah Jane Schwytzer, MSN, RN-BC, CEN

COPING: ANXIETY

Normal (Adaptive)
- Universal adaptive response to danger

Abnormal
- Maladaptive response to a stimulus that does not present danger
- Associated with disturbance in neurotransmitters

Factors Affecting the Severity of Anxiety
- Strength and intensity of stressors
- Duration of stressors
- Individual coping abilities
- Individual's perceived sense of helplessness

Variables Affecting Coping Abilities
- Culture
- Religion
- Education
- Past experiences

Variables Affecting the Development of Anxiety
- Perceived threat to biological integrity
- Perceived threats to self-esteem
- Frustration of needs or motives
- Inability to control or influence meaningful events
- Mental association with previous anxiety-producing events

Assessment of Anxiety
- Mild
  - Alert, attentive, confident
  - Open to new experiences
  - Good problem-solving abilities
  - Can deal with more than one issue at a time
  - Can apply coping mechanisms
- Moderate
  - Narrowed perceptual fields
  - Lessened ability to problem-solve
  - Increased respirations, heart rate, muscle tension
  - Dry mouth, clammy palms, palpitations
  - Restlessness
- Severe
  - Impaired cognition
  - Narrowed perceptual fields
  - Focus on only one detail at a time
  - Decreased ability to concentrate
  - Unable to learn
  - Pacing, sweating, hyperventilation
  - Tremors, numbness, tingling
  - Nausea, headache, dizziness
- Panic
  - Chest pain, breathlessness, tachycardia
  - Feeling of impending death
  - Closed perceptual fields
  - Unrealistic perceptions
  - Inability to communicate clearly
  - Need for rapid resolution

Nursing Diagnosis
- Risk for anxiety due to knowledge deficit
- Risk for anxiety due to stress of surgery

Interventions
- Identify knowledge level.
- Determine coping mechanisms.
- Include support person in pre-op teaching.
- Determine patient's wishes regarding care.
- Assess for level of anxiety: scale 1 to 10.
- Limit demands on patient.
- Reduce sensory stimuli.

- Utilize patient's present coping mechanisms.
- Focus on present and short-term goals.
- Teach ways to stop anxiety:
  - Guided imagery
  - Relaxation
  - Controlled breathing
- Avoid interaction with others who are anxious.
- Provide clear, consistent communication.
- Allow expression of feelings: *listen.*
- Pharmacological therapy if needed.

POSTTRAUMATIC STRESS DISORDER

- Anxiety disorder following a life-threatening or traumatic event
  - Natural disaster
  - Accidents
  - Conflict: war, murder, abuse, rape

Symptoms
- Reexperiencing the event
  - Dreams
  - Intrusive thoughts
- Avoidance of situations that trigger memories of the event
- Avoidance of feelings related to the event
- Numbing of feelings
- Lack of enjoyment
- Hypervigilance
  - Startles easily
  - Difficulty sleeping

Interventions
- Refer for specialty care.
- Build trusting relationships.
- Explore trauma and its meaning.
- Increase coping strategies.

BODY IMAGE DISTURBANCE

- Body image is how we internally view our physical selves.

Causes of Body Image Disturbance
- Eating disorders
- Body dysmorphic disorder
- Loss of body part
- Changed body part

Nursing Interventions

- Acknowledge denial, depression, anger as normal ways to cope.
- Do not rush sharing of feelings.
- Encourage attractive clothing to de-emphasize loss or changed body part.
- Facilitate gradual exposure to loss or changed body part.
- Involve patient in his or her own care; maximize abilities.
- Be aware of your own nonverbal behaviors.

DEPRESSION

- Predictable response to illness and hospitalization
- Often accompanies loss and grief
- Neurobiological disorder
- Has significant morbidity and mortality; contributes to suicide, illness, disruption in interpersonal relationships, substance abuse, and lost work time

Table 5–1. DSM-IV Criteria to Diagnose Major Depression

One of the first two symptoms in Cluster 2 for 2 or more weeks plus any 4 of the remaining symptoms

Cluster 1	Cluster 2
Sleep disturbances	Psychological or psychosocial symptoms
Attention or concentration problems	Depressed mood
Energy level change; fatigue	Reduction in pleasure or interest
Psychomotor disturbances	Feelings of guilt
Physical or neurovegetative symptoms	Suicidal thoughts

Gillman, P (2007). Retrieved from ANCC Medical-Surgical Nurse Certification Review Seminar, Module 8.

Risk Factors for Suicide

- Male
- 55 years or older
- White
- Concurrent medical illness
- Social isolation
- Family history of depression or suicide
- Command hallucinations
- Access to firearms
- Depression with melancholy or delusions
- Family violence

Signs for Concern

- Feelings of hopelessness, worthlessness
- Withdrawal from social activities

- Changes in sleeping or eating patterns
- Feelings of rage, anger, need for revenge
- Feelings of exhaustion
- Frequent physical complaints
- Trouble with concentration
- Academic issues
- Feelings of listlessness, irritability
- Regular or frequent crying
- Reckless, impulsive behaviors
- Physical neglect

Nursing Interventions
- Validate the presence of depression.
- Provide emotional support through empathetic listening.
- Encourage expression of feelings.
- Avoid cheerfulness and false reassurance.
- Encourage involvement in self-care.
- Assist in goal-setting and problem-solving.
- Assess for suicidal ideation.
- Consult for psychotherapy or pharmacological therapy.

Crisis Intervention
- Methods used to offer immediate, short-term help to individuals who experience an event that produces emotional, mental, physical, and behavioral distress.
- Crisis: any situation in which the individual perceives a sudden loss of ability to use effective problem-solving and coping skills.
  - Natural disasters
  - Sexual assault
  - Criminal victimization
  - Medical or mental illness
  - Thoughts of suicide or homicide
  - Loss of or drastic changes in relationships

Purpose of Crisis Intervention
- Reduce intensity of patient's reaction to crisis.
- Assist patients to return to pre-crisis level of functioning.
- Prevent development of long-term problems.
- Maintain safety of the person experiencing the crisis.

Crisis Intervention Services
- Family doctors
- Mental health specialists
- Religious leaders or counselors
- Health maintenance organizations
- Community mental health centers
- University- or medical school–affiliated programs
- State hospital outpatient clinics
- Social service agencies
- Private clinics and facilities

- Employee assistance programs
- Local medical or psychiatric societies
- Hospital psychiatry departments or outpatient clinics

END-OF-LIFE CARE

- End-of-life decisions can be difficult and complex.
- Satisfaction with choices depends on the information received and the way in which the information is presented.
- Patient's views and wishes for end-of-life care should be respected.

Palliative Care

- Interdisciplinary care that focuses on symptom management for the individual and family suffering from life-limiting disease.
- Goal is to prevent or relieve suffering and support best quality of life regardless of the stage of the disease.
- Should be provided when cure or reversibility is unlikely and treatment burden is high.
- Examples: stroke, cancer, renal disease, end-stage cardiac disease, liver failure, dementia.

Hospice

- Multidisciplinary care for patient and family throughout the dying process.
- Provides comprehensive medical and support services.
- Focus on symptom management and quality of life.
- Included under the umbrella of palliative care.
- Begins when patient prognosis is 6 months or less.
- Regards dying as a normal part of life and provides support for peaceful and dignified death.

Cultural Considerations

- Sensitive communication
- Use interpreter for objective verbal communication
- Personal space
- Eye contact: avoiding shows respect in some cultures
- Touch: determine patient comfort
- View of healthcare professionals
  - Hispanic or Latino
    - Catholicism: predominant religion
    - May avoid eye contact
    - Family: often extended; may make decisions
    - May not complain of pain
    - Prayer and folk remedies common
    - Strong belief in afterlife
  - Black
    - Displays of emotion acceptable
    - Discuss issues with eldest family member
    - Pain reported, but fearful of addiction
    - Often do not report depression
    - Home remedies common
    - Strong belief in afterlife

- Chinese-American
  - Buddhist and Christian religions
  - Avoid eye contact
  - Family may make decisions; patient passive
  - Communication with family may appear loud and argumentative
  - May not report pain
  - Chinese medications and acupuncture common
  - Belief in afterlife varies
- Native American
  - May not openly express religion
  - Belief systems vary among tribes
  - Stoicism common; complaints vague
  - Avoid eye contact
  - Traditional medicines common
  - Some avoid eye contact with the dying

GRIEF AND LOSS

- Grief: emotional response to loss and its accompanying changes
- Grieving: internal process used by the person to work through the loss
- Mourning: actions or expressions (outward manifestations) of grief
- Loss: actual or potential situation in which there is a loss or change of an object, persons, body part, or emotion

Kübler-Ross: Stages of Grief

- Denial: shock and disbelief
  - Serves as buffer in helping to mobilize defenses to cope with situation.
- Anger: resistance to loss
  - May be directed at family or healthcare workers.
- Bargaining: attempt to postpone the loss
  - Expresses willingness to do anything to postpone the loss.
- Depression: realization of full impact of the loss
  - May talk freely or withdraw.
- Acceptance: emotional pain is gone and hope returns
  - Patient may appear devoid of emotion.
- Sequence of stages may vary.
- Not all stages may occur.

Physical Changes at the End-of-Life

- Pain: physical, psychological, or spiritual
- Changes in mental status
- Failure to eat and drink
- Failure to respond to the presence of others
- Guarding
- Resisting care
- Rapid heartbeat, diaphoresis, change in baseline vital signs

Table 5-2. Symptom Management Strategies for the Patient at the End of Life

Problem	Intervention
Constipation	Stimulant laxatives and enema after 3 days without bowel movement Bowel regimen to prevent constipation for patients on narcotics
Delirium	Treat other symptoms: pain, fever, social isolation No restraints Anti-anxiety medications if patient is safety risk Sitters
Dyspnea	Opioids to decrease work of breathing Anti-anxiety medications to manage respiratory-related anxiety Humidified oxygen, fans for airflow
Cough	Cough suppressants Elevate head of bed
Congestion (terminal secretions)	Anticholinergics (scopolamine patch [Transderm], atropine eye drops sublingual) dry up secretions Side-lying position with head elevated
Anorexia	Hourly mouth care Treat constipation, nausea, and vomiting Offer favorite foods and fluids
Nausea & vomiting	Antiemetics Complementary therapies
Fatigue	Frequent rest periods
Anxiety	Antidepressants, anti-anxiety agents for sleep and relaxation Provide emotional and spiritual support
Pain	Narcotic analgesics, NSAIDs for bone pain, provide support

Table 5-3. Emotional or Spiritual Symptoms of Approaching Death

Symptom	Intervention
Withdrawal	Communicate as usual or provide reassurance
Vision-like experiences	Reassurance
Restlessness	Listen Give permission to die
Decreased socialization	Express support Give permission to die
Unusual communication	Verbalize what needs to be said Kiss, hug, cry

Physical Symptoms That Indicate Death Is Imminent
- Shallow respirations with periods of apnea
- Upper respiratory congestion
- Mottled extremities
- Weak or absent peripheral pulses
- Decreased or absent urine output
- Disorientation or decreased consciousness

Nursing Interventions at the Time of Death
- Document time and any related data.
- Provide support for family; allow expression of grief.
- Provide open, honest dialogue.
- Allow loved ones time to view, touch, and hold the body.
- Report death to organ donation center (identify tissue donation).
- Prepare body for transport to funeral home or morgue.
- Refer loved ones to chaplain, social services, support groups for grief counseling.

CULTURAL OR ETHNIC BELIEFS AND PRACTICES

Cultural Overview
- The understanding and implementation of culturally competent care is necessary for the provision of quality patient and family care in today's healthcare settings.
- Culturally competent care requires that the nurse be sensitive to cultural needs and be able to respond to them. This sensitivity is based on the recognition of cultural diversity and respect for cultures different than the nurse's own. It also requires that the nurse be willing to modify care based on the health beliefs, practices, language, communication styles, values, and role of family and community in the patient's culture.
- Knowledge of specific cultural and ethnic variations can relieve patient anxiety, facilitate understanding, and enhance likelihood of a successful outcome. It is important for the nurse to be aware that customs vary within a population as well as between populations.
- The nurse can assess the cultural needs of the patient and family by asking questions, interviewing the patient and family, and observing practices and behaviors.

Selected Concepts of Cultural Importance

Communication
- Language is essential for effective communication. It is not safe to assume that the knowledge of a few English words will be sufficient for the understanding of care requirements and concerns. It is essential that the nurse use someone other than family members as interpreters if needed to enhance the exchange of information. Culturally and linguistically appropriate signs and translation materials should be made available.
- The style of speech such as tone, intensity, and pacing can influence the reception and understanding of communication both negatively and positively. Loud, repetitive speech patterns may be used for clarification or may indicate anger in some cultures.

- Use of silent, nonverbal, and contextual cueing communication such as eye contact, gestures, posture, and touch can be interpreted differently across cultures. Long eye contact may signify rudeness, inattention, or disrespect in some cultures while signaling respect and attention in others. Touch is welcomed and conveys a sense of concern and compassion in some cultures, unwelcome in others, and welcomed but prohibited on some parts of the body or between genders in other cultures, or a particular sequence of touch may be prescribed.
- The cultural background, age, gender, or role of the healthcare provider can influence the patient's ability to interact effectively.

Health Beliefs and Practices

- It is important to know the patient's views of health and illness and their related cultural practices. Does the patient's culture view illness as a curse for some action? Does their culture have health remedies that can be included in the current health treatment regimen? Does the patient's culture include health practices that are harmful and signify a need for education and change, such as the ingestion of potentially toxic substances?
- Health beliefs and practices must also be considered when planning for preventive and restorative care. Cultures that believe health is externally controlled and not within the control of the individual may not be receptive to health promotion activities.
- Some cultures have health topics that are considered taboo, not to be discussed in public, with certain family members, or with persons of the opposite gender. An understanding of these beliefs can facilitate the presence of appropriate individuals should these health topics need to be addressed.
- An understanding of dietary practices, home remedies, and spiritual beliefs surrounding illness, health, and even death will assist the development of a culturally appropriate plan of care.
- Cultural beliefs also can impact the expression of disease symptoms such as pain and fatigue or the reaction to death. The nurse must be familiar with the patient's and family's approach to these events and prepare for appropriate interactions.

Space

- Personal space is an important and culturally sensitive issue. Some cultures prefer specific distances for certain interactions while others have no preferences. Isolation may be an issue in the care of individuals from cultures that value the intimate and personal zones of interaction.
- The concept of space also can be a factor when viewed as the environmental space or the patient's immediate surroundings. Strong religious or ethnic beliefs may require that certain objects or persons be present in the room or that furniture be arranged in a particular way.

Time Orientation

- Time orientation such as valuing past, present, or future time frames can impact health practices and planning for interventions. People who believe in the impact of ancestral intervention or interpersonal interactions may have a hard time planning for the future, while people who live for the future may have a hard time resting and recovering in the present.
- The nurse must recognize the time orientation of the patient and family and communicate clearly about any time-sensitive tests or activities.

Diet

- Understanding a person's meaning of food, dietary requirements, and practices can be a significant factor in ensuring appropriate interactions. Knowledge of cultural and religious dietary restrictions and practices is required to provide and adapt appropriate care.
- Dietary restrictions or preferences can be met by allowing family members to select meal items or bring particular food items that are desired by the patient.

Family and Social Relationships

- The social relationships of the patient are very important. Knowledge of the role of elders, community or cultural leaders, community support, and family are important to understand when addressing healthcare decisions and understanding patient behaviors. Does the individual assume responsibility for his or her own care when ill, or do family or community members assume responsibility?
- Interpersonal relationships can affect the patient's behaviors, decision-making, and interaction with healthcare providers.

Specific Cultural Considerations

- Chinese-American
  - Communication
    - Often shy and reserved. Tone of voice may be viewed as loud at times but is due to the expressive nature of the language.
    - Eye contact with someone older or considered superior is a sign of disrespect. Slight bow is form of greeting and respect.
    - Negative feelings such as anger or hostility are not displayed openly.
    - Smiling is the major expression of many emotions in Asian cultures. It can mean happiness and agreement but can also be used to express anger, frustration, embarrassment, or a lack of understanding.
    - Interpreters can be used for complicated health issues but be aware of the need to use an interpreter of appropriate gender for topics of modesty.
    - Patient should be addressed as Mr. or Mrs. unless advised otherwise.
  - Health practices
    - Believe that health is based on a harmony with nature; thus, illness is being out of balance. The concepts of "hot" (Yang) and "cold" (Yin) and their assignment to certain foods, activities, and so on are used to maintain a healthy balance.
    - The body is a gift that must be maintained and cared for. One example is the belief that blood donations are a sign of disrespect to ancestors and that blood contains a person's "life energy."
    - Pain, discomfort, and hunger are tolerated in silence because of the belief that nothing should be accepted the first time offered. The nurse should observe physical signs and offer relief methods as needed.
    - Chinese medical practices of acupuncture, acupressure, and herbs are common adjuncts to medical care. Patients may not admit to using these for fear of disapproval.
    - The rubbing of coins on the body is a cultural treatment for illness. This practice can leave dark scratches and welts that have occasionally been misinterpreted as signs of abuse.
    - A traditional period of "lying-in" is practiced for 7 days following childbirth. Because of the belief that the woman is weak after giving birth and susceptible to "outside forces" that may cause illness and pain, the woman is only to rest, stay warm, and avoid exercise and bathing during this time.

- An apparent lack of interest in and bonding with a new baby is based in a cultural belief that drawing attention to the new baby can entice "spirits" to "steal" the infant by causing its death. Despite appearances, however, the baby is the center of the family's attention.
- Personal hygiene is important. Patients generally prefer toilet to bedpan because bodily elimination is viewed as unclean and should not be performed in bed.
- Space and privacy
  - Avoid unnecessary physical contact.
  - Keeping respectful distance is important.
  - Very private and modest.
- Time orientation
  - Past-oriented.
  - Being on time is less valued in many Asian cultures than in the United States. Healthcare providers must be aware of this and reinforce the need for compliance with appointment times.
- Diet
  - Food is important in maintaining balance of Yin and Yang. Certain foods are considered important for the maintenance of good health or to cure illness. Families should be encouraged to bring in special foods.
  - Drinking hot liquids such as teas and soups when sick helps to maintain health balance.
- Family and social relationships
  - Cultural norm is that the needs of the group take precedence over the needs of the individual.
  - Males are more highly respected than females.
  - Children are expected to respect their elders. The oldest male in the family often is involved in care decisions.
  - Family members may assist with care, particularly of elder males. The caring role is generally the responsibility of a female member of the family.
  - Large, extended family social networks means a large number of visitors may come to the hospital and bring food.
- Black
  - Communication
    - Affection is communicated through touch, frequent handshakes, being close, and hugging as a greeting as well as during times of need.
    - Eye contact is maintained to show respect and trust.
    - Patients should be addressed as Mr. or Mrs. until advised otherwise.
    - Literacy may be an issue when asked to sign forms. Ask what level of school was completed before assuming informed consent and orally explain to patient and family satisfaction.
    - "Black English," which includes different meanings for some words, may be used. Healthcare providers must make sure that understanding is achieved.
  - Health practices
    - The cause of physical illness may be attributed to natural or supernatural causes, or God's punishment, or exposure to cold or wind.
    - Mental illness is believed to be due to a lack of spiritual balance.
    - Family and relatives are expected to help with care during illness.
    - Magic and voodoo are sometimes used in rural areas. Folk medicine such as teas, herbs, warm compresses, and talismans may be used by folk healers. Home remedies are usually tried before seeking care elsewhere.

- Patient experiencing pain may remain stoic so as not to bother the nurse, or may openly express pain but avoid pain medications for fear of addiction.
- Patients tend to rely on older women of the family for assistance and advice during pregnancy and birth.
- Family frequently cares for dying patient until death is imminent. Patients are then transferred to the hospital, because death in the home is believed to bring bad luck to the home.
- Loved ones will openly show emotions at patient's death.
- Space and privacy
  - Respect privacy.
  - Will provide information if trust is established.
  - Affection displayed through close contact.
- Time orientation
  - Present-oriented; do not like to wait.
  - Life issues take priority over keeping appointments.
  - Assistance in prioritizing healthcare and health promotion activities can be beneficial for the patient.
- Diet
  - Usual meal pattern is three meals per day with the inclusion of hearty meals of cold drinks, meats and cooked greens, red and yellow vegetables, and fresh fruits.
  - May have religious restrictions on foods and drinks, such as Muslim and Seventh Day Adventist dietary laws.
  - Lactose intolerance is common.
- Family and social relationships
  - Family is very important.
  - Many extended family members are possible and may be included in decision-making.
  - Religion and religious behaviors are valued.
  - Elders are held in high esteem.
  - Funerals are often celebrations of passing to a better place.
- Hispanic or Latino
  - Communication
    - Many dialects and levels of speech and writing skills; healthcare providers must provide clear oral and visual instructions for understanding.
    - Nonverbal communication based on respect; little direct eye contact with perceived authority such as healthcare providers.
    - Typically will stand when healthcare providers enter a room.
    - Silence may show disagreement with plan of care.
    - Nonverbal clues needed to detect presence of pain because patient generally will not complain.
    - Therapeutic touch acceptable; touch by strangers can be viewed as disrespectful or unwelcome.
    - Handshaking is viewed as polite.
    - Warm and expressive with family and close friends.
    - Same-gender translators generally acceptable.
    - Should be addressed as Mr. or Mrs. until advised otherwise.
  - Health practices
    - Health is feeling well and being able to maintain role.
    - Religion is major influence on healthcare practices.
    - Believe in hot and cold theory of disease prevention.

- Traditional folk healers may be involved in care. Folk remedies have prominence in this culture. "Evil eye," hex, or bad spirits may be the believed basis for diseases.
- Illness viewed as family crisis and must be dealt with as a family. Major healthcare decisions made by head of household, but will require family consultation.
- Importance of family assisting in care.
- Prevention activities restricted because of belief that future is in God's hands.
- The ill patient prefers to be cared for at home by family members and will seek medical assistance when no improvement in condition or disease interferes with role expectations.
  - Space and privacy
    - Immediate family is involved in care; visitors are expected to be quiet, concerned, and stay out of the way.
    - Modesty is very important, especially in females.
  - Time orientation
    - Present-oriented; may arrive late for appointments because of different cultural perceptions of the importance of being on time and of what "on time" means; little planning ahead.
    - Not responsive to a hurried pace.
  - Diet
    - Food is primary form of socialization.
    - Three meals per day; prefer to eat meals as a family.
    - Traditional food beliefs may be based on Galan's humoral theory of body's humors: blood, phlegm, yellow bile, and black bile must be kept in balance. Diseases caused by disruption of the hot and cold balance of these humors are treated with heat, cold, moisture, and dryness.
    - Fresh fruits, vegetables, beans, and rice are common staples. The family may be encouraged to bring food to the patient.
    - Soup and herbal teas used to speed recovery.
  - Family and social relationships
    - Extended family and children are valued.
    - Traditional family is the foundation of society. Older adults and authority are to be respected.
    - Strong religious community, connections, and support.
- Native American
  - Communication
    - Avoid eye contact as a sign of respect.
    - Requests are generally carefully considered before made.
    - Generally quiet and stoic; however, at times of grieving, demonstrative behaviors may be exhibited.
  - Health practices
    - Health and illness are related to harmony with nature. A holistic perspective on life and health influences the integration of spiritual, physical, social, and psychological approaches.
    - Folk healers (shamans) are frequently involved in care.
    - Medicine bundles or a bag filled with herbs blessed by a medicine man or woman during a healing ceremony is worn frequently.
    - Tribal rituals and taboos impact healthcare decisions. Tribal rituals may be performed as well as medical care regimens. Encourage inclusion of both in care.

- Immediate family involved in decisions; however, children are not expected to impose their wishes in end-of-life decisions.
- Space and privacy
  - Respect privacy
  - Keep respectful distance
  - Light touch handshakes acceptable
- Time orientation
  - Present-oriented
  - Feel that time is flexible
- Diet
  - Generally light breakfast; number of meals depends on social activities.
  - Enjoy sharing food with family and visitors due to strong sense of hospitality and respect for visitors.
  - Foods may be blessed per religious tradition. Staff should respect traditions.
- Family and social relationships
  - Personal autonomy very important.
  - Pride in culture and tribal nation.
  - Religion is a way of life.
  - Tribal elders are authority.
  - Respect and value for children, who are seen as helpers for the family, particularly with the elderly.

SEXUALITY

Assessment
- Sexual health history
  - Physical relationships
    - Number of lifetime partners
    - Number of current partners
    - Same sex, opposite sex, or both
    - Current relationship
  - Functional relationships
  - Lifestyle
    - Drug use—including illicit—marijuana, cocaine
    - Alcohol use: amount, frequency
  - Self-esteem factors
  - History of sexually transmitted infections (STIs)
  - History of sexual dysfunction
- Factors affecting sexual desire
  - Illness
  - Stress
  - ETOH
  - Abuse history
  - Risk of pregnancy
  - Financial issues
- Assess patient's developmental state with regard to sexuality
- Perform physical assessment of urogenital area
- Determine patient's sexual concerns

- Assess impact of high-risk behaviors, safe sex practices, use of birth control
- Assess medical conditions and medications that affect sexual function

Common Female Problems
- Orgasmic dysfunction
  - Results from:
    - Endometriosis
    - Menopause
    - Vaginal scarring
    - Psychological trauma
    - Medications: SSRIs
- Vaginismus
  - Painful penetration secondary to contraction of the vaginal muscles
- Dyspareunia
  - Painful intercourse
- Lack of desire
  - Lack of lubrication

Common Male Sexual Dysfunction
- Erectile dysfunction
  - Inability to achieve or sustain an erection firm enough for intercourse
  - Caused by:
    - Illness
      - Diabetes
      - Stroke
      - Atherosclerosis
      - Spinal cord injury
      - Prostate surgery
    - Psychological factors
      - Guilt
      - Depression
      - Performance anxiety
      - Fear of intimacy
    - Smoking
    - Drug or alcohol use
      - Diuretics
      - Metoclopramide
      - Beta blockers
      - ACE inhibitors
- Premature ejaculation
- Delayed ejaculation

Care Planning
- Create atmosphere in which patient can discuss sexual concerns.
- Refer to appropriate resources for sexual concerns.
- Explore patient's beliefs, attitudes, understanding of sexuality and sexual functioning.
- Provide education on safe sex, sexually transmitted diseases, and family planning.

Psychological Responses

STRESS

- A condition or feeling experienced when a person perceives that demands exceed the personal and social resources the person is able to mobilize, while recognizing that there is an intertwined instinctive stress response to unexpected events.

Components
- Stressor: stimulus
- Stress perception: recognition of the stressor in the brain
- Stress response: activation of the fight, flight, or fright system

Types of Stressors
- Internal: originate within the person
  - Lifestyle choices
  - Precipitated by physiological or psychological stimuli (cancer, depression, anxiety)
- External: originate outside the body and are precipitated by changes in the external environment
  - Bright light, rudeness, deadlines, sudden death, hurricanes, daily issues
- Acute: brief and tangible, readily identified
- Chronic: of longer duration, may be intangible and not readily identified
  - May pose serious health threat if not managed
- Developmental: occur at various points throughout the life span; predictable
  - Getting married, adjusting to retirement
- Situational: precipitated by various situations, unpredictable
  - Positive or negative
    - Illness, new job

GENERAL ADAPTATION SYNDROME

- Physical responses to stress

Alarm Stage
- Initiation of fight or flight response

Shock phase
- Stressor may or may not be perceived
  - Adrenaline and cortisone are released
  - Lasts 1 to 24 hours

Countershock Phase
- Reversal of the body changes produced in shock phase
  - Body prepared to react
  - Symptoms
    - Increased blood pressure, pulse, respirations
    - Decreased gastrointestinal motility

- Pupil dilation
- Increased perspiration
- Anxiety
- Anorexia
- Fatigue
- Nausea

Resistance Stage
- Reflects the individual's adaptation to the stressor.
- Body attempts to cope with and limit stressor.
- Expends energy in order to adapt.
- Symptoms disappear.

Exhaustion
- Occurs only if stress is overwhelming, not removed, or if coping is ineffective.
- May end with death if outside sources not available.
- Symptoms may reappear.
- End of this stage depends on adaptive energy resources, severity of stressor, and external adaptive resources provided.

Risk Factors for Stress
- Women in general
- Working mothers
- Family caregivers
- Less educated persons
- Divorced or widowed
- Unemployed
- Isolated persons
- Persons discriminated against or targets of bigotry
- Uninsured persons
- City dwellers

Gerontological Considerations
- The ability to achieve relaxation response to stress is decreased as one ages.
- Older adults have reduced resiliency.
- Chronic stress enhances the aging process; stress responses become inefficient.

Stress Responses Influenced by Lack of Coping Resources
- Coping resources
  - Social support
  - Problem-solving skills
  - Material resources
  - Medical problems
- Stress-reduction techniques
  - Maintain healthy lifestyle
  - Utilize relaxation techniques
  - Use cognitive-behavioral methods to decrease stress
  - Use positive coping strategies
  - Verbalize feelings

- Have positive outlook
- Use humor
- Seek professional help

SUBSTANCE USE DISORDERS

- Substance: agent ingested to alter mood or behavior for nonmedical reasons
- Diagnosis of substance abuse (one or more of the following occur within a 12-month period):
  - Recurrent substance use resulting in failure to fulfill major role obligations
  - Recurrent substance use in situations that are physically hazardous
  - Substance use causes legal problems
  - Substance use despite having persistent or recurrent social or interpersonal problems
- Substance dependence (three or more of the following occur within a 12-month period):
  - Tolerance, withdrawal, use in larger amounts over a longer period than intended
  - Persistent desire or unsuccessful efforts to cut down
  - Great deal of time spent in activities necessary to obtain the substance
  - Reduction in social, occupational, or recreational activities because of substance use
  - Substance use continues despite knowledge of problems
- Types of substances abused:
  - Stimulants: cocaine, amphetamines
  - Hallucinogens: LSD, DMT, PCP, ecstasy
  - Depressants: barbiturates, benzodiazepines, meprobamate, chloral hydrate
  - Opioids: morphine, heroin, oxycodone (Oxycontin), hydromorphone (Dilaudid)
  - Inhalants: nitrous oxide, amyl nitrate, butyl nitrite, toluene, acetone, airplane glue
  - Steroids
  - Prescription drugs: methadone, hydrocodone, soma
  - Alcohol
  - Nicotine
- How use affects medical-surgical care:
  - Physical presence of the drug
  - Complications due to withdrawal
- Screening: CAGE questionnaire for alcohol abuse (Ewing, 1984):
  - C: Cut down
  - A: Annoyed by criticism of your drinking
  - G: Guilty about drinking
  - E: Eye-opener in the morning
  - Most frequently used for the detection of alcoholism in the clinical setting
  - If two or more responses are "yes," a complete alcohol use disorder assessment should be completed
- Substance abuse interview questions (Osborn, Wraa, & Watson, 2010):
  - How many packs of cigarettes do you smoke daily?
  - Do you take any prescription drugs now?
  - Do you drink alcohol each day? If so, do you drink a pint or about a quart?
  - Do you drink a pint or a quart of alcohol or more on occasion?
  - When was your last drink?
  - Do you have a drug habit?
  - What drugs do you use?
  - What is your daily cost?
  - When did you last drink more than you intended to?

Violence

DOMESTIC VIOLENCE

- Infliction of threat or physical harm upon an intimate partner

Risk Factors
- History is not compatible with the exam
- Repeat visits for the same complaint
- Delay in seeking care
- Many symptoms with negative physical findings
- Any injury during pregnancy
- Depression
- Interactions with partner suggest interpersonal problems

Nursing Interventions
- Ask directly about domestic violence, apart from the partner
- Accurately document allegations in patient's own words
- Address safety regards: returning home vs. leaving home
- Report to authorities
- Partner violence screen (Feldhaus, Koziel-McLain et al., 1997)
    - Have you been hit, kicked, punched, or otherwise hurt by someone in the past year?
    - Do you feel safe in your current relationship?
    - Is there a partner from a previous relationship who is making you feel unsafe now?

ELDER ABUSE

Types of Elder Mistreatment
- Neglect (caregiver)
    - 50% of all cases
    - Intentionally or unintentionally fails to provide for elder's basic needs
- Physical
    - 25% of all cases
    - Intentional physical force resulting in bodily injury
    - Hitting, shaking, improper use of restraints
- Emotional
    - 30% of all cases
    - Infliction of anguish, pain, distress
    - Isolation, threats, humiliation, intimidation, yelling
- Sexual
    - Any form of nonconsensual sexual behavior
    - Rape, molestation, sexual harassment
- Financial
    - Mismanagement or misuse of elder's resources or property
    - Unexplained monetary expenditures, lack of money for personal necessities

- Self-neglect
  - Personal disregard or inability to perform self-care
  - Poor hygiene, unkempt home environment
- Abandonment
  - Desertion or willful forsaking of an elder
  - Dropping off in emergency department and leaving
- Institutional mistreatment
  - An elder with contractual arrangement for care suffers abuse or neglect
  - Any combination of examples above

Risk Factors
- Over 75 years of age
- Dependent functional status
- Poor social network
- Poverty
- Minority
- Cognitive impairment
- Living with one individual
- Less than 8th grade education
- Female
- Living alone or with abuser
- History of family violence

Abuser Characteristics
- Mental illness
- Substance abuse
- History of family violence
- Legal or financial issues
- Poor social network
- Dependency on older adult

Nursing Interventions
- Watch for caregiver role strain and provide support
- Complete thorough assessment using valid tool, such as Elder Assessment Instrument (EAI)
- Assess for physical abuse
  - Fractures, bruises in regular patterns
  - Burns on soles of feet or buttocks
  - Unusual hair loss
- Assess for neglect
  - Pressure ulcers, contractures, body odor, dehydration, malnourishment, depression
- Report neglect and abuse to the authorities
- Maintain safety for patient; use referral services

REFERENCES

Advameg Inc. (2011). Crisis intervention. In *Encyclopedia of mental disorders*. Retrieved from http://www.minddisorders.com/Br-Del/Crisis-intervention.html

D'Avanzo, C. (2007). *Mosby's pocket guide to cultural health assessment* (4th ed.). St. Louis, MO: Mosby.

Feldhaus, K. M., Koziel-McLain, I., Amsbury, H. L., Norton, I. M., Lowenstein, S. R., & Abbott, J. T. (1997). Accuracy of 3 brief screening questions for detecting partner violence in the emergency department. *JAMA, 277,* 1357–1361.

Fulmer, T. (2008). Elder mistreatment assessment. *Try This, 15,* 1–2. Retrieved from http://consultgerirn.org/uploads/File/trythis/try_this_15.pdf

Giger, J. N., & Davidhizar, R. E. (2008). *Transcultural nursing: Assessment and intervention* (5th ed.). St. Louis, MO: Mosby.

Mauer, F. A., & Smith, C. M. (2005). *Community public health nursing practice: Health for families and populations* (3rd ed.). St. Louis, MO: Elsevier.

National Institute of Mental Health. (2009). *Where to get help*. Retrieved from http://www.nimh.nih.gov/health/publications/men-and-depression/where-to-get-help.shtml

National Institute of Mental Health. (2010). *How to find help*. Retrieved from http://www.nimh.nih.gov/health/topics/getting-help-locate-services/index.shtml

Osborn, K. S., Wraa, C. E., & Watson, A. B. (2010). *Medical-surgical nursing: Preparation for practice*. Upper Saddle River, NJ: Pearson.

6

Delivery of Care

Nancy Henne Batchelor, MSN, RN-BC, CNS,
& Eileen Werdman, MSN, RN-BC, CNS

STRATEGIES FOR COST-EFFECTIVE CARE

Length of Stay (LOS)
- Number of days a patient stays in a healthcare facility.
- Used to assist in determining cost savings.

Utilization Review
- Evaluating necessity, appropriateness, and efficiency of healthcare services for a specific patient population.
- Can be preformed either by the third-party payer or by a department of a hospital.

Clinical Pathways
- Assists in evidence-based practice.
- Developed by interdisciplinary team.
- Protocols agreed to by physician can be implemented automatically without an order.

Clinical Practice Guidelines
- Designed to decrease cost and increase quality.
- Can be used in conjunction with clinical pathways.
- Provide diagnosis-based, step-by-step intervention for providers to follow in an effort to promote quality care.
- Also called standardized clinical guidelines.

Demand Management (Care Management)
- Approach used my managed care organizations.
- Decrease members' (enrollees') demand for health services.
- Encourage members (enrollees) to maintain good health and a healthy lifestyle.

Standards of Care
- Minimum accepted actions expected from professionals and healthcare organizations.
- Developed by professional organizations, Nurse Practice Acts, and other regulatory agencies.

Benchmarking
- Identifies best practice.
- Continuously comparing one's performance with that of the industry's leader.

Total Quality Management (TQM)
- Also known as Continuous Quality Improvement (CQI).
- Developed by W. Edward Deming.
- Based on the premise that the individual is the focal element on which production and service depend.
- Focused on doing the right things the right way the first time, and problem-prevention planning, not retrospective and reactive problem-solving.

Health Promotion, Disease and Illness Prevention
- Encourages people to become partners in maintaining their own health.
- Education is the key.

Evidence-Based Practice
- Identifies high-quality, clinically relevant research that can be applied to clinical practice and the development of health policy.
- Patient care is based on the best evidence available.
- Integrated problem-solving technique using:
  - Literature review and critical appraisal of the research
    - Systematic reviews of randomized clinical trials
    - Descriptive and qualitative studies
  - Use of one's own expertise
  - Patient's preferences and values
- Formulating the clinical question
  - PICO (Patient population, Intervention, Comparison, & Outcome)
    - Patient: age, gender, race, ethnicity, values, problem
    - Intervention: treatment or diagnostic test
    - Comparison: comparing one intervention against similar interventions
    - Outcome: end result
- Literature review
  - Databases (e.g., CINAHL, MEDLINE, Cochrane Database)
  - Search strategy
    - Formulate question
    - Determine database
    - Determine best study design to answer question
    - Determine subject heading and key words (using PICO)
    - Search and apply inclusion and exclusion criteria

- Critically examine the literature
- Applying the evidence: change personal practice or seek channels to institute change

RESEARCH

Nursing Process
- Conceptual phase
  - Identify the problem.
- Designing and planning phase
  - Select design of the study.
  - Identify study population.
  - **Determine sampling method.**
  - **Finalize plan.**
  - Pilot study.
- Empirical phase
  - Collect data.
- Analysis phase
  - Analyze data.
- Dissemination phase
  - Communicate findings.

Research Utilization
- Select a problem.
- Retrieve relevant literature.
- Read theories and studies.
- Critique studies.
- Decide on use of each study in data synthesis.
- Implement practice change.
- Evaluate change and modify practice as needed.

Models of Research Utilization in Nursing
- CURN Project: Conduct and Utilization of Research in Nursing, 1975–1980
  - Developed clinical protocols to direct the use of selected research findings in practice.
  - Encouraged collaborative practice.
- Stetler Model of Research Utilization
  - Outlines a series of steps to assess and use research findings.
  - Facilitates evidence-based practice (EBP).
  - Practitioner-focused.
  - Emphasizes critical thinking.
- Iowa Model for Research in Practice
  - Provides framework for nurses to make day-to-day decisions.
  - Infuses research into practice to improve quality of care.
  - Develop question, search literature, determine quality of results, conduct study if not happy with the results, develop guidelines, compare recommended practice to current practice.
  - Make changes using principle of planned change.
- Rosswurm and Larrabee
  - Guides practitioners through EBP process.

- Used in primary care settings.
- Adopted as standard of care (SOC) in acute-care settings.
- Nurses find this model easy to understand (resembles the Nursing Process).

NURSING-SENSITIVE QUALITY INDICATORS

- 1994: Nursing-sensitive quality indicators for acute-care settings (American Nurses Association's [ANA's] Safety and Quality Initiative)
- Purpose: to highlight strong linkages between nursing actions and patient outcomes
- 1988: ANA funded the National Database of Nursing Quality Indicators (NDNQI)
- Indicators
  - Mix of RN, LPN, unlicensed staff
  - Total nursing care hours provided per patient day
  - Pressure ulcers
  - Patient fall
  - Patient satisfaction with
    - Pain management
    - Educational information
    - Overall care
    - Nursing care
  - Nosocomial infection rate
  - Nurse staff satisfaction

CONTINUITY OF CARE

- An interdisciplinary process that includes patients, families, and significant others in the development of a coordinated plan of care.
- Facilitates patient's transition between settings and healthcare providers, based on changing needs and available resources.
- Nursing Scope and Standards of Practice.
- For additional information, go to the American Nurses Association (http://www.nursingworld.org/) or your state board of nursing.

DIFFERENTIATED NURSING PRACTICE

- Models of clinical nursing practice that recognize the level of education and clinical skills.
- Outcomes include but are not limited to organizations capitalizing on the varied education programs leading to RN licensure.
- Focuses on the division of labor needed to meet patient needs and to provide distinctive level of practice.

PATIENT CLASSIFICATION SYSTEMS

- Grouping of patients according to specific characteristics.
- Hours of nursing care assigned for each patient classification.
- Unique to a specific institution.

- Ongoing review is critical.
- Internal or external forces affecting the unit influence the classification system.

MEANS TO ORGANIZE PATIENT CARE

- Care delivery models change for a variety of reasons (e.g., economic factors, staff shortages or excess, philosophy, tasks, technology)
- Care delivery models
  - Total patient care
    - Oldest method
    - Nurse assumes total responsibility for meeting the needs of all assigned patients during his or her shift
  - Functional nursing
    - Evolved as a result of World War II
    - Uses relatively unskilled workers who have been trained to complete certain tasks
  - Team and modular nursing
    - Ancillary personnel collaborate to provide care to a group of patients under the direction of a professional nurse
    - Requires extensive team communication and regular team planning conferences
  - Primary nursing
    - Originally designed for an all-RN staff
    - Primary nurse assumes 24-hour responsibility for planning of care for one or more patients from start of hospitalization to discharge
    - During work hours, the primary nurse provides direct care for those patients
  - Case management
    - Collaborative process that assesses, plans, implements, coordinates, monitors, and evaluates options and service to meet an individual's health needs through communication and use of available resources to promote quality, cost-effective outcomes (Gillman, 2007; Glettler & Leen, 1996)
    - Coordinates care throughout an episode of illness
    - Focuses on individual patient, not population of patients

How to Choose the Most Appropriate Organization Mode to Deliver Patient Care

- Skill and expertise of the staff
- Availability of registered professional nurses
- Economic resources of the organization
- Acuity of the patients
- Complexity of the tasks to be completed
- The ultimate aim is maintenance of a therapeutic and safe environment for the patient.

Multidisciplinary Team

- Nurses are responsible for coordinating the efforts of a multidisciplinary team.
- To provide highest quality of care, the goals and priorities for each individual patient need to be considered.

Multidisciplinary Action Plans (MAPS)
- Combination of critical pathways and a nursing care plan that indicates when nursing interventions should occur.
- Promotes care management and interdisciplinary collaboration.
- Commonly used in case management to facilitate expected outcomes and to document variances.

Delegation
- "Achieving performance of care outcomes for which you are accountable and responsible by sharing activities with other individuals who have the appropriate authority to accomplish the work" (Yoder-Wise, 2003).

PAIN MANAGEMENT

Epidemiology
- Pain is a problem of epidemic proportions.
- 1 in 3 people living in the United States will experience some type of pain.
- 2 of 3 people experiencing acute pain will suffer from unrelieved pain.
- 50% to 75% of people experiencing chronic pain will be partially or totally disabled, temporarily or permanently.
- The person experiencing pain is the only one who can accurately define and describe it.

Theories of Pain
- Gate control theory
  - Gating mechanism in the spinal cord either permits or prevents pain information transmission to the brain.
  - Pain is modulated at the substantia gelatinosa in the dorsal horn.
  - Nociceptive neurons transmit pain signals.
- Neuromatrix theory
  - A widely distributed neurologic network in the brain: body-self neuromatrix.
  - Matrix made up of somatosensory, limbic, thalamocortical components, synaptic architecture of which is determined by genetic and sensory influences.

Variables Influencing the Patient's Perception of Pain
- Pain perception
  - Awareness of a feeling of pain
- Pain threshold
  - The point at which the person feels and reports pain
  - Influenced by environmental and social factors
- Pain tolerance
  - Ability to endure pain
  - Influenced by age, gender, sociocultural background

Types of Pain
- Acute
  - Sudden onset, temporary, and usually localized
  - Has identified cause (e.g., trauma, surgery, inflammation)
  - Lasts 6 months or less

- Warns of actual or potential injury to tissue
- Initiates fight or flight response

Table 6-1. Types of Pain

Type	Description
Somatic	Arises from nerve receptors in skin or close to body surface Sharp, well-localized, or dull and diffuse
Visceral	Arises from body organs Dull, poorly localized Associated factors: nausea, vomiting, hypotension, restlessness Radiates or referred
Referred	Perceived at site distant from stimulus May occur with visceral pain Felt over the skin in any body part sharing the same spinal nerve

- Characteristics of acute pain
  - Tachycardia
  - Shallow, rapid respirations
  - Dilated pupils
  - Pallor
  - Increased blood pressure
  - Sweating
- Chronic pain
  - Prolonged pain lasting longer than six months
  - Not always associated with an identified cause
  - Often unresponsive to conventional medical treatment
  - Dull, aching, diffuse

Table 6-2. Categories of Chronic Pain

Type	Description
Recurrent acute	Relatively well-defined episodes interspersed with pain-free episodes (e.g., migraine, sickle cell crisis)
Ongoing time-limited	Identified by a defined time period (e.g., cancer, burns)
Chronic nonmalignant	Non–life-threatening; persists beyond expected time for healing (e.g., chronic lower back pain); most common type of chronic pain
Chronic intractable nonmalignant syndrome	Similar to chronic nonmalignant; patient unable to cope well with pain Accompanied by physical, social, and/or psychology disability

- Common chronic pain conditions
  - Chronic low back pain
  - Neuralgias
  - Reflex sympathetic dystrophies

- Hyperesthesias
- Myofascial pain syndrome
- Cancer
- Chronic postoperative pain
- Central pain
  - Related to lesion in the brain spontaneously producing high-frequency bursts of impulses perceived as pain.
  - Perception of body position and movement may be lost.
  - Causes: tumor, vascular lesion, trauma, inflammation.
- Phantom pain
  - Occurs after amputation.
  - May be due to stimulation of severed nerves at amputation site.
  - Symptoms: itching, twisting, pressure, tingling, burning, stabbing, cramping.
- Psychogenic pain
  - Experienced in the absence of any diagnosed physiologic cause or event.
  - Emotional needs prompt pain sensations.
  - Physiologic changes may occur.
  - May result from interpersonal conflicts, need for support, or desire to avoid traumatic or stressful event.

Factors Affecting Response to Pain

- Age
  - Older adults have decreased perception and higher pain tolerance due to physiological aging changes.
  - Older adults perceive pain as a normal consequence of aging.
  - Older adults are hesitant to take pain medication because of potential for addiction.
- Sociocultural influences
  - Response to pain is strongly influenced by family, community, and culture.
  - Sociocultural influences affect an individual's pain tolerance, interpretation, and verbal and nonverbal reaction to pain.
  - Responses to pain vary greatly among cultures.
  - Nurses must have cultural competence when assessing and managing pain.
- Emotional status
  - Factors that increase pain:
    - Anxiety
    - Fear
    - Other conditions or symptoms occurring simultaneously
    - Fatigue
    - Lack of sleep
    - Depression
- Past experiences with pain
- Source and meaning
- Knowledge

  HISTORY
  - Pain onset
  - Description
  - Localization
  - Intensity
  - Quality

- Pattern
- Factors that relieve or intensify
- Patient's reaction to the pain

Pain Intensity Rating Scales

- Numeric Rating Scale (NRS, 0–10)
  - Used in clinical settings.
- Visual Analog Scale (VAS, 0–100)
  - Used in research settings.
- Visual Analog Scale with Anchors
  - Horizontal or vertical line with anchors: "no pain" to "pain as bad as it could be."
- FACES
  - Used primarily in pediatric population; can be used with adults.
- FLACC Scale (0–10)
  - Observer-rated scale; originally used for children.
  - Can be used for the nonverbal and dementia patient.
  - Five areas observed: face, legs, activity, crying, and consolability.
- PAINAD (Pain Assessment in Advanced Dementia, 0–10)
  - Adapted from the FLACC and Discomfort Scale for Dementia of the Alzheimer's Type (DS-DAT) tools.
  - Assesses five areas for possible indicators of pain in patients with severe dementia:
    - Breathing
    - Vocalization
    - Facial expression
    - Body language
    - Consolability

Nursing Management

PHARMACOLOGIC TREATMENT
- Nonnarcotic analgesics (nonsteroidal anti-inflammatory drugs [NSAIDs])
  - Acetaminophen, aspirin, ibuprofen
  - Used for mild to moderate pain and in combination with narcotics for moderate to severe pain
  - Act on peripheral nerve endings; minimize pain by interfering with prostaglandin synthesis
- Opioid analgesics
  - Codeine, hydrocodone, morphine, tramadol, oxycodone, fentanyl, methadone
  - Used for moderate to severe pain
  - Bind to opiate receptors within and outside central nervous system (CNS)
  - When taken as recommended, risk of addiction is low
  - When pain is not adequately treated, client may seek more narcotic relief, thus increasing risk of tolerance
- Adjuvant medications
  - Antidepressants (tricyclics) act on the retention of serotonin in the CNS and inhibit pain sensation
    - Used for neuropathic pain in cancer patients
  - Local anesthetics
    - Benzocaine, lidocaine
    - Block initiation and transmission of nerve impulses in local area, blocking pain

- Anticonvulsants
  - Gabapentin (Neurontin), phenytoin (Dilantin), carbamazepine (Tegretol)
  - Treat neuropathic pain by reducing neuronal hyperactivity and suppressing paroxysmal discharge
- Steroids
  - Prednisone, dexamethasone (Decadron)
  - Used for neuropathic pain in cancer patients with tumor infiltration or compression
- Nerve blocks
  - Steroid injections

COGNITIVE-BEHAVIORAL INTERVENTIONS
- Cutaneous stimulation: heat, cold, massage, transcutaneous electrical nerve stimulation (TENS)
- Relaxation: simple strategies such as slow, rhythmic breathing
- Distraction: focusing attention on nonpainful stimuli
- Imagery: using imagination to develop mental pictures
- Biofeedback: process that makes person aware of body functions and promotes modification of these functions at a conscious level

Evaluation
- Determine whether relief has been achieved.
- Determine most effective interventions.
- Set realistic goals (complete relief may not be obtainable); determine level of pain patient can tolerate and maintain quality of life.
- Reassess as needed.

Patient and Family Teaching
- The use of narcotics to treat severe pain is unlikely to cause addiction.
- Abstain from alcohol when taking narcotics.
- Check with healthcare provider before taking over-the-counter agents.
- Increase fluids and fiber to prevent constipation.
- Side effects include dizziness, drowsiness, impaired thinking; use caution when driving or making important decisions.
- Report decreased effectiveness or increased side effects to healthcare provider.

Gerontological Considerations When Using Pain Medications
- Start low and go slow.
  - Increased risk of adverse reactions because of age-related differences in pharmacokinetics and pharmacodynamics.
  - Watch for delirium; ensure that drug-induced cognitive and behavioral changes are not managed with additional medications.
- The older adult may not report pain over fear of addiction when narcotics are prescribed.
- Older adults are more likely to take multiple medications regularly, which increases the risk of adverse effects.
- Regular medication assessments—including over-the-counter, herbal, and nutraceuticals— should be conducted in primary care.

ALTERNATIVE AND COMPLEMENTARY THERAPIES

- Based on holistic nursing: caring for the mind, body, and spirit
- Evidence-based and integrative
- Enhance the health and quality of life for those who choose to practice
- Complementary therapy: therapy used in addition to conventional therapy
- Alternative therapy: unconventional therapy used instead of conventional therapy
- Best used as complementary therapies, along with conventional therapies
- Emphasize "natural mode" of healing

Types of Therapies
- Biologic-based
  - Dietary therapies
    - Dietary approaches and special diets that are applied for risk factors or chronic diseases
      - Atkins, Pritikin, vegetarian
  - Herbal medicine
    - Plant-derived preparations used for therapeutic and preventive purposes
      - Garlic, St. John's Wort, chamomile
  - Mega-vitamins
- Mind-body
  - Meditation
    - Naturally occurring rest state in order to heal, energize, integrate, assimilate
    - Facilitates sense of being centered
    - Improves overall sense of well-being
  - Biofeedback
    - Use of electronic equipment to read brain wave patterns, muscle tension, or electrical skin resistance
  - Aromatherapy
    - Use of pure essential oils to heal emotional and physical imbalances
  - Music
    - Reduces stress and anxiety
    - Involves hands, voice, emotions, mind, and spirit
    - Active: playing instruments or singing
    - Passive: listening to music to relax, stimulate, motivate, or soothe the body and mind
  - Imagery
    - Mind–body intervention to ease stress and promote sense of peace and tranquility during a stressful time
    - Used as adjunct in post-operative pain control
  - Guided imagery
    - Uses directed mental images to promote physical healing or changes in attitude or behavior
    - Visualization exercises are used as self-help tool
    - Primary aim is to guide the individual to state of a calm, silent, and still mind.
- Manipulation or body-based
  - Chiropractic
    - Manual adjustment or manipulation of the vertebral column and extremities
    - Uses direct hand contact and mechanical and electrical treatment modalities

- Massage
  - Kneading or manipulating muscles and soft tissue to improve health and comfort
  - Increases blood circulation
- Craniosacral therapy
  - Manual manipulation aimed at remedying supposed distortions in the structure and function of the brain and spinal cord, bones of skull, sacrum, and interconnected membranes.
- Reflexology
  - Pressure applied to specific points on hands and feet that are alleged to correspond to certain organs, glands, and body parts.
  - Similar to acupressure (see below)
  - Used for sinus congestion, headaches, asthma, premenstrual syndrome
- Energy-based
  - Healing touch
    - Hands-on and energy-based technique intended to balance and align human energy field, accelerate wound healing, relieve pain, promote relaxation, prevent illness, and ease the dying process
  - Reiki
    - Light hand placement intended to channel healing energies to the recipient
  - Acupuncture
    - Insertion of thin, flexible needles into the skin along alleged energy meridians to stimulate and influence physiological, psychological, and emotional functions in the mind and body
    - Goal is to restore overall energy balance.
    - Used in treatment of low back pain, arthritis, tendonitis, Ménière's disease
    - Most widely used for pain relief
  - Acupressure
    - Finger pressure along alleged energy meridians to manipulate soft tissue at specific points
    - Used to treat arthritis, tension, stress, aches, pains

SAFETY AND ENVIRONMENTAL ASSESSMENT

Patient Safety
- National Patient Safety Goals
  - Developed by the Joint Commission
  - Require healthcare facilities to focus on specific safety practices
- Hospital Report Cards
  - Consumer-oriented reports cards available to the public.
  - Information on
    - Quality outcome measurements
    - Hospital's experience in providing care
- Rapid Response Teams/Medical Emergency Teams (RRT/MET)
  - Intervene when the patient is beginning to decline.
  - Do not replace the code team.

Disaster Preparedness
- A plan to ensure the organization can respond and function under extreme circumstances
- Required by licensing and accreditation agencies
- Internal and external plans
- Any situation that may overwhelm hospital resources
  - Internal
    - Hospital fire
    - Power failure
    - Water shortage
  - External
    - Airplane crash
    - Terrorist attack
    - Natural disaster
    - Structural collapse

Sources of Injury
- Falls
  - Assess risk and monitor closely.
  - Falls are the leading cause of injury that results in death in older patients.
  - Prevention is key.
    - Physical assessment
    - Home assessment
- Restraints
  - Use alternative methods first.
  - Follow institutional policy and monitor patient.
- Medications
  - Five Rights or Six Rights (includes documentation)
    - Five Rights
      1. Right patient
      2. Right time and frequency of administration
      3. Right dose
      4. Right route of administration
      5. Right drug
    - Six Rights
      1. Right medication
      2. Right route
      3. Right time
      4. Right client
      5. Right dosage
      6. Right documentation
  - Know patient allergies and reactions.
  - Question unusual orders.
  - Inadequate patient education:
    - Assess knowledge before and after teaching.
    - Use return demonstration when possible.

- Abandonment
  - Be clear when transferring care.
    - ICARE
      - Introduction
      - Chief complaint or current status
      - Assessment
      - Results
      - Evaluate
      - Disposition
    - SBAR
      - Situation
      - Background
      - Assessment
      - Request or recommendation
  - Document completion of treatment.
- Malfunctioning equipment
  - Check equipment regularly.
  - Notify appropriate persons regarding malfunction equipment.

Risk Management

- Identification of risks, real or perceived (by employees, patients, and public)
- Occurrence or incident reports
  - Completed following untoward event, regardless of injury.
    - Medication errors
    - Falls
  - Should be detailed, objective, and factual.
    - No opinions, assumptions or accusations

REFERENCES

Dunham-Taylor, J. M., & Pinczuk, J. Z. (2010). *Financial management for nurse managers: Merging the heart with the dollar* (2nd ed.). Sudbury, MA: Jones & Bartlett.

Eliopolous, C. (2010). *Gerontological nursing* (7th ed.). Philadelphia: Lippincott Williams & Wilkins.

Finkelman, A. W. (2006). *Leadership and management in nursing.* Upper Saddle River, NJ: Pearson Prentice Hall.

Flaherty, E. (2008). Using pain rating scales with older adults. *AJN: American Journal of Nursing, 108*(6), 40–47.

Gillman, P. (2007). *ANCC Medical-Surgical Nurse Certification Review Seminar,* Silver Spring, MD: American Nurses Credentialing Center.

Horgas, A. (2008). *Pain: Nursing standard of practice protocol: Pain management in older adults.* Retrieved from http://consultgerirn.org/topics/pain/want_to_know_more

Ignatavicius, D. D., & Workman, M. L. (2010). *Medical-surgical nursing: Patient-centered collaborative care* (6th ed.). St. Louis, MO: Saunders Elsevier.

Jackson, M. (2002). *Pain: The fifth vital sign.* New York: Crown.

Jacox, A., Carr, D. B., Payne, R., Berde, C. B., Breitbart, W., Cain, J. M. ... Weissman, D. E. (1994). *Management of cancer pain: Clinical practice guideline No. 9* (AHCPR Publication No. 94–0592). Rockville, MD: Agency for Health Care Policy and Research, U.S. Department of Health and Human Services.

Jacques, E. (2009). *FLACC Scale—Pain Assessment Tool.* Retrieved from http://pain.about.com/od/testingdiagnosis/ig/pain-scales/Flacc-Scale.htm

Keegan, L. (2001). *Healing with complementary and alternative therapies.* Albany, NY: Delmar.

Marquis, B. L., & Huston, C. J. (2009). *Leadership roles and management functions in nursing, theory and application.* Philadelphia: Wolters Kluwer Health/Lippincott Williams & Wilkins

Matzo, M. L., & Sherman, D. W. (Eds.). (2001). *Palliative care nursing: Quality care to the end of life.* New York: Springer.

McCaffery, M. (1979). *Nursing management of the patient with pain.* Philadelphia; Lippincott.

Melnyk, B. M., & Fineout-Overholt, E. (2005). *Evidence-based practice in nursing & healthcare. A guide to best practice.* Philadelphia: Lippincott Williams & Wilkins.

National Institutes of Health. *Pain intensity scales.* Retrieved August 13, 2010, from http://painconsortium.nih.gov/pain_scales/index.html

Osborn, K. S., Wraa, C. E., & Watson, A. B. (2010). *Medical-surgical nursing: Preparation for practice.* Upper Saddle River, NJ: Pearson.

Roussel, L., Swansburg, R. C., & Swansburg, R. (2006). *Management and leadership for nurse administrators* (4th ed.). Sudbury, MA: Jones & Bartlett.

Tabloski, P. A. (2010). *Gerontological nursing* (2nd ed.). Upper Saddle River, NJ: Pearson.

Yoder-Wise, P. S., & Kowalski, K. E. (2006). *Beyond leading and managing: Nursing administration for the future.* St. Louis, MO: Mosby Elsevier.

7

Nursing Process

Deborah Jane Schwytzer, MSN, RN-BC, CEN

NURSING PROCESS OVERVIEW

- Systematic, dynamic, purposeful sequence of steps designed to gather patient-, family-, significant other-, and community-focused data to be analyzed and used by the professional nurse to develop a patient-centered plan of care.
- It uses knowledge of the scientific method to develop a goal-directed plan of care that is based on specific nursing interventions with measurable outcomes, using a common language for practice: the nursing diagnosis.
- It is a patient-centered, goal-directed process developed in collaboration with the patient and/or family and other healthcare professionals.
- Promotes the involvement of the patient, family, significant other, and community in the planning and implementation of care that will enhance positive outcomes.
- Steps of the Nursing Process include:
  - Assessment: develop patient-specific database.
    - Data obtained from primary and secondary sources in the areas of medical, psychosocial, cultural, self-care, and environmental status as well as physical assessment.
    - Data obtained are both subjective (communicated) and objective (observable or measurable).
    - Data collected through the use of appropriate communication and interviewing methods that establish a rapport and full disclosure of information.
    - Data organized and verified for accuracy.
    - Data documented in a clear and concise manner for communication.

- Diagnosis and analysis: use critical thinking skills to analyze data collected and to identify health risks, health needs, and strengths, and to identify appropriate nursing diagnosis.
  - Diagnosis formulated based on the North American Nursing Diagnosis Association (NANDA).
  - Actual and potential needs are identified.
  - Needs and diagnoses are prioritized and categorized as those that are managed by nursing and those that require a collaborative and interdisciplinary approach.
- Planning: identify appropriate interventions and measurable patient outcomes or goals intended to promote, maintain, and restore health.
  - Nursing diagnoses must be prioritized to ensure patient safety.
  - Collaborative short-term and long-term outcomes or goals must be developed with appropriate interventions and time frames based on evidence-based practice.
  - Plan of care must be documented to allow for continuity and updating.
- Implementation: nursing plan of care is initiated.
  - Daily goals and interventions are determined and clearly communicated with patient/family/significant other.
  - Care activities are appropriately delegated as needed.
  - Ongoing assessment and documentation must occur.
- Evaluation: determination of achievement and effectiveness of developed plan of care.
  - Ongoing data are collected on the effects of prescribed interventions.
  - Patient progress and achievement of goals and desired outcomes are assessed.
  - Plan of care is evaluated, modified, and communicated as needed.

Assessment

HISTORY
- Subjective information gathered from patient and significant others through interviews or a written screening tool that collects data on the present and past health of the patient. It includes health strengths, responses to past illnesses, and current health concerns.
- Biographical data: name, address, age, gender, marital status, ethnic origin, primary language, occupation
- Reason for seeking care: patient's self-report of why she or he is seeking health care
- History of present health concern: symptom analysis
  - Location: precise location of pain or concern
  - Character or quality: description of pain or concern such as sharp, dull, achy, burning
  - Severity or quantity: description of intensity of pain using a visual or numerical pain scale, or may quantify amounts (e.g., drainage, discharge, blood)
  - Timing: onset of symptoms, how long they have been present, and/or how often the symptoms occur
  - Setting: what causes the symptoms to occur or what was the patient doing at the time of occurrence or when the symptoms recurred
  - Aggravating or relieving factors: what makes the symptoms better or worse: For instance, does a change in weather cause a change in the symptoms, or does rest or heat decrease symptoms? What treatments has the patient tried and was there any change in symptoms?
  - Associated factors: Are there any other symptoms related to the chief complaint? For example, do they experience blurred vision or nausea with their headache?

- Patient's perception: How does the symptom affect the patient's daily activities or what does the patient think the symptom may mean? Does the patient see it as a threat to long-term health?
- Sample mnemonics for symptom analysis are given in Table 7–1.

Table 7-1. Symptom Mnemonics

PQRSTU	OLD CART	COLD SPA
P: Provocation or Palliative	O: Onset	C: Characteristics
Q: Quality or Quantity	L: Location	O: Onset
R: Region or Radiation	D: Duration	L: Location
S: Severity Scale	C: Characteristics	D: Duration
T: Timing	A: Alleviating symptoms	S: Severity
U: Understand patient's perception	R: Relieving factors	P: Pattern
	T: Treatment	A: Associated factors

- Past medical and surgical history: past childhood and adult illnesses, immunization history (tetanus, diphtheria, and pertussis [Td/Tdap]; measles, mumps, and rubella [MMR], influenza, pneumococcal), past surgeries, obstetric history, accidents, allergies, medications, last physical examination.
- Family history: age of parents, living or deceased; genetic or past illnesses in family members including parents, grandparents, aunts, uncles, children. A genogram may be helpful to illustrate relationships.
- Social history: exercise habits, social activities, sleep pattern, family and social relationships, type of work, stressors, recreational drugs, alcohol intake, nicotine and caffeine, education, finances, coping strategies, developmental level, environmental risks, religious affiliation, culture, values and belief systems.
- Functional and lifestyle history: purpose is to assess the patient's ability to perform activities of daily living through discussion of health promotion activities and daily self-care activities such as toileting, feeding, dressing, bathing, cleaning, shopping, and mode of transportation. Assessment tools such as the Functional Independence Measure Scale or the Katz Index of ADLs as well as a thorough assessment of risk for falls can be used to determine need for assistance or ability to care for self. What is patient's perception of his or her health and ability to function?
- Review of systems: purpose is to evaluate the past and present health status of each body system, evaluate health promotion activities, and verify data collected during the previous health history. This area is patient self-report, not objective findings of the examiner. The examiner will inquire about:
  - General health state: Patient's perception of his or her general health status. Note any recent weight gain or loss, nutritional intake, recent appetite change, fatigue, fever, chills, malaise. 24-hour nutritional assessment also can be completed.
  - Skin: History of skin diseases; changes in skin pigmentation, texture, or moisture; jaundice, bruising, rashes; appearance of moles, lesions, or sores; odors; excessive sweating; changes in nail texture; amount of sun exposure, use of sun screens; typical skin care methods.

- Hair: Changes in hair distribution, growth patterns, or texture. Usual care products and practices, coloring products.
- Head and neck: Recent head or neck trauma. History of headaches, vertigo, syncope, pain, tenderness, stiffness, difficulty swallowing, areas of swelling.
- Eyes: Use of glasses or contacts, vision changes, pain, double vision, blurring, night blindness, halos, spots or "floaters," excessive tearing or drainage, glaucoma, or cataracts. Date of last eye exam.
- Ears: Use of hearing assistive devices, hearing changes, drainage, earaches, tinnitus (ringing in the ears), vertigo, frequent ear infections, excessive cerumen (earwax). Date of last hearing exam and method of cleaning ears.
- Nose and sinuses: Recent colds, nosebleeds, sinus pain, pressure sensation, drainage, stuffiness, polyps, obstructions, difficulty breathing, known allergies, hay fever symptoms, or change in sense of smell.
- Mouth and throat: Dentures; caries; toothaches; gum bleeding or swelling; lesions in mouth, on tongue, or in throat; dysphagia; hoarseness, voice changes; change in taste; tonsillectomy; throat pain or swelling; enlarged thyroid. Date of last dental exam and usual daily dental care activities.
- Breasts: Noted lumps, drainage from breasts or nipples, pain or tenderness, dimpling or changes in size or appearance, swollen or tender axillary lymph nodes. Date of last mammogram and whether patient performs monthly breast self-exams.
- Respiratory: Any shortness of breath, activity tolerance, breathing pattern changes, chronic cough, sputum production or change in color, bloody sputum, pain, frequent colds and respiratory infections. Date of last chest x-ray.
- Cardiac: Any areas of noted edema or history of edema, number of pillows used at night, chest pain or pressure, murmurs, arrhythmias, palpitations. Date of last blood pressure check and ECG.
- Gastrointestinal: Any indigestion, stomach or abdominal pains, difficulty swallowing, nausea, vomiting, gastric reflux, gas, jaundice, hernias, bowel habit changes, diarrhea, constipation, abdominal swelling.
- Urinary: Frequency; any dysuria, nocturia, difficulty maintaining or decrease in urine stream, hesitancy, polyuria, bedwetting, incontinence, history of frequent urinary tract infections or kidney stones.
- Genital
  - Male: Presence of discharge, testicular pain, testicular lumps, infertility, difficulty with erections, impotence, hernias, enlarged prostate. Use of safe sex practices and regular testicular self-examination.
  - Female: Onset of menarche, date of last menstrual period, premenstrual symptoms, irregular or painful menstrual bleeding, vaginal discharge, history of STIs. Use of birth control, safe sex practices, or hormone replacement therapy. Date of last Pap smear.
- Peripheral vascular: Noted varicosities; calf or leg pain; pain when walking, climbing stairs, or sitting; leg, calf, or hand cramping; blood clots in legs, arms, or ankles; swelling in extremities; changes in temperature or sensation in hands or feet.
- Anal, rectum, and prostate: Pain with defection, hemorrhoids, blood in stool, constipation. Enlarged prostate, difficulty with or frequent urination, incomplete bladder emptying.
- Musculoskeletal: Pain in joints or changes in range of motion, stiffness, swelling, deformities, bone tenderness, gout, arthritis, spontaneous fractures, muscle atrophy, or spinal disc herniation.

- Neurological: mood, behavior changes, depression, anger, head trauma, headaches, loss of strength or coordination, memory problems, thought process changes, difficulty speaking or expressing ideas, seizure.
- Hematological: fatigue, bruising, bleeding, clotting, problems, anemia, sickle cell anemia, blood transfusions, blood reactions.
- Endocrine: fatigue, intolerance of temperature extremes, bulging eyes, weight changes, thirst, changes in urine production, change in hair distribution, swelling in anterior neck, diabetes mellitus, hormone replacement therapy.
- Psychiatric: depression, irritability, tension, feelings of excessive stress, disturbances in thought processes, suicidal or homicidal ideations, difficulty concentrating.

PHYSICAL EXAM
- Objective examination of patient using the four physical assessment techniques.
  - Inspection: direct observation of general appearance and all areas of the body; size, shape, symmetry, color, position. Also use sense of smell to detect odors.
  - Palpation: use of fingertips to examine organs and tissues of the body to assess temperature, moisture, texture; detect masses, consistency, size, and shape; pulsations, crepitus, and tactile discrimination.
    - Best performed on relaxed patient.
    - Light palpation using gentle, light touch with finger pads to assess superficial surfaces, masses, fluid and tender areas.
    - Deep palpation with firm fingertips and hands to assess tenderness and deeper organs and body structures 2 to 3 cm deep.
    - Ballottement using fingers to assess floating masses in fluid-filled spaces, return to normal position, and tenderness related to rebound of masses.
  - Percussion: short tapping or striking of one object against another to determine organ size, shape, density, content, tenderness of underlying structures.
    - Five types of sounds can be generated depending on composition or content of structure
      - Flatness: heard over dense tissues such as bone
      - Dull: normal over solid organs such as liver
      - Resonance: normal in areas of part air and part solid such as lung
      - Hyperresonant: heard over areas of mostly air such as lungs with emphysema
      - Tympanic: heard over areas of air-filled organs such as gastric bubble or puffed cheek
  - Auscultation: using sense of hearing to assess sounds produced by the organs and body systems.
    - Direct auscultation: use of ear alone to detect sounds such as wheezing and hyperactive bowel sounds
    - Indirect auscultation: use of a listening device such as a stethoscope or Doppler to detect pulses, heart, lung, or normal bowel sounds
      - Bell of stethoscope: best used to hear low-pitched sounds such as vascular bruits
      - Diaphragm of stethoscope: best to hear high-pitched sounds such as bowel and heart sounds
- Components
  - General appearance: overall appearance
    - Appears stated age
    - Level of consciousness
    - Skin color

- Nutritional status: obese, anorexic, well-nourished
- Posture and mobility: uses an assistive device?
- Facial expression: smile, frown
- Mood or affect: friendly, inquisitive, appropriate for situation
- Speech: articulation, appropriate, preferred language
- Hearing: any deficiencies noted
- Personal hygiene and attire: cleanliness and attire appropriate for season
- Measurements
  - Height
  - Weight
  - Body mass index
    - Weight $\div$ height^2 $\times$ 703
    - Normal BMI: 18.5 to 24.9 kg/m^2
    - Underweight: < 18.5 kg/m^2
    - Overweight: 25.0 to 29.9 kg/m^2
    - Obesity: 30.0 to 39.9 kg/m^2
    - Extreme obesity: $\geq$ 40.0 kg/m^2
  - Snellen Eye Chart for vision
  - Temperature
  - Pulse
    - Usually radial pulse
    - Normal range: 60 to 100 beats/minute
    - Tachycardia: > 100 beats/minute
    - Bradycardia: < 60 beats/minute
  - Respirations
    - Normal range 10 to 20 breaths/minute
  - Blood pressure
- Skin and nails
  - Inspect general skin color throughout body.
  - Palpate skin and note texture, moisture, and temperature.
  - Describe location and characteristics of any lesions or masses.
  - Use Braden Scale for predicting pressure sore risk in at-risk patients.
  - Inspect and palpate nails for coloration and texture.
- Head and face
  - Inspect and palpate scalp, hair, and cranium. Note hair distribution and texture. Record any areas of scalp asymmetry.
  - Inspect and palpate face for symmetry of facial structures, facial expression, movement, and areas of tenderness.
  - Palpate the temporomandibular joint for crepitus or tenderness when patient opens and closes mouth.
- Eyes
  - Inspect external eye structures, conjunctivae, sclera, cornea, and iris.
  - Test visual fields by confrontation.
  - Test extraocular muscles with corneal light reflex and six cardinal positions of gaze.
  - Test pupils for response to light and accommodation.
  - Perform ophthalmoscope exam to inspect fundus, red reflex, optic disc, and vessels.
- Ears
  - Inspect and palpate external ears for symmetry, skin coloration, tenderness and condition, and auditory meatus.

- Perform otoscope exam to inspect ear canal and tympanic membrane for color, integrity, and landmarks.
- Perform hearing tests with voice and tuning forks for hearing acuity and lateralization.
- Nose
  - Inspect and palpate external nares for symmetry, lesions, and tenderness.
  - Test patency of each nostril.
  - Inspect nares mucosa, septum, and turbinates with speculum.
- Mouth and throat
  - Inspect mouth, tongue, teeth, gums, floor of mouth, upper palate, tonsils, and uvula for structure, color, and presence of any lesions or swelling.
  - Note movement of uvula when patient says "ahh."
  - Test for presence of gag reflex.
  - Palpate mouth and tongue for lesions and texture changes.
- Neck and neck vessels
  - Inspect neck for symmetry, pulsations, jugular venous distention (JVD), and lumps.
  - Palpate cervical lymph nodes, carotid pulses, trachea, and thyroid gland.
  - Auscultate carotid pulses for bruits.
  - Test range of motion (ROM) and strength of shoulder, neck, and head muscles.
- Chest
  - Inspect anterior and posterior surfaces of chest for structure, symmetry, respiratory effort, pulsations, heaves, and skin for lesions.
  - Palpate bilateral expansion, tactile fremitus, and tenderness.
  - Palpate posterior spinous processes for tenderness.
  - Palpate for point of maximal impulse (PMI) at heart apex.
  - Percuss lung fields, diaphragmatic excursion, costovertebral angle tenderness.
  - Auscultate lung fields for adventitious sounds.
  - Auscultate for heart sounds and any murmurs. Note rate and rhythm.
- Breasts: female and male
  - Inspect for symmetry, mobility, and any dimpling.
  - Palpate breast tissues including tail of Spence region in axillae for lumps and texture changes.
  - Palpate regional lymph nodes and nipples for discharge.
- Abdomen
  - Inspect contour, symmetry, umbilicus, inguinal area, pulsations, and skin color and texture.
  - Auscultate bowel sounds in all quadrants and vascular sounds over aorta and renal arteries.
  - Percuss all quadrants, liver span, and spleen.
  - Palpate all quadrants using light and deep palpation.
  - Palpate liver, spleen, aorta, femoral pulses, and inguinal lymph nodes.
- Extremities: upper and lower
  - Inspect bilateral size, symmetry, color, joints, skin texture, and hair distribution.
  - Palpate pulses: radial, brachial, femoral, popliteal, posterior tibial, and dorsalis pedis.
  - Palpate skin temperature, turgor, and for edema.
  - Palpate joints and muscles for tenderness.
  - Test passive and active range of motion and muscle strength.

- Female genitalia and rectum
  - Inspect genital region for hair distribution, color, lesions, swelling, and discharge.
  - Inspect perianal region for lumps, lesions, rashes, redness, discharge, and fissures.
  - Palpate external rectal sphincter for tenderness, lumps, characteristics of stool. Test feces if present for occult blood.
- Male genitalia and rectum
  - Inspect penis and scrotum for hair distribution, color, lesions, swelling, and discharge.
  - Inspect perianal region for lumps, lesions, rashes, redness, discharge, and fissures.
  - Palpate penis, scrotum, and testis for shape, tenderness, nodules, and presence of discharge.
  - Palpate external rectal sphincter for tenderness, lumps, characteristics of stool. Test feces if present for occult blood.
- Neurologic exam
  - Mental status: appearance, behavior, facial expression, speech, mood, orientation, attention span, recent memory, remote memory, thought processes, and perceptions
  - Cranial nerves (see Table 7–2)

Table 7–2. Cranial Nerves

Cranial Nerve	Name	Type	Function	Test to Be Performed by Nurse
CN 1	Olfactory	Sensory	Smell	Identify sample—strong-smelling item held under each nostril separately
CN 2	Optic	Sensory	Vision	Visual acuity: Snellen/ Rosenbaum chart and visual fields
CN 3	Oculo-motor	Motor	Extraocular eye movement; papillary constriction; upper eyelid elevation	Cardinal positions of gaze—upward, downward, and inward eye movement; pupil response to light
CN 4	Trochlear	Motor	Extraocular eye movement	Cardinal position of gaze—downward and inward eye movement
CN 5	Trigeminal	Sensory	Face and head; corneal reflex	Sensation of soft and sharp object against face
		Motor	Chewing; biting; lateral jaw movement	Clenching teeth and opening jaw against resistance
CN 6	Abducens	Motor	Extraocular eye movement	Cardinal position of gaze—outward eye movement

CN 7	Facial	Sensory	Taste	Place sour, sweet, bitter, and salty liquid on tongue
		Motor	Facial muscle movement	Open and close mouth, open and squeezing eyes closed
CN 8	Acoustic	Sensory	Hearing; balance	Weber and Rhinne tests; ability to walk a straight line
CN 9	Glosso-pharyngeal	Sensory	Taste; sensations in throat	Gag reflex
		Motor	Swallowing	Swallowing and saying "ah"
CN 10	Vagus	Sensory	Sensations in throat, larynx, thoracic, and abdominal viscera such as heart, lungs, and GI tract	Gag reflex
		Motor	Swallowing, gag reflex, heart rate, and GI peristalsis	Swallowing and symmetrical rise of uvula as patient says "ah"
CN 11	Spinal accessory	Motor	Shoulder movement; head rotation	Shrug shoulders against resistance; turn head from side to side against resistance
CN 12	Hypo-glossal	Motor	Tongue movement	Symmetry of tongue movement from side to side; clear speech of sounds of letters "l", "t", "d", "n"

- Motor system: gait, balance, coordination, skilled movements such as rapid alternating movements
- Sensory system: pain, touch, vibration, position, fine touch, stereognosis, graphesthesia, point location and discrimination
- Common laboratory test results
  - Each laboratory has its own set of "normal range" or "reference range" on the lab report. These values depend on the equipment or method used to determine and report the results.
  - Test results can be affected by a variety of factors, including age, gender, underlying or preexisting disease, the time of day when the sample was taken, active infections, and medications.
  - Results must be interpreted in the context of all other information available.

Table 7-3. Complete Blood Count

Complete Blood Cell Count	Normal Range	Function	Potential Causes of Elevation	Potential Causes of Decrease
Hematocrit (Hct)	Male: 42%–52% Female: 37%–47%	Percent of total blood volume made up of RBCs	COPD Congenital heart disease Polycythemia vera Severe dehydration	Anemia Cirrhosis Hemolytic reaction Hemorrhage Leukemia Pregnancy
Hemoglobin (Hgb)	Male: 14–18 g/dL Female: 12–16 g/dL	Transports oxygen and carbon dioxide	COPD Congestive heart failure Dehydration High altitude	Anemia Hemorrhage Kidney disease Neoplasm Sarcoidosis
Red blood cell count (RBC)	Male: 4,700,000–6,100,000/mcL Female: 4,200,000–5,400,000/mcL	Total number of circulating RBCs	Congenital heart disease High altitude Polycythemia vera Dehydration	Hemorrhage Anemia Leukemia Renal failure Dietary deficiency Overhydration
Platelet count	150,000–400,000/mcL	Essential to blood clotting	Malignancy Iron deficiency anemia Rheumatoid arthritis	Hemorrhage Disseminated intravascular coagulation (DIC) Chemotherapy
White blood cell count (WBC)	5,000–10,000 cells/mL	Fight infection and react to foreign tissues and bodies	Infection Trauma Stress Tissue necrosis Inflammation	Autoimmune disease Drug toxicity Overwhelming infection

Table 7-4. White Blood Count Differential

WBC Differential	Normal Range	Function	Potential Causes of Elevation	Potential Causes of Decrease
Neutrophils	55%–70%	Initial phagocytosis of bacteria	Acute infection Inflammation Acute appendicitis	Anemias Leukemias Viral diseases
Eosinophils	1%–4%	Involved in allergic reactions	Allergies Cancer	Burns Shock

Basophils	0.5%–1%	Promote healing	Inflammation Wound healing Leukemia	Stress Pregnancy Hypersensitivity
Monocytes	2%–8%	Phagocytosis of bacteria over extended time	Viral disease Cancer	Aplastic anemia
Lymphocytes	20%–40%	Involved in immune reactions		Cancer Leukemia Renal failure

Table 7–5. Metabolic Panel

Test	Normal Range	Function	Potential Causes of Elevation	Potential Causes of Decrease
Albumin	3.5–5.0 g/dL	Blood protein that maintains colloidal osmotic pressure	Dehydration	Alcoholic cirrhosis Malnutrition Nephrotic syndrome Leukemia Cystic fibrosis
Ammonia	10–80 mcg/dL	Byproduct of protein catabolism	Liver disease Reye's syndrome Hepatic encephalopathy Congestive hepatomegaly	Malignant hypertension
Amylase	30–100 u/L	Catabolism of carbohydrates	Acute pancreatitis Alcohol ingestion Renal disease Peptic ulcer disease Cholecystitis	Liver damage Pancreatic destruction
Bilirubin, total	0.2–1.2 mg/dL	Breakdown product of hemoglobin	Hepatitis Cirrhosis Toxins Hemolysis	Iron deficiency anemia
Calcium	8.7–10.7 mg/dL	Used in bone and teeth formation, muscle contraction, and blood clotting	Chronic renal failure Primary hyperthyroidism Metastatic bone tumors Osteoporosis Paget's disease	Hypoparathyroidism Decreased vitamin D ingestion Hypomagnesemia Chronic renal failure Acute pancreatitis

cont.

Table 7–5. Metabolic Panel (cont.)

Carbon dioxide	23–30 meq/L	Maintains metabolic acid–base balance	Respiratory acidosis Compensated metabolic acidosis Emphysema Severe vomiting	Respiratory alkalosis DKA Starvation Lactic acidosis Renal failure Dehydration
Chloride	99–107 meq/L	Maintain electrical neutrality	Diarrhea Hyperalimentation	DKA Vomiting
Creatinine	0.5–1.1 mg/dL	Byproduct of muscle catabolism	Renal failure CHF Neoplasm	Pregnancy Muscle mass destruction
Glucose (fasting)	60–109 mg/dL	Converts glucose to glycogen for storage	Diabetes mellitus Stress Cushing's syndrome Acute pancreatitis Corticosteroid use	Hypothyroidism Addison's disease Insulin overdose Starvation
Lipase	10–52 u/L	Converts triglycerides into fatty acids	Acute pancreatitis Renal failure Pancreatic cancer	
Magnesium	1.6–2.7 mg/dL	Assists in muscle contraction, protein and carbohydrate metabolism	Renal failure Severe dehydration Lithium intoxication Hypothyroidism Addison's disease	Hyperthyroidism Hyperalimentation Malabsorption Diuretics Chronic dialysis
Phosphorus	2.5–4.6 mg/dL	Assists in metabolism of fats, carbohydrates and proteins and energy transfer as ATP	Hypoparathyroid-ism Renal failure Bone disease Excessive vitamin D intake Addison's disease	Alcoholism Diabetes Acidosis Diuretics
Potassium	3.4–5.3 meq/L	Protein synthesis, glucose storage and electrical activity of heart muscles and others	Acute renal failure Metabolic acidosis Anuria Oliguria	Dehydration Vomiting or diarrhea Starvation Stress DKA
Protein, total	6.4–8.3 g/dL	Maintains colloid osmotic pressure, supplies amino acids	Dehydration Nausea Vomiting Excessive exercise Malnutrition	Starvation Malabsorption syndrome Burns Chronic renal failure

Sodium	137–147 meq/L	Maintains extracellular volume, cardiac and skeletal muscle contraction through sodium-potassium pump	Diabetes insipidus CHF Hepatic failure Severe nausea and vomiting	Vomiting Diarrhea SIADH Burn injury Renal failure
TSH	0.410–5.90 µIU/mL	Stimulates release of T3 and T4 for metabolic processes; controls rate of metabolism, growth, and development and neurological maturity	Thyroid gland malfunction	Hypothyroidism Renal failure Strenuous exercise
Urea nitrogen (BUN)	8–21 mg/dL	End product of protein metabolism	Dehydration Renal insufficiency Diabetes mellitus Sepsis High-protein diet	Severe liver disease Malnutrition Overhydration Pregnancy Low protein intake

Table 7–6. Clotting Studies

Test	Normal Range	Function	Potential Causes of Elevation	Potential Causes of Decrease
Prothrombin time (PT)	11.1–13.3 sec	Clotting mechanism of extrinsic pathway	Disseminated intravascular coagulation (DIC) Liver disease Coumadin therapy	High-fat diet
Activated partial thromboplastin time (aPTT)	23–33 sec	Clotting mechanism of intrinsic pathway	Hemophilia Cirrhosis Vitamin K deficiency DIC Heparin administration	Cancer Early DIC
Fibrinogen	190–395 mg/dL	Clotting mechanism	Acute inflammation Trauma CAD CVA Peripheral arterial disease	Liver disease Fibrinolysis Malnutrition Cancer Large-volume blood transfusions

Table 7-7. Urinalysis

Test	Normal Range
Specific Gravity	1.002–1.030
pH	5–8
Protein	< 30 mg/dL
Bilirubin	Negative
Urobilinogen	0.2–1 EU/dL
Glucose	Negative
Ketones	Negative
Occult blood	Negative
Leukocyte esterase	Negative
RBCs	0–5
WBCs	0–5
Bacteria	Negative
Casts	0–4

Table 7-8. Arterial Blood Gases

Test	Normal Range
pH	7.35–7.45
pCO_2	35–45 mm Hg
pO_2	83–108 mm Hg
Bicarbonate (HCO_3)	19–24 mmol/L
O_2 Saturation	95%–98%

pH	pCO_2	HCO_3	Disturbance	Potential Causes
↓	↑	Normal	Respiratory acidosis	Respiratory depression, CNS trauma, pneumonia, COPD, pulmonary disease
↑	↓	Normal	Respiratory alkalosis	Hyperventilation, pain, overventilation
↓	Normal	↓	Metabolic acidosis	Diabetes, shock, renal failure
↑	Normal	↑	Metabolic alkalosis	Vomiting, nasogastric drainage, sodium bicarbonate overdose

- Common diagnostic tests
  - Electrocardiography (ECG): noninvasive examination of electrical activity of the heart
  - Computed tomography (CT): noninvasive radiographic examination of body tissues noting density changes
  - Doppler studies: noninvasive study of tissues using ultrasound beam to create a three-dimensional picture of the structure
    - Cardiac Doppler studies examine cardiac structure and valves for abnormalities.
    - Vascular Doppler examines the peripheral vessels to examine structural malformation, blood flow or occlusion.
  - Magnetic resonance imaging (MRI): noninvasive study that creates images of body structures in planes through the use of radiofrequency waves in a magnetic field
  - Endoscopy: invasive direct observation of body area through the use of a flexible fiberoptic tube; areas studied include bronchi, colon, esophagus, bile duct
  - Radiography (x-ray): noninvasive examination using radiation to visualize underlying structures, primarily but not exclusively bone
  - Ultrasound: noninvasive procedure using high-frequency sound waves to create images of underlying structures to detect abnormalities or contents of the structures; areas include abdomen, spleen, liver, uterus, gallbladder

Diagnosis and Analysis

- Diagnostic reasoning is used to interpret the data gathered from the assessment step to identify patient-specific needs and strengths.
- Needs are identified based on the interpretation of the data as actual health problems present or areas of potential need or risk.
- Nursing diagnosis components:
  - Problem statement: diagnostic label that defines the health need.
  - Etiology: the related factor that is the probable cause of the health need.
  - Defining characteristics: identifies the need based on signs and symptoms.
    - Example: Acute pain related to inflammation of right leg as manifested by verbal report of pain and guarding of right leg.
- The NANDA taxonomy list is commonly used as the internationally recognized list of nursing diagnoses.

Planning

- During the planning step, in collaboration with the patient and the interdisciplinary healthcare team, the nurse will:
  - Prioritize selected nursing diagnoses based on hierarchy of needs theory.
  - Develop measurable patient goals or outcomes that describe the desired result of the nursing care.
  - Develop individualized specific interventions or nursing orders to achieve these patient goals in a specific time frame.
- Planned goals and interventions are culturally sensitive and include patient autonomy and wishes. Goals and interventions are *patient*-driven and not nursing goals to be achieved.
- The written plan is communicated to the patient, family members, caregivers, and all healthcare providers to ensure continuity and accuracy.

Implementation

- During this step, the written nursing plan of care is executed. Interventions may be delegated and supervised as appropriate with the expectation that any observed changes or needs be reported to the RN immediately.
- The plan of care is continually assessed, data are collected, and plan is modified as needed during this step by the RN with input from all members of the healthcare team caring for the patient as well as from the patient.
- Documentation, including specific actions and patient responses, is essential during this step. This written documentation should be focused toward achievement of goals and ensuring continuity of care among providers, family, and others.

Evaluation

- During this step, the entire written nurse care plan is assessed for the achievement of goals and the success of interventions but also the need for modifications in the plan of care.
- Reassessment of the patient is completed to note any changes in the patient's needs and incorporate any new goals and interventions.
- The evaluation step is essential to the success of the nursing process because it incorporates the assurance of quality, appropriate, and effective nursing care to meet the identified patient needs.

REFERENCES

Ackley, B. J., & Ladwig, G. B. (2008). *Nursing diagnosis handbook: An evidence-based guide to planning care* (8th ed.). St. Louis, MO: Mosby Elsevier.

Doenges, M. E., Moorhouse, M. F., & Murr, A. C. (2008). *Nursing diagnosis manual: Planning, individualization, and documenting patient care* (2nd ed.). Philadelphia: F.A. Davis.

Jarvis, C. (2008). *Physical examination & health assessment* (5th ed.). St. Louis, MO: Saunders.

Pagana, K. D., & Pagana, T. J. (2009). *Mosby's diagnostic and laboratory test reference* (9th ed.). St. Louis, MO: Mosby Elsevier.

Wallace, M., & Shelkey, M. (2008). Monitoring functional status of hospitalized older adults. *American Journal of Nursing, 108*(4), 64–71.

Weber, J., & Kelley, J. H. (2010). *Health assessment in nursing* (4th ed.). Philadelphia: Wolters Kluwer Health/Lippincott Williams & Wilkins.

8

Health Promotion and Wellness

Nancy Henne Batchelor, MSN, RN-BC, CNS

HEALTH MAINTENANCE AND WELLNESS PRINCIPLES

Focus of Health Care
- Goes beyond treatment of illness and injury
- Includes prevention and wellness promotion
- Includes comprehensive plan of care that will guide patient and family toward healthy lifestyle and away from risk factors
  - Healthy People 2020
    - Mission
    - Identify nationwide health improvement priorities
    - Increase public awareness and understanding of determinants of health, disease, and disability and the opportunities for progress
    - Provide measurable objectives and goals applicable at the national, state, and local levels
    - Engage multiple sectors to take action to strengthen policies and improve practices that are driven by the best available evidence and knowledge
    - Identify critical research, evaluation, and data collection needs
  - Overarching goals
    - Attain high-quality, longer lives free of preventable disease, disability, injury and premature death
    - Achieve health equity, eliminate disparities, and improve health of all groups
    - Create social and physical environments that promote good health for all

- Promote quality of life, healthy development, and healthy behaviors across all life stages
- Foundational health measures that indicate progress toward goal achievement
- General health status
  - Life expectancy
  - Healthy life expectancy
  - Years of potential life lost
  - Physically and mentally unhealthy days
  - Self-assessed health status
  - Limitations of activity
  - Chronic disease prevalence
- Health-related quality of life and well-being
- Physical, mental, and social health–related quality of life
- Participation in common activities
- Determinants of health
- Range of personal, social, economic, and environmental factors that influence health status
  - Biology
  - Genetics
  - Individual behavior
  - Access to health services
  - Environment in which people are born, live, learn, work, play, and age
- Disparities—Measures of disparities and inequity include differences based on
  - Race/ethnicity
  - Gender
  - Physical and mental ability
  - Geography
- New topic areas for 2020
  - Adolescent health
  - Blood disorders and blood safety
  - Dementias, including Alzheimer's disease
  - Early and middle childhood
  - Genomics
  - Global health
  - Health care–associated infections
  - Health-related quality of life and well-being
  - Lesbian, gay, bisexual, and transgender health
  - Older adults
  - Preparedness
  - Sleep health
  - Social determinants of health
  - Immunization and infectious diseases
- Infectious disease remains a major cause of illness, disability, and death
- Immunization recommendations for the United States target 17 vaccine-preventable diseases across the life span
- Goals for immunization and infectious disease focus on technological advancements and ensuring that states, local public health departments, and nongovernmental organizations, together with the nation attempt to control the spread of infectious diseases

- Essential components for reducing infectious disease transmission
  - Disease awareness
  - Completion of prevention and treatment courses
  - Vaccine-preventable diseases that are leading causes of illness and death in the United States
  - Viral hepatitis
  - Influenza
  - Tuberculosis
- Tools in the fight against newly emerging and re-emerging infectious disease
  - Disease surveillance
  - Proper use of vaccines
  - Antibiotics
  - Screening and testing guidelines
  - Scientific improvements in diagnosis of infectious disease-related health concerns
  - Immunizations
- The most cost-effective clinical preventive services
- Core component of preventive services package
  - Routine immunizations
  - Save 33,000 lives
  - Prevent 14 million cases of disease
  - Reduces direct healthcare costs by $9.9 billion
  - Saves $33.4 billion in indirect costs
- Infectious diseases
- Respiratory diseases
  - Includes influenza and pneumonia
  - 8th leading cause of death in the United States (56,000/year)
- Hepatitis and tuberculosis
  - Resources to support prevention efforts are not always available
  - Need to provide information about healthy lifestyles and prevention
- Emerging issues in immunization and infectious diseases
  - Shifting demographics require protection of the growing needs of increasing diverse and aging population
  - Detection of new infectious agents and diseases
    - International travel and trade
    - Migration
    - Importation of food and agricultural practices
    - Threats of bioterrorism
  - Inappropriate antibiotic use and environmental changes increase potential for worldwide epidemics

Risk Modification
- American Heart Association
  - Smoking
  - Physical inactivity
  - Cholesterol
  - Blood pressure
- American Cancer Society
  - Environmental risks
  - Diet

- Nonmodifiable risk factors
  - Age
  - Gender
  - Race and ethnicity
  - Family history
- Types of prevention
  - Primary: action to prevent disease or make environment less harmful
  - Secondary: screening and early detection of asymptomatic disease
  - Tertiary: manage disease to prevent late complications
- Screening
  - Useful when disease can be detected before clinical manifestation at a reasonable cost
  - Sensitivity: ability of a test to correctly identify persons with a disorder
  - Specificity: ability of a test to identify persons without the disease

Table 8-1. Common Screening Recommendations

Exam	Frequency	Source
Blood pressure	Every exam, 1–2 years	USPSTF, AHA
Breast exam	Annually, age > 40 (ACS); every 2 years, age > 50 (USPSTF)	ACS, USPSTF
Mammogram	1–2 years, ages 50–69 1–3 years, ages 70–85 (as willing and appropriate)	ACS, USPSTF
Pelvic exam and pap smear	Begin at 18 or if sexually active Pap every 2–3 years after 3 negative; can decrease or d/c, > age 65–69	ACS, USPSTF
Cholesterol	20 years and > every 5 years > 2 years of age if high risk	NCEP, USPSTF
Rectal exam & fecal occult blood	Annually, age > 50	ACS, AHCPR
Colonoscopy	Every 5 years, age > 50	ACS
Visual Acuity	Annually, age > 50	AARP
Hearing	Every 2–5 years	AARP
Mouth, nodes, testes, skin, heart, lungs	Annually	ACS, AHA
Glucose	Every 3 years	USPSTF, ADA
Thyroid Function	Every 5 years for women 35 & >	USPSTF
Electrocardiogram (ECG)	Age > 40–50	AHA
Glaucoma	With annual eye exam	USPSTF
Mental status	As needed: be alert to decline	USPSTF
Bone mineral density	Women: age 50 Men: age 70 Every 2 years	USPSTF

| Breast self-exam | Monthly (women) | ACS, AARP |
| Dental exam and cleaning | Exam annually, every 2 years with dentures; cleaning every 6 months | AARP |

Note. AARP = American Association of Retired Persons; ACS = American Cancer Society; AHA = American Heart Association; USPSTF = United States Preventive Services Task Force; ADA = American Dietetic Association; NCEP = National Cholesterol Education Program.

From *ANCC Medical-Surgical Nurse Certification Review Seminar*, Module 10, by P. Gillman, 2007, Silver Spring, MD: American Nurses Credentialing Center.

- Immunizations
  - Prevent infectious disease and disability caused by the disease
  - Protect the individual and society

Table 8-2. National Guidelines for Immunizations for Adults in the United States

Vaccine	Dose Requirements	Age/When to Get
HPV	3 doses (0, 2, 6 months)	Age 13–26 Ideally pre-sexual activity HPV4: males age 9–26
Varicella	2 doses (0, 4–8 weeks)	All adults without evidence of immunity (unless contraindicated because pregnant or immune-compromised)
Pneumococcal	1–2 doses with certain risk factors (ages 19–64 years) 1 dose, age > 65	Revaccinate 5 years later for persons at high risk or first immunization before age 65
Influenza	1 dose, annually	Age > 50 Younger persons if high risk
Meningococcal	1 or more	Asplenia or first-year college students in dorms
Hepatitis B	3 doses (0, 1, 6 months)	Persons at high risk
Hepatitis A	2 doses (0, 6–18 months)	Prior to travel or work outside U.S. Persons at high risk
Tetanus, diphtheria	1 dose every 10 years after 3-dose primary series (0, 1–2, 4–6 months)	Sub 1 dose Tdap between ages 19–64 yrs
Herpes zoster	Single dose	Age > 60 years regardless of prior episodes of zoster

Adapted from *Immunizations* by the Centers for Disease Control and Prevention, 2010, retrieved from http://www.cdc.gov/vaccines

- Smoking cessation
  - Smoking is a risk factor associated with
    - Cardiovascular disease
    - Respiratory disease
    - Cancer
  - Secondhand smoke increases risk for
    - Bronchitis
    - Asthma
    - Heart disease
    - Respiratory disease
  - Guidelines for smoking cessation: The Five A's
    - Ask about smoking every visit
    - Advise all smokers to stop
    - Assess willingness to stop
    - Assist patient with quitting
    - Arrange for follow-up
- Obesity
  - Increases risk of premature death
  - Magnitude of risk is same as between smokers and nonsmokers
  - 20% of cancer deaths in women and 14% in men are caused by obesity
  - 30% of cancer deaths are tobacco-related; 25% related to diet, physical inactivity, and weight
  - Goals for weight loss
    - Reduce body weight by about 10% in 6 months
    - May attempt further weight loss if successful
    - Reasonable rate of loss: 1 to 2 pounds per week
    - Diet
      - Weight loss: 10 calories per pound of ideal body weight (IBW)
      - Maintenance: 12 calories per pound of current weight
  - Special populations with low rates of physical activity
    - Women
    - Low income
    - Low education
    - Hispanic
    - Black
    - Northeast and Southern states
    - Persons with disabilities
  - Perceived barriers to exercise
    - Lack of time
    - Lack of access to convenient facilities
    - Lack of safe environment
    - Perceived physical limitations
    - Lack of knowledge about how and why exercise should be done
    - Lack of motivation
  - Actual benefits of exercise
    - Reduces mortality and morbidity
    - Increases functional level of other areas in life
    - Improves mood
    - Improves body composition

- Improves blood sugar, blood pressure, high-density lipoprotein, cholesterol
- Increases metabolic rate
- Burns more calories, aiding weight loss
- Improves bone density
- Improves cognitive function
- Types of exercise
  - Isotonic (aerobic)
    - Uses oxygen
    - Much more efficient in production of energy
    - Uses large muscle groups in rhythmic motion
  - Isometric (anaerobic)
    - Less efficient, done without oxygen
    - Contraction of muscle without movement
  - Activities combining aerobic and anaerobic
    - Walking while carrying groceries
    - Riding a bicycle while gripping handlebars tightly
- Exercise guidelines
  - Start slow and go slow
  - Walking is excellent exercise; use pedometer to count steps
  - Weight training or resistance exercise builds muscle and improves cardiac expenditure
  - Goal: 30 to 60 minutes on most days of the week
  - Can be divided into short sessions (10 minutes x 3)

THEORETICAL MODELS FOR USE IN HEALTH PROMOTION

Health Belief Model
- Explains why healthy people use health-protecting and disease-preventing services
- Identifies benefits of changing behavior
- Identifies barriers to changing behavior
- Explores ways to overcome barriers, enhance benefits
- Identifies media cues that influence the person
- Guides program development to increase likelihood of success
- Application of the model
  - Explore person's beliefs
  - Identify benefits of changing behavior—personally meaningful reason
  - Identify barriers
  - Explore ways to overcome barriers and enhance benefits
  - Identify media cues that may influence the person
  - Use information to develop mutually acceptable goals for health-related behaviors such as diet, exercise, and smoking

Pender's Health Promotion Model
- Focus on health-seeking behaviors and prevention, not disease
- Assesses barriers, benefits, modifying factors, cues to action
- Similar to Health Belief Model

Transtheoretical Model
- Designed for use across health professions
- Identifies stages of change
- Matches intervention to the stage of change
- Basis for National Institutes of Health guidelines for smoking cessation
- Stages:
  - Precontemplation: no intention to change
    - Introduces notion of change
  - Contemplation: acknowledges need for change but ambivalent or anxious
    - Provide information to motivate
  - Preparation: explores options
    - Provide details
  - Action: behavior changes
    - Modify plan and revise as needed
  - Maintenance: continues the change
    - Monitor for relapse
  - Termination: revise self-image
    - Behavior is no longer a threat

Adult Learning Theory
- Adults are self-directed.
- Adults are interested in information that will benefit them.
- Adults use a wide variety of resources.
- Principles related to learning styles:
  - Identify learning styles of teacher and learner.
  - Teachers should be cautioned about using their preferred style.
  - Most effective teaching occurs when teaching is done using learner's style.
  - Different learning styles should always be encouraged.
  - Learning styles can be learned and developed with practice and direction by teacher and learner.

Adult Education
- Includes education of the adult and family or caregiver
- Adults want knowledge that serves a specific needs or solves a problem.
- Barriers can include
  - Cognitive or mood impairment
  - Decreased vision
  - Decreased hearing
  - Fatigue, physical debilitation
  - Lack of learner readiness
- Factors affecting the teaching-learning process
  - Educational level
    - Sixth grade reading level
  - Socioeconomic status
    - Assist with accessing resources
  - Support systems
    - Identify and include them
  - Age
    - Impacts information processing

- Culture
  - Incorporate beliefs, language needs, health practices
- Adult education theories tell us learning is best when
  - The learner is involved.
  - It is relative to the learner.
  - Multisensory approach is used.
    - Auditory
    - Visual
    - Kinesthetic
  - It is repetitious.
- Consider appropriate educational material according to
  - Age
  - Gender
  - Culture
  - Language
- Learning and the older adult: key points
  - New learning should relate to what the patient already knows.
  - Environmental factors affect the learning process.
    - Lighting
    - Background noise
    - Overstimulation
  - Motivation and desire to learn new information need to be considered.
  - Learner should be in control of what and how much is learned in each session.
  - Ability to learn should be considered.
    - Literacy: reading comprehension, problem-solving
    - Ability to apply information
  - Congruence of language is important for successful adult learning.
    - Language barriers
    - Understanding of information
  - Learning can be affected by physical wellness or illness.
  - Teacher/learner ratio should be low when dealing with the older adult.
  - Learning environment should be comfortable.
  - Learner wants new and pertinent information.
  - Common physical changes that affect learning and the older adult
    - Decreased vision
    - Decreased hearing
    - Impaired cognition
    - Depression
    - Stress
    - Chronic Illness

Patient Education Process
- Assess
  - Knowledge
  - Motivation
  - Readiness to learn
  - Physical or sensory impairments

- Determine nursing diagnosis
  - Knowledge deficit
  - Ineffective coping
- Identify goal-setting behavioral objectives
  - Affective, cognitive, psychomotor
- Teaching strategies
  - Role-playing
  - Guided discussion
  - Demonstration with return demonstration
- Evaluation, reteaching, and documentation
- Patient education and the older adult
  - Allow additional time.
  - Help learner identify associations between items.
  - Promote physical comfort.
  - Eliminate distractions.
  - Ensures glasses and hearing aids are on and working.
  - Set realistic mutual goals.
  - Encourage verbal response and allow time.
  - Reinforce correct responses and provide immediate feedback.
  - Use examples relating to learner's life and experience.
  - Use simple, black-on-white, large-letter visuals.
  - Include family member or caregiver when possible and appropriate.
  - Provide new information in writing, at appropriate reading level.
  - Always treat the learner with respect and dignity.
  - Incorporate techniques for effective communication.

Lifestyle Management and Anticipatory Guidance

- Assessment of health patterns
  - Can determine current health status.
  - Access to health maintenance.
  - Identify patient healthcare beliefs.
    - Prevention practices
    - Diet
    - Exercise
    - Lifestyle practices
- Assessment of cultural beliefs and practices
  - Cultural identity can determine how patient views self and how he or she seeks healthcare services.
  - Identify how spiritual or religious beliefs affect health care.
  - Identify home care remedies.
  - Identify holistic remedies.
- Assessment of spiritual beliefs
  - Assess to determine how individual's beliefs affect health.
  - Inquire about advance directives.
- Enhancing adherence
  - Frame teaching to match patient's perceptions.
  - Inform patient of expected effects and the time frame of effects.
  - Suggest small rather than large changes.
  - Be specific: establish contracts.

- It may be easier to add new behaviors than to eliminate established ones.
- Promote self-management and encourage active participation.
- Reduce barriers; mobilize support.
- Elicit and respond to patient concerns.
- Modify treatment plan to increase possibility of adherence.
- **Persist, encourage, support.**

REFERENCES

Centers for Disease Control and Prevention. (2010). *Immunizations.* Retrieved from http://www.cdc .gov/vaccines

Eliopolous, C. (2010). *Gerontological nursing* (7th ed.). Philadelphia: Lippincott Williams & Wilkins.

National Institutes of Health. (2009). *NIH news in health: Thyroid disease.* Retrieved from http:// newsinhealth.nih.gov/2009/February/feature2.htm

Osborn, K. S., Wraa, C. E., & Watson, A. B. (2010). *Medical surgical nursing: Preparation for practice.* Upper Saddle River, NJ: Pearson.

U.S. Department of Health and Human Services. (2010). *About Healthy People 2020.* Retrieved from http://www.healthypeople.gov/2020/about/default.aspx

U.S. Department of Health and Human Services. (2010). *About Healthy People 2020: Foundation health measures.* Retrieved from http://www.healthypeople.gov/2020/about/tracking.aspx

U.S. Department of Health and Human Services. (2010). *About Healthy People 2020: Immunization and infectious diseases.* Retrieved from http://www.healthypeople.gov/2020/topicsobjectives/2020/ overview.aspx?topicid=23

U.S. Department of Health and Human Services. (2010). *About Healthy People 2020: What's new for 2020.* Retrieved from http://www.healthypeople.gov/2020/about/new/2020.aspx

U.S. Department of Health and Human Services. (2011). Centers for Disease Control and Prevention *Recommended adult immunization schedule- United States 2011.* Retrieved from http://www.cdc .gov/vaccines/schedules/downoads/adult/mmwr-adults-schedule.pdf

9

Management and Leadership

Eileen Werdman, MSN, RN-BC, CNS

QUALITY AND PERFORMANCE IMPROVEMENT

Quality
- Focuses on structure, process, and outcomes
- Healthcare facilities worked to improve quality after pressure from external sources (e.g., third-party payers)

Quality Improvement
- Focus on ongoing quality
- Always room for improvement

Quality Assurance
- Old term no longer used
- Difficult to assure quality
- Focused on existing quality

Total Quality Management (TQM)
- Now referred to as TQI: total quality improvement
  - Continuously improving system
  - Main principles
    - Customer focus
    - Identify key process to improve quality
    - Include everyone involved in problem-solving

- Developed by Dr. W. Edward Deming
  - Doing it right the first time
  - FOCUS: Find, Organize, Clarify, Understand, Select; PDCA: Plan, Do, Check, Act
- Hallmark of Japanese management system
- Problem prevention and planning lead to quality
- Involve everyone in every aspect of quality for every product and service
- Empowers employees

Toyota Production System
- More contemporary
- Customer focus
- Philosophy: solving individual problems immediately, one at a time and at the point of origin
  - Requires change in culture, commitment of leadership time and resources
  - Offset by results
    - Greater quality of care
    - Improved patient safety
    - Decrease in cost
    - Increased job satisfaction (Thompson, Wolf, & Spear, 2003)

Malcolm Baldrige National Quality Award
- Uses integrative approach to improve practice performance
- In health care, creates a performance improvement process driven by the customers—
patients, clinicians, insurers—and the data

Quality Control
- Everyone should be involved.
- Provide feedback to employees about current quality.
- Quality care does not equal patient satisfaction.
- Patient satisfaction reflects whether the nurse met patient expectations.
- Quality control programs
  - Most organizations have one.
  - Cost containment plays a role.

External Forces on Quality
- Medicaid and Medicare
  - When first introduced, there was no need to justify care or quality.
  - Payment was based on cost incurred.
  - Changed when costs increased and the government wanted justification.
- Professional Standards Review Organizations
  - Professional Standards Review Board legislation (PL 92–603, 1972): one of the first efforts
  to look at cost containment and quality.
  - Mandated certification of need, review of care, and evaluation of care as well as
  care providers.
  - Changes made in healthcare facilities because Medicaid and Medicare population is
  a large proportion of business. Facilities that did not or could not make the necessary
  changes closed.
- Prospective Payment System (PPS)
  - Payments based on Diagnosis-Related Groups (DRGs).
  - Increased the need for organizations to watch costs yet provide quality care.

- PPS pays fixed amount for care regardless of actual costs.
- Issues
  - Decreased length of stay, questionable quality, increased acuity of patient (patients tend to wait longer to see healthcare provider)
  - Increased dissatisfaction by nurse with their job
- Joint Commission
  - Private nonprofit organization that audits healthcare organizations and programs
  - Voluntary accreditation
  - Has undergone multiple name changes over the years
- Centers for Medicare and Medicaid Services (CMS)
  - Active role in setting standards
  - Medicare Quality Initiative (MQT)
    - 4 components
      - Survey and conduct regulation and enforcement activities
      - Information made available to all
      - Ongoing community-based improvement programs
      - Collaboration and partnership among all stakeholders
    - Involved in new benchmarking and measuring health outcomes
- National Committee for Quality Assurance (NCQA)
  - Private nonprofit organization
  - Accredits managed care organizations
  - Voluntary
- Maryland Hospital Association Quality Indicator Project
  - Research project
    - Not intended to establish performance thresholds or standards of care
    - Is looking at benchmark indicators and measurements
- Multistate Nursing Home Case Mix & Quality demonstration
- Report card
  - Makes performance information about an organization available
- Quality and Safety Education for Nurses (QSEN)
  - Funded by Robert Wood Johnson Foundation
  - Goal: to improve nursing care
  - 6 levels
    - Patient-centered care
    - Teamwork and collaboration
    - Evidence-based practice
    - Quality
    - Safety
    - Informatics
- Institute of Medicine (IOM)
  - 5 levels
    - Patient-centered care
    - Teamwork and collaboration
    - Evidence-based practice
    - Quality improvement and safety
    - Informatics

Medical Errors and Quality

- Many reports suggest medical errors are on the rise in health care.
  - Institute of Medicine (IOM)
    - *To Err Is Human* (1999)
      - 44,000 to 98,000 people die per year due to medical errors.
      - Medical errors are 8th leading cause of death.
      - Looks at types of errors.
      - Medication errors on the rise due to individual behavior and flaws in the system.
      - "The focus was to prevent mistakes by designing health systems to make it harder for people to make mistakes, easier to do things correctly" (Tomey, 2009 p. 46).
  - Patient Safety and Quality Improvement Act (2005)
    - Treats medical errors voluntarily submitted to new private organizations as confidential, prohibits from subpoena or legal discovery.
  - Leapfrog Group
    - Coalition of public and private organizations that provide healthcare benefits.
    - Growing group of nonhealthcare organizations committed to modernizing current healthcare system.
      - CPOE (computer physician order entry)
      - HER (evidence-based hospital referral)
      - Intensive care unit physician staffing
      - Leapfrog self-practice score
      - Also endorses use of bar codes in medication administration

Critical Event Analysis (CEA)

- A method used to review causes of adverse events.
- Requires data collection, investigation, determining, and reporting the cause.
- Implementing of corrective actions and then monitoring for sustainability.

Root Cause Analysis

- A method designed to uncover the problem that resulted in a patient adverse event.
- Similar to CEA.

Accountability

- Types
  - Personal: morally responsible for the consequence of one's own actions
    - One person cannot be accountable for another
  - Fiscal: to the organization for appropriate staffing per negotiated budget
    - Staff level: being stewards of the resources

CONFLICT RESOLUTION

Conflict

- "[D]efined as the internal or external discord that results from differences in ideas, values or feelings between two or more people" (Marquis & Huston, 2009, p. 487).
- Neither good nor bad; when handled well, can be constructive and move issues forward.

Categories of Conflict
- Intergroup: two or more groups
- Intrapersonal: within one person
- Interpersonal: two or more different opinions (values, goals, or beliefs)

Management (Resolution)
- Creating a win-win situation
- Strategies (Thomas-Kilmann Conflict Model): key to success, match strategy with conflict (Yoder-Wise & Kowalski, 2006)
  - Compromise: each party gives up something of equal value
  - Competing: one pursues what one wants at another's expense
  - Cooperating or accommodating: opposite of competing; problems are usually not solved
  - Smoothing: decreases emotional component of the conflict and focuses on the agreement versus the differences
  - Avoiding: aware of the conflict but choosing not to acknowledge it
  - Collaborating: assertive and cooperative, usually results in a win-win situation
  - Strategies for use on a unit
    - Confrontation
    - Third-party consultation: neutral party
    - Behavior changes
    - Structure changes
    - Soothing

DELEGATION
- Critical leadership skill
- Function of the professional nurse
- Check with local state board regarding legal implications
- Ability to have work done though others
  - RN working with unlicensed assistive personnel (UAP)
    - The Omnibus Budget Reconciliation Act of 1987 established minimum hours of education and practice for UAP.
    - **RN holds ultimate responsibility and accountability for care provided.**
  - Manager to RN
- Consistent with the nursing process

Common Errors
- Under-delegating: false assumption that delegating is interpreted as a lack of ability to complete the job.
  - Lack of trust in subordinates to do the job right
- Improper delegating: tasks delegated at wrong time, to wrong person, for wrong reason.
  - Delegating items beyond person's capability
- Over-delegating: delegating too much.

Effective Delegation
- Plan ahead.
- Identify necessary skills and level of skill required to complete the task.
- Select most capable person.

- Communicate goal clearly.
- Empower the person to get the job done.
- Set deadline and monitor progress towards deadlines.
- Model role and provide guidance.
- Evaluate performance.
- Reward accomplishment.

ASSERTIVENESS

- Behavior: communicating allows people to express themselves in direct, honest, and appropriate ways that do not infringe on another's rights.
- Use of "I" statements.
- Carries rights and responsibilities.
- Assertiveness and aggressiveness are not interchangeable.
- Remember diversity; be sensitive of person's culture.

ADVOCACY

- Standing up for what one believes in.
- Most vital and basic role of the nurse.
- Advocate for profession, patient, and staff.
- Advocacy is a standard for nurse administrators.
- Helping others to grow (many skills are needed).
  - Risk-taking
  - Vision
  - Self-confidence
  - Ability to articulate needs
  - Assertiveness

Workplace Advocacy
- Environment is both safe and conducive to professional and personal growth.
- Whistle-blowers
  - Looked at with distrust; considered disloyal
  - Important advocacy role

Professional Advocacy
- Leadership
- Must be involved in the profession to better it
- Legislation and public policy
  - Important issues: healthcare reform and scope of practice for nurses in the state

PROFESSIONAL DEVELOPMENT

Role Model
- Someone worthy of imitation
- Experienced and competent employees
- Passive role versus preceptor role, which is active and purposeful

Mentors
- Experienced individual who befriends and provides professional guidance to a person
- Conscious and purposeful relationship that extends a number of years
- Leads by example
- Mentors freely choose whom to mentor
- Four stages
  - Initiation: relationship established
  - Cultivation: coaching, protection, sponsor
  - Separation
  - Redefinition
- Separation and redefinition are difficult but necessary if the mentor has done a good job

COMPETENCY
- Having the abilities to meet the requirements of the role
- What is used to determine competency:
  - State board license
  - Certification
  - Performance review
  - Checklist and audits
  - Peer evaluation
  - Assessment
    - A piece of performance review
    - A piece of career planning and development of learning needs
  - Collaboration
    - Win-win strategy
    - Key concepts (Finkelman, 2006)
    - Partnership
    - Interdependence
    - Collective ownership and responsibility

REFERENCES

Dunham-Taylor, J., & Pinczuk, J. Z. (2010). *Financial management for nurse managers: Merging the heart with the dollar* (2nd ed.). Sudbury, MA: Jones & Bartlett.

Finkelman, A. (2006). *Leadership and management in nursing.* Upper Saddle River, NJ: Prentice Hall.

Finkelman, A., & Kenner, C. (2009). *Teaching IOM: Implications of the Institute of Medicine reports for nursing education.* Silver Spring, MD: American Nurses Association.

Institute of Medicine. (1999). *To err is human: Building a safer health system.* Washington, DC: Author.

Marquis, B. L., & Huston, C. J. (2009). *Leadership roles and management functions in nursing: Theory and application.* Philadelphia: Wolters Kluwer Health/Lippincott Williams & Wilkins.

Thompson, D., Wolf, G., & Spear, S. (2003). Driving improvement in patient care: Lessons learned from Toyota. *Journal of Nursing Administration, 33*(11), 585–595.

Tomey, A. M. (2009). *Guide to nursing management and leadership* (8th ed.). St. Louis, MO: Mosby Elsevier.

Yoder-Wise, P. S., & Kowalski, K. E. (2006). *Beyond leading and managing: Nursing administration for the future.* St. Louis, MO: Mosby Elsevier.

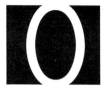

Legal and Ethical Issues

Eileen Werdman, MSN, RN-BC, CNS

LEGAL ASPECTS OF NURSING

Licensure
- Receiving a license to practice nursing is a privilege, not a right.
- Graduating from accredited nursing school and passing NCLEX does not equal license.
- Intended to provide public safety, examination determines minimum competency.
- Must be knowledgeable of the state Nurse Practice Act
- Many states require continuing education to renew license.

Authority
- Comes from the law.
- Nurse Practice Act is the single most important piece of legislation for the nurse.
  - Defines scope of practice
  - Lists acts and tasks that are prohibited and the consequences
  - Describes how and when to renew your license
  - Defines the educational requirements for entry into practice
  - Provides definitions and the scope of practice for each level of nursing practice
  - Describes the process by which individual members of the board of nursing are selected and the categories of membership
  - Outlines the appeal steps if the nurse believes the disciplinary actions taken by the board are not fair or valid

Scope of Practice

- Defines the actions and duties allowed by the profession.
  - Describes who, what, where, when, why, and how of nursing practice
  - Describes responsibilities for which its practitioners are accountable
    - Held accountable to the standard of care in existence at the time of care
- When the courts or legislation increases the nursing role, the legal responsibility of the nurse increases as well.

Regulatory Guidelines

- Regulators are organizations and agencies that set rules, regulations, and/or standards that healthcare providers must follow if the providers want to continue providing care.
- Standards used by regulators come from many sources.
  - Consumers
  - Providers
  - Payers
  - Professional organizations
  - State, local, and federal laws
- Federal
  - Centers for Medicare and Medicaid Services (CMS)
    - Utilization review
      - Preadmission certification
      - Concurrent review
      - Discharge planning
      - Case management
      - Second surgical opinion
    - Handicap access standards
    - Medicare
      - Federal health insurance program
      - For people ages
      - 65 years and older
      - Also for people younger than 65 years with long-term disabilities
    - Medicaid
      - Jointly funded state-federal health insurance program
      - For eligible low-income people
      - Coverage varies by state but meets federal requirements
      - No age restrictions
    - Occupational Safety and Health Administration (OSHA)
      - Implemented to ensure safe, healthy workplaces
      - Provides national leadership in occupational safety and health
      - Enforced by the Department of Labor
      - Violations incur a citation and/or a fine and if serious enough, the workplace can be closed.
    - Health Insurance Portability and Accountability Act of 1996 (HIPAA)
      - Regulations greatly expand patient's right to confidentiality in all healthcare settings
      - One of the most important reasons for the act was the concept that patients retained a right to their own medical information.
      - Limits how information will be used or shared
      - Mandates safeguards for the protection of health information
      - Shifts control of health information from providers to the patient

- National
  - Joint Commission (formerly known as the Joint Commission for Accreditation of Healthcare Organizations, JCAHO)
    - Nonprofit organization
    - Mandates all hospitals have quality assessment programs
    - Focuses on organizational performance or outcomes based on predetermined standards
    - Maintains a list of accredited organizations and survey results, which are available to the public
  - Agency for Healthcare Research and Quality (AHRQ)
    - Engages in the testing and reporting of safety improvement strategies
    - Funds research to determine the best evidence for safe and effective practice guidelines
    - Houses the National Clearinghouse for Quality Measures
  - Professional organizations
    - Examine professional scope of practice and professional standards
- Most states have laws regarding dissemination of quality performance data in the form of Health Care Quality Report Cards.
  - Insurance programs
    - Medicare (see above)
    - Medicaid (see above)
    - Federal Employee Health Benefit Program
      - Covers about 10 million federal employees and their dependents
      - Voluntary, contributory program open to all federal employees
    - Private health insurance
      - Carriers such as Blue Cross Blue Shield, Anthem, Prudential, Metropolitan
      - Traditional fee-for-service plans
  - Managed care
    - Basic reimbursement on historical area change data, relative value scales, and actuarial data
    - Majority pay providers "capitated" fee
      - Fee paid monthly based on number of enrollees who have selected provider as primary care provider

NURSING LANGUAGE

- Nursing Minimum Data Sets (NMDS)
  - Standardize the collection of nursing data
  - The minimum data sets required for electronic charting
- Nursing Interventions Classifications (NIC)
  - Links nursing interventions and patient outcomes
  - Research-based classification system that provides a common, standardized language
  - All specialties and settings
- Nursing Diagnosis Taxonomy
- NANDA International (formerly North American Nursing Diagnosis Association; www.nanda.org)
- Nursing diagnosis is the end product once all of the assessment data are collected and analyzed

STANDARDS OF PRACTICE AND MALPRACTICE

Nurse Practice Act (see above)
- Varies from state to state.
- Each nurse is responsible to know the parameters of practice and the state's rules and regulations.
- Ignorance is not an acceptable defense.

Sources of Laws
- Constitution
  - Fundamental principles that govern a nation, society, or corporation
- Statutes
  - Documented rules for living, both state and federal
  - Deal with relationships to others
    - Ethics of society in writing
  - Nurse Practice Act is an example
- Administrative agencies
  - Given authority to act by legislative bodies
  - Create rules and regulations that enforce statutory laws
    - State Boards are an example
  - Only valid to the extent that they are within the scope of the authority granted to them by the legislative body
- Court decisions
  - Judicial decisions are made by the courts to interpret legal issues that are in dispute

Classification of Legal Action
- Criminal
  - Considered harmful to society as a whole
    - Murder
    - Drug violations
    - Some violations of the Nurse Practice Act
      - Misuse of narcotics
      - Abuse
      - Neglect
  - Felonies: imprisonment
  - Misdemeanor: fine, no jail
- Civil
  - Private interest and rights between persons involved in case
  - Known as torts
    - Civil wrong or injury resulting from a breach of a legal duty that exists by virtue of society's expectations
    - Unintentional
      - Is a civil wrongdoing resulting from the defendant's negligence
    - Intentional
      - Deliberate breach of an individual's rights
        - Assault: act that places patient in fear of harmful or offensive touching
        - Battery: touching without justification or permission

- Defamation: communication of false information orally (slander) or in writing (libel) that damages reputation
- Invasion of privacy: giving unauthorized access to patient or patient's information
  - Example: taking patient's photo without permission
- False imprisonment: unjustifiable restriction of movement
- Quasi-intentional
  - Lacking intent but a willful action and direct causation
    - Examples: defamation of character and invasion of privacy (breach of confidentiality)
- Malpractice and negligence
  - Malpractice
    - A tort committed by a professional action in a professional capacity
    - Failure to act as a reasonable, prudent nurse in the same or similar situation would
    - Professional negligence
  - Negligence
    - General term meaning carelessness either by omission (not doing something) or commission (doing something that should not be done)
    - Failure to act as an ordinary person would in same or similar situation
    - Remember, taking no action is considered an action
    - Categories of negligence
      - Failure to follow standards of care
      - Failure to use equipment in a reasonable manner
      - Failure to communicate
      - Failure to document
      - Failure to assess and monitor
      - Failure to act as a patient advocate
      - Components of negligence (Gillman, 2007)
      - Duty
      - Breach of duty
      - Causation
      - Injury or harm
- Source of liability
  - Personal
    - Each person is accountable for his or her own actions.
  - Physician and other independent practitioners
    - Each professional is accountable and responsible for actions under his or her individual scope of practice.
  - Supervisory
    - Expected to act as a reasonable supervisor under the same or similar circumstances would.
      - Task properly assigned to a worker who is competent to safely perform it.
      - Adequate supervision is provided if the worker needs it.
      - The nurse provides appropriate follow-up and evaluation of delegated task.
  - Institutional
    - *Respondeat superior:* meaning the hospital is responsible for the actions of its employees.
      - Many exceptions apply and each nurse is still responsible and accountable for his or her own actions or failure to act.

- Student and instructor
  - Nursing students have responsibility for their own actions and can be held liable.
  - Students are held to the same standard as an RN.
  - Instructors have supervisory liability.
- Specialty areas
  - Critical care, obstetrics, emergency care, and mental health are examples where nurses are held to additional standards based on the setting.

PATIENT'S RIGHTS

- The Patient Care Partnership (formerly the Patient's Bill of Rights)
  - What the patient can expect
    - High-quality care
    - A clean and safe environment
    - Involvement in his or her own care
      - Discussing medical condition
      - Discussing treatment choices
      - Understanding healthcare goals and values
      - Understand who should make decisions when the patient cannot
    - Protection of privacy
    - Help when leaving the hospital
    - Help with billing claims (American Hospital Association, 2003)
- Privacy and confidentiality (see HIPAA above)
- Consent
  - Oral or written: unless specified, oral and written are equally valid
  - Key to consent is patient comprehension
  - Types
    - Express
      - Consent given by direct words
    - Implied
      - Inferred by the patient's conduct, such as holding out arm for blood pressure
      - Legally implied or presumed: in an emergency situation
    - Informed
      - The person giving consent must fully understand the
        - Procedure to be performed
        - Risks involved
        - Expected or desired outcomes
        - Expected complications or adverse reactions
        - Alternative treatments
      - Consent may be given by
        - A competent adult
        - A legal guardian or person holding durable power of attorney
        - An emancipated or married minor
        - Mature minor (varies by state)
        - Parent of a minor child
        - Court order
    - Revocation
      - Consent can be revoked by the patient

- The Patient Self-Determination Act
  - Right to refuse care
    - Right to be left alone
      - Can refuse any treatment, including medications, except when actively violent to self or others
  - Advance directives
    - Legal document (name varies by state)
    - States patient's wishes regarding life-sustaining medical care if the patient is unable to make decisions
    - Cure, stabilize function or prepare for dignified death (Richerson & Watson, 2010)
    - Documents healthcare wishes or selecting a person to make decisions regarding health care
    - A copy of the directive is placed in the medical record
  - Access medical records in a reasonable time frame, to extent permitted by law
  - To be free from restraints that are not medically required

ETHICS

- The science relating to moral actions and individual value systems (Osborn, Wraa, & Watson, 2010, p. 66)
  - Nursing perspective: ethics is concerned with motives and attitudes and the relationship of these attitudes to the overall care of the patient (Osborn, Wraa, & Watson, 2010, p. 66)
  - Dilemma: nurses often are placed in situations where they are expected to be agents simultaneously for the patient, physicians, and the organization, all of which may have conflicting needs, wants, and goals (Marquis & Huston, 2009, p. 70)
  - Ethical frameworks (examples) assist in determining personal values and beliefs
    - Teleological theory (utilitarianism or consequentialist)
      - Good or bad
      - Greatest good for the greater number of people
        - Example: insurance company that meets the needs of many but may refuse to cover organ transplant
      - End justifies the means
  - Deontological theory
    - Right or wrong regardless of consequence
    - Principles
      - Duty-based: a duty to do something or not do something
      - Rights-based
        - Rights are different from needs, wants, or desires
- Ethical principles
  - Autonomy: personal freedom, right to choose
  - Beneficence: actions should promote good
  - Nonmaleficence: do no harm
  - Veracity: honesty
  - Justice: equal and fair treatment
  - Paternalism: allows one to make decisions for another
  - Fidelity: keeping commitments
  - Respect of others: incorporates all the above

- Ethical dilemmas and decision-making
  - Who should make the decision?
  - What are the possible options or courses of action?
  - What are the available and reasonable alternatives?
  - What are the consequences for all options?
  - Which rules, obligations, and values should direct the choices?
  - What are the desired goals and outcomes in the given situation? (Osborn, Wraa, & Watson, 2010, p. 69)
- Ethics committee: makes decisions in the clinical area
  - Provides structure and guidelines
  - Serves as an open forum
  - Functions as a patient advocate
- Examples of potential ethical dilemmas
  - Religious
    - Beliefs, rituals, customs
  - Cultural
    - Culture refers to integrated patterns of behavior developed over time (way of life)
    - Cultural diversity: differences among people
    - Cultural competence: respecting all differences
    - Cultural sensitivity: being aware of and appreciating the differences among people
  - Resources
    - Access to care: healthcare reform
    - Limited by circumstances such as lack of transportation, high cost of care, fear and distrust, or poor communication
  - Organ transplant
    - Insurance companies not covering the surgery
  - End of life
    - Self-determination
    - See discussion in end of life section of Chapter 4

DOCUMENTATION

- Recording information collected by the nurse and making it available to the rest of the healthcare team.
- Medical record is a legal document.

Documentation Standards

- Accreditation standards
  - Joint Commission
    - Standard abbreviations, acronyms, symbols, and dose designations not to be used
  - State, federal and professional standards
    - Health Care Financing Administration
    - Insurance companies
    - Professional organizations such as American Nurses Association (ANA)
    - Institutional policies
    - Nurse Practice Act

Documentation Principles

- Write legibly
- Date and time each entry
- Use approved abbreviations to reduce errors; avoid unapproved abbreviations
  - For example:
    - IU for international unit
    - QD for daily
    - QOD for every other day
    - MS for morphine sulfate
  - Do not use a trailing zero (use 10 mg instead of 10.0 mg)
  - Do use a leading zero (use 0.5 mg instead of .5 mg)
- Document in chronological order.
- Document objectively, just the facts.
  - What you see, hear, and do.
- Follow institutions policies on documentation.
- Identify all patient problems, actions, and responses.
  - Do not document a patient problem without an action and patient response.
- Document variances from established plan and rationale.
- Sign all entries and include credentials.
- Never

    Document procedures or medication administration in advance.

    Chart for another person.

    Add information at a later date without indicating date of addition.

    - Changing a patient record after the fact is tampering.
  - Add inaccurate information.
  - Refer to staff conflicts or staffing problems.
  - Document that you filed an "incident report."
  - Destroy records.
- Situations where special documentation is required:
  - Consent forms
  - Advance directives
  - Restraints: follow institution policy
  - Leaving against medical advice (AMA)
    - The chart should reflect that the patient is aware he or she is leaving AMA, understands the risks of leaving, and understands that he or she can come back.

- Document the following:
  - People notified of patient's decision
  - Information provided to patient such as risks and or instructions
  - Name of anyone accompanying patient
  - Patient's destination if known
- Incident reports
  - Not a piece of the medical record.
  - Written documentation of an unusual occurrence.
  - Factual.
  - If multiple persons involved, each fills out a separate form.
  - Include problem, actions, follow-up, and patient's response.

REFERENCES

American Hospital Association. (2003). *The patient care partnership*. Retrieved from
http://www.aha.org/aha/issues/Communicating-With-Patients/pt-care-partnership.html

Dunham-Taylor, J., & Pinczuk, J. Z. (2010). *Financial management for nurse managers: Merging the heart with the dollar*. (2nd ed.). Sudbury, MA: Jones & Bartlett Publishers.

Finkelman, A. W. (2006). *Leadership and management in nursing*. Upper Saddle River, NJ: Pearson Prentice Hall.

Gillman, P. H. (2008). Legal and ethical issues. In *Medical-surgical nursing certification review seminar*. Silver Spring, MD: American Nurses Credentialing Center.

Ignatavicius, D. D., & Workman, M. L. (2010). *Medical-surgical nursing: Patient-centered collaborative care* (6th ed.). St. Louis, MO: Saunders Elsevier.

The Joint Commission. (2010). *Facts about the official "do not use" list*. Retrieved from
http://www.jointcommission.org/assets/1/18/Official_Do_Not_Use_List_6_111.PDF

Marquis, B. L., & Huston, C. J. (2009). *Leadership roles and management functions in nursing: Theory and application*. Philadelphia: Wolters Kluwer Health/Lippincott Williams & Wilkins.

Osborn, K. S., Wraa, C. E., & Watson, A. B. (2010). *Medical-surgical nursing: Preparation for practice*. Boston: Pearson.

Richerson, K., & Watson, A. (2010). Health care trends and regulatory aspects of health care delivery. In Osborn, K.S., Wraa, C.E., & Watson, A.B. (2010). *Medical-surgical nursing: Preparation for practice*. Upper Saddle River, NJ: Pearson Prentice Hall.

Roussel, L., Swansburg, R. C., & Swansburg, R. (2006). *Management and leadership for nurse administrators* (4th ed.) Sudbury, MA: Jones & Bartlett Publishers.

Cardio-Pulmonary System

Paula Harrison Gillman, MSN, RN-C, ANP-BC, GNP-BC

GENERAL APPROACH

- The cardiovascular system, together with the pulmonary system, is responsible for the delivery of oxygenated blood to all of the body's organs and tissues. Dysfunction in one system usually leads to dysfunction in the other.
- Cardiac output (CO) (L/min) is the product of heart rate (HR) x stroke volume (SV; amount of blood ejected with each beat). Normal values are 4 to 8 L/min.
- Cardiac index is the cardiac output corrected for body surface area.
- Stroke volume is influenced by 3 factors:
  - Preload: The amount of blood returning to the heart, determining ventricular end-diastolic volume and thus fiber stretch
  - Afterload: The resistance that the ventricles must pump against to eject their blood volume
  - Contractility: The actual contractile strength of the muscle fibers in the ventricles, which is also influenced by preload through the Frank-Starling Law:
    - Increased filling of the ventricles will cause a more vigorous cardiac contraction, up to the point that the ventricles are overfilled and contraction will then weaken.
- Heart rate and stroke volume are influenced by sympathetic and parasympathetic nervous control.
  - Norepinephrine released via the sympathetic nervous system affects B1 receptors, causing an increase in HR (positive chronotropic effect) and contractility of the heart (positive inotropic effect). In addition, venous constriction increases blood return to the heart, thus increasing ventricular filling.

- Acetylcholine released via the vagus nerve of the parasympathetic nervous system produces a decrease in HR (negative chronotropic effect).
- Sympathetic stimulation can increase cardiac output up to several times the resting value. Endurance athletes and patients in early shock may have a cardiac output of 30 L/min.
- From 1996 to 2006, the death rate from coronary heart disease declined 36.4%, but cardiovascular disease remains the number one cause of mortality in the United States, accounting for about 27% of deaths.
- 12% of noninstitutionalized adults have a diagnosis of heart disease.
- Four million hospital discharges annually have heart disease as the primary diagnosis, with an average length of stay of 4.4 days.
- Heart disease costs nearly $500 billion annually.
- A number of risk factors are common to all cardiovascular disease and many of these are modifiable, making the disease largely preventable.

RED FLAGS

- It also should be noted that diabetes mellitus, although a disease of the endocrine system, grossly affects the progression and outcomes of cardiovascular disease. Adults with diabetes have death rates from cardiovascular disease that are 2 to 4 times higher than among adults without diabetes. Even patients with impaired glucose metabolism, being classified as having the metabolic syndrome but not diabetes, have more rapid progression of atherosclerosis.
- Certain groups have more atypical presentations of heart disease. Older persons, women, and people with diabetes are among those who may present with an "angina-equivalent" rather than typical substernal chest pain. These atypical symptoms may include:
  - Shortness of breath
  - Fatigue
  - Dizziness
  - Nausea
  - Other nonspecific symptoms
- Hypertension, a major risk factor for cardiovascular disease, is often silent in presentation until damage occurs to the brain, heart, eyes, or kidneys.

Common Disorders of the Cardiovascular System

HYPERTENSION (HTN)

Description
- Defined as a systolic blood pressure (SBP) over 140 mm Hg and/or a diastolic blood pressure (DBP) over 90 mm Hg on three or more occasions.
- Normal BP is < 120/80 mm Hg.
- Prehypertension is defined by SBP 130 to 139 mm Hg and/or DBP 90 to 99 mm Hg.

Etiology
- Primary, essential, or idiopathic HTN accounts for 95% to 99% of cases.
- Secondary HTN results from another condition such as renovascular disease, renal failure, sleep apnea, pregnancy, or drugs or substances that can elevate BP such as alcohol, nonsteroidal anti-inflammatory drugs (NSAIDs), and decongestants.

Incidence and Demographics
- Approximately 30% of the U.S. population has high blood pressure.
- Incidence is about 50% higher in Blacks as compared to White or Mexican Americans.
- Prevalence increases with age, and by the 7th or 8th decade of life, more than 70% of persons have HTN.
- Due to the epidemic of childhood obesity, incidence in preadolescents, teens, and young adults is on the rise.

Risk Factors
- Smoking
- Abnormal lipids
- Diabetes mellitus
- Age > 60 years
- Sex
- Family history
- Obesity
- Physical inactivity

Prevention and Screening
- Screening is recommended every 2 years in adults with normal BP (< 120/80) and every 1 year for persons with prehypertension.
- All persons with any elevation in BP should be educated about lifestyle modifications that can reduce their BP, such as
  - Losing weight
  - Increasing physical activity
  - Limiting alcohol consumption
  - Stopping smoking
  - Managing stress
  - Following the DASH diet

Assessment

HISTORY
- Previous BP readings
- History of diabetes mellitus
- Concurrent comorbid conditions such as
  - Hyperlipidemia
  - Coronary artery disease
  - History of stroke
  - Peripheral artery disease
  - Renal disease
- Dietary assessment focusing on sodium intake and alcohol consumption
- Current medications that can raise BP: NSAIDs, decongestants, oral contraceptives, erythropoietin, corticosteroids, cyclosporine, tacrolimus, antidepressants that inhibit the reuptake of norepinephrine such as Effexor, Cymbalta, and Pristiq
- Use of herbal products, such as bitter orange, ephedra
- Illegal substances that raise BP: anabolic steroids, cocaine, amphetamines
- Family history of HTN or other cardiovascular, renal disease, or diabetes mellitus
- Symptoms are rare with moderately elevated BP, but it is prudent for the nurse to question the patient about the following symptoms
  - Vision changes

- Headache, dizziness
- Shortness of breath
- Chest pain, palpitations
- Swelling

PHYSICAL EXAM
- Measure BP in both arms; the higher arm should be taken as most reflective of systemic arterial pressure
- Height, weight, waist circumference
- Funduscopic exam evidence of hypertensive retinopathy:
  - Arterial-venous nicking
  - Cotton wool spots (ischemic infarcts in retina)
  - Retinal hemorrhages
  - Papilledema
- Neck: carotid bruits, jugular venous distension, thyroid
- Heart: Irregular rhythm, murmurs, or gallop (an S4 gallop often occurs in persons with longstanding HTN who develop a thickened left ventricle [LVH], which causes a late diastolic or presystolic sound when the ventricle is filling)
- Lungs: Adventitious sounds
- Abdomen: Aortic or renal artery bruits
- Extremities: Pulses, edema
- Neurological: Focal changes that might indicate prior stroke (altered speech, one-sided weakness, facial droop, etc.)

DIAGNOSTIC STUDIES
- Urinalysis to assess for blood, protein, and glucose
- Urine microalbumin
- Hematocrit
- Blood chemistries including sodium, potassium, and calcium
- Renal and liver function tests
- Thyroid function tests (if hyperthyroidism is suspected)
- Uric acid (often associated with hyperuricemia)
- ECG to assess cardiac rhythm, evidence of prior myocardial infarction, voltage criteria for LVH
- Echocardiogram to assess for left ventricular thickness and function

Nursing Management

NONPHARMACOLOGIC TREATMENT
- Lifestyle modifications
  - Weight loss in persons who are overweight or obese
  - DASH (Dietary Approaches to Stop Hypertension), a diet high in potassium and calcium and low in sodium
  - Mediterranean diet, a diet that emphasizes plant-based foods like fruits, vegetables, whole grains, nuts and legumes; healthy fats (olive oil and canola oil); fish and poultry at least twice/week and drinking red wine in moderation (optional)
  - Increased physical activity
  - Limiting alcohol consumption to no more than two drinks per day in most men and one drink per day in women and lighter-weight men; a "drink" is defined as a 12-oz. beer, 5-oz. glass of wine, or 1 oz. of liquor

PHARMACOLOGIC TREATMENT
- Lowering blood pressure with medications significantly reduces the complications of HTN. Many classes of medications are available. Treatment guidelines suggest selecting treatment based on other comorbid conditions, when present. Moderate to severe elevations in blood pressure require more than one agent to reduce BP to a normal range.
- Table 11–1 lists the classes of medication, examples within each class, and common side effects.

Table 11–1. Antihypertensive Medications

Drug Class	Medications	Side Effects
Diuretics	HCTZ Chlorthalidone	Electrolyte imbalances (low K^+, low Na^+, high Ca^{++}) Orthostatic hypotension Hyperuricemia
Beta blockers	Metoprolol Atenolol Bisoprolol Carvedilol	Bradycardia Heart block Fatigue Nightmares/insomnia Congestive heart failure Bronchospasm Sexual dysfunction
Calcium channel blockers	Amlodipine Nifedipine Nisoldipine Felodipine Verapamil Diltiazem	Peripheral edema Headache Constipation Diarrhea Tachycardia Heart block Dizziness Flushing
Angiotensin-converting enzyme inhibitors (ACEIs)	Lisinopril Enalapril Monopril Ramipril	Dry hacking cough Hyperkalemia Angioedema Acute renal failure Fetal malformations
Angiotensin receptor blockers (ARBs)	Losartan Irbesartan Candesartan Valsartan	Hyperkalemia Angioedema (rarely) Acute renal failure Fetal malformations
Direct renin inhibitors	Aliskiren	Hyperkalemia Angioedema Diarrhea Acute renal failure Fetal malformations
Alpha blockers	Doxazosin Terazosin	Orthostatic hypotension Fatigue Dry mouth

cont.

Table 11–1. Antihypertensive Medications (cont.)

Central adrenergic inhibitors	Clonidine Guanfacine	Sedation Dry mouth Rebound HTN with sudden withdrawal
Direct-acting vasodilators	Hydralazine Minoxidil	Tachycardia/palpitations CHF, angina Headache Nausea, vomiting, diarrhea Systemic lupus erythematosus (hydralazine)

Special Considerations

- Many patients claim to have "white-coat hypertension": a blood pressure that is only elevated in the healthcare setting. True white-coat HTN is actually rare. Most people who have BP elevations in situations of stress experience high blood pressure throughout each day, for example, when they are driving in traffic, late for a deadline, arguing about something, or during any of the other stressful encounters that most people experience each day. A 24-hour ambulatory BP monitor is the only modality to diagnose this condition.
- Home monitoring of blood pressure can be useful in some situations, but causes stress and anxiety in others.
- Lowering BP too rapidly (even to high normal levels) can cause dizziness and fatigue in an ambulatory person.
- The approach to managing BP on a chronic basis differs from acute management during critical illness, when rapid reduction of BP is often needed to prevent bleeding or other complications. In these circumstances, intravenous agents often are used to allow for rapid titration.
- Elderly persons most commonly have an elevation in systolic BP with a normal diastolic reading (isolated systolic hypertension). Medications given to treat HTN will lower both systolic and diastolic readings. If diastolic BP is lowered too much (in an effort to normalize SBP), older persons may experience dizziness, falls, or chest pain, necessitating an alteration in the "goal" BP.
- Cost and complexity of the pharmacologic regimen must be minimized to enhance adherence.
- Patients most commonly stop medications for the following reasons; thus, education is of utmost importance:
  - "Unexpected" side effects; thus, patients should be informed of potential side effects and advised how to avoid or whether they are transient.
  - Lack of understanding that therapy is chronic, not short-term, and that regular follow-up with a healthcare provider is essential.

Follow-up

EXPECTED OUTCOMES
- Patient will have a BP within normal range (< 120/80) or at goal for that individual.
- Patient will have minimal or at least tolerable side effects from his/her medication regimen.
- Patient will verbalize understanding that treatment of HTN, either by lifestyle modifications or pharmacologic interventions, is lifelong, in order to prevent complications and reduce the risk of cardio- and cerebrovascular disease.

COMPLICATIONS
- Untreated HTN leads to damage of target organs.
  - Eyes: retinal damage and potential blindness
  - Heart: left ventricular hypertrophy, heart failure, arrhythmias, ischemic heart disease
  - Brain: stroke or transient ischemic attack
  - Kidneys: nephrosclerosis leading to chronic kidney disease
  - Peripheral arterial disease
- Complications can also result from over-treatment of blood pressure or from side effects of medications: falls, fractures, electrolyte imbalances, heart failure, bradycardia, allergic reactions, bronchospasm, constipation, or rebound hypertension to name a few.

ISCHEMIC HEART DISEASE

Description
- Ischemic heart disease results from atherosclerosis of the coronary arteries that supply the myocardium with oxygen. Plaque accumulation causes narrowing of the vessel lumen and compromises blood flow. This process occurs gradually over time, and often causes symptoms of angina pectoris.
- Angina pectoris refers to the exertional substernal chest pain that occurs when a mismatch between oxygen demand of the myocardium and oxygen supply occurs. Angina pectoris is relieved by either rest (decreases oxygen demand) or nitroglycerine (increases oxygen supply).
- Rupture of a coronary plaque can cause subtotal (unstable angina or a myocardial infarction [MI] without ST segment elevation) or total occlusion of a coronary vessel. This condition is called acute coronary syndrome (ACS). Total occlusion without intervention leads to an acute transmural myocardial infarction, causing ST-segment elevation on the electrocardiogram (ECG).

Etiology
- Atherosclerotic progression is accelerated by three processes: endothelial dysfunction, inflammation, and thrombosis.
- Advanced lesions usually have a thicker fibrous cap and thus are less prone to rupture.
- Plaques at risk for rupture leading to ACS are those with a lipid core and a thin fibrous cap containing collagen. Plaque rupture exposes the collagen matrix, which is highly thrombogenic.

Incidence and Demographics
- About 17.6 million Americans have coronary heart disease.
- Myocardial infarctions occur at a rate of about 1 every 30 seconds.

Risk Factors
- Nonmodifiable
  - Male sex
  - Older age
  - Family history
  - Postmenopausal status
  - Race (Blacks, Native Americans, and Hispanics are more likely to have disease than Whites)

- Modifiable
  - Smoking
  - High LDL cholesterol (see Table 11–5)
  - Low HDL cholesterol
  - Uncontrolled hypertension
  - Uncontrolled diabetes
  - Physical inactivity
  - Obesity
  - Uncontrolled stress

Tables 11–2 through 11–5 outline the classification of lipid abnormalities according to the National Cholesterol Education Panel (NCEP) guidelines.

Table 11–2. Total Cholesterol Classification

< 200	Desirable
200–239	Borderline high
> 240	High

Adapted from *Third report on detection, evaluation and treatment of high blood cholesterol in adults (Adult Treatment Panel III)*, by National Cholesterol Education Panel (NIH Publication 01-3670), 2001, Bethesda, MD: NHLBI Health Information Center.

Table 11–3. LDL Classification

< 100	Optimal
100–129	Near optimal
130–159	Borderline high
160–189	High
≥ 190	Very high

Adapted from *Third report on detection, evaluation and treatment of high blood cholesterol in adults (Adult Treatment Panel III)*, by National Cholesterol Education Panel (NIH Publication 01-3670), 2001, Bethesda, MD: NHLBI Health Information Center.

Table 11–4. HDL Classification

< 40	Low
≥ 60	High

Adapted from *Third report on detection, evaluation and treatment of high blood cholesterol in adults (Adult Treatment Panel III)*, by National Cholesterol Education Panel (NIH Publication 01-3670), 2001, Bethesda, MD: NHLBI Health Information Center.

Table 11–5. Triglyceride Classification

< 150	Optimal
> 150	High

Adapted from *Third report on detection, evaluation and treatment of high blood cholesterol in adults (Adult Treatment Panel III)*, by National Cholesterol Education Panel (NIH Publication 01-3670), 2001, Bethesda, MD: NHLBI Health Information Center.

Prevention and Screening

- More emphasis should be placed on prevention of coronary heart disease. As noted above, many risk factors may be modified by lifestyle changes or pharmacologic interventions, thereby reducing the morbidity and mortality associated with this disease.
- Benefits of screening asymptomatic persons with one or no risk factors by exercise treadmill testing or electron beam CT are not supported by the literature. False positive (particularly in women) and false negative test results are both possible.
- Advancing age (and accumulation of risk factors) increases lifetime risk of an event and improves the sensitivity of screening tests. A calculator to estimate CHD risk is available online at http://hp2010.nhlbihin.net/atpiii/calculator.asp.

Assessment

HISTORY
- Subjective symptoms, including substernal chest pressure that may radiate to the back, jaw, or left arm; nausea; diaphoresis; shortness of breath at rest or with exertion; or profound fatigue.
- Risk factors and comorbid conditions should be assessed.
- History of other conditions that can cause chest pain, such as gastroesophageal reflux (GERD), lung disease, chest wall pain, or costochondritis.
- Family history of premature coronary disease: first-degree male relative before age 55 or first-degree female relative before age 65.

PHYSICAL EXAM
- Vital signs: elevated or low BP, slow or accelerated pulse
- Skin: xanthelasma or xanthomas, pallor or cyanosis
- Funduscopic exam for changes of hypertension
- Neck: carotid bruits or jugular venous distention
- Chest: palpation of chest wall for tenderness
- Heart: rate, rhythm, murmurs, S3 or S4 gallop, palpate point of maximal impulse (PMI) for increased or decreased intensity and localization
- Lungs: adventitious or absent sounds (in bases with pleural effusion)
- Abdomen: bruits
- Pulses: quality and character (diminished peripheral pulses occur with decreased cardiac output)
- Neurological: altered mental status with decreased cerebral perfusion

DIAGNOSTIC STUDIES
- Differential diagnoses: Numerous other medical conditions can cause chest pain that is similar to coronary ischemia. Consideration must be given to the quality, character, duration, and intensity of the pain, as well as precipitating factors, in order to differentiate causes of chest pain. Specific tests may be needed to rule out other causes of chest pain.
  - GERD or esophageal spasm: barium swallow or esophagogastroduodenoscopy (EGD)
  - Pericarditis: ECG shows ST elevation in all leads
  - Chest wall pain: based on physical exam
  - Pulmonary embolus: CT scan or V/Q scan
  - Aortic dissection: chest CT
  - Bronchospasm: spirometry
  - Spontaneous pneumothorax: chest X-ray
  - Anxiety: suspected based on history
- Acute
  - 12-lead ECG
  - Cardiac enzymes/troponin
  - CXR
  - Cardiac catheterization
- Subacute
  - Exercise electrocardiography (exercise treadmill test): inexpensive test that is recommended for persons having an intermediate pretest probability of having disease; patient must be able to walk on treadmill.
  - Radioisotope imaging (nuclear): used in conjunction with treadmill testing or pharmacologic stress testing to look at myocardial function or flow.
  - Stress echocardiography: two-dimensional echo can detect wall motion abnormalities that may correspond to ischemia or prior myocardial damage; also can be used in conjunction with treadmill testing or pharmacologic agents.
  - Pharmacologic stress testing: used when patients are unable to reach an adequate workload by exercise.
  - Electron-beam computed tomography (EBCT) or calcium scoring: detects calcium in coronary arteries as an early marker of atherosclerosis; can detect clinically insignificant disease to "warn" about the necessity of risk factor reduction.
  - Coronary angiography: considered the "gold standard" in diagnosing ischemic heart disease; reveals distribution and severity of obstructive lesions.

Nursing Management

NONPHARMACOLOGIC TREATMENT
- Lifestyle modifications
  - Weight loss in persons who are overweight or obese
  - Two servings of fish/week for omega-3 fatty acids
  - Diet low in saturated, trans fats, and cholesterol and high in fiber
  - Moderate alcohol consumption (1 to 3 drinks/day) reduces CAD mortality by 20% in persons who do not experience an elevation in BP related to drinking.
  - Increased physical activity improves exercise tolerance and raises HDL cholesterol.
  - Smoking cessation

PHARMACOLOGICAL TREATMENT
- Medical management of ischemic heart disease has long-term outcomes equal to interventional therapies in certain groups of patients, such as those with normal left ventricular function.
  - Nitrates
    - Increase coronary blood flow, decrease myocardial oxygen demand and peripheral resistance
    - Short-acting agents may be taken sublingually to relieve acute angina pectoris
    - Long-acting preparations may be given daily, taking care to provide for a nitrate-free period in order to prevent tolerance (for example, a nitrate patch is worn for only 12 hours/day)
    - Side effects may include headache, orthostatic hypotension, and syncope
  - Beta-blocking agents
    - Decrease heart rate, myocardial contractility, and systemic blood pressure, thereby decreasing myocardial oxygen demand
    - Improve survival after an MI
    - Side effects may occur: congestive heart failure in patients with reduced ejection fraction, bradycardia or heart block, bronchospasm (noncardioselective agents), fatigue, erectile dysfunction, depression, sleep disturbances
  - Calcium channel blockers
    - Decrease the influx of calcium into slow channels of heart and smooth muscle, thereby causing coronary vasodilation, preventing coronary vasospasm, and causing systemic vasodilation
    - Side effects may occur: dizziness, flushing, headache, hypotension, peripheral edema, constipation, diarrhea, rebound tachycardia; AV block, and heart failure with verapamil and diltiazem
  - Antiplatelet drugs
    - Reduce platelet aggregation by various actions
    - Aspirin (81 to 325 mg) is least expensive agent and given unless contraindicated
    - Plavix (clopidogrel) 75 mg is an alternative for those who can't tolerate aspirin; also given in combination with aspirin following percutaneous coronary intervention
    - Side effects may occur: increased risk of bleeding and skin rash
  - Angiotensin-converting enzyme inhibitors (ACEIs)
    - Decrease mortality after MI
    - Most beneficial with left ventricular dysfunction
    - Side effects may occur: dry, hacking cough; hyperkalemia; angioedema; acute renal failure; fetal malformations
  - HMG-CoA reductase inhibitors (statins)
    - Reduce cholesterol production in the liver, thereby lowering LDL cholesterol; in some cases, also lower triglycerides and raise HDL cholesterol
    - Lowering cholesterol reduces rate of plaque formation and extreme lowering can cause plaque reversal.
    - Statin drugs also stabilize plaques and reduce inflammation.
    - Cholesterol treatment guidelines recommend an LDL < 100 mg/dL as "optimal" in everyone, but drug therapy is initiated based on other risk factors for atherosclerosis (see Table 11–6).
    - Target LDL for persons with multiple poorly controlled risk factors and established coronary disease is < 70 mg/dL.

- Optimal triglyceride level is < 150 mg/dL.
  - Optimal HDL cholesterol level is > 45 mg/dL.
- Table 11–6 identifies target levels for lifestyle and drug treatment according to NCEP guidelines. TLC refers to therapeutic lifestyle choices, which is the terminology used to describe the standard lifestyle changes of weight loss, exercise, and low-fat, low-cholesterol diet.

Table 11–6. LDL Treatment Goals

Risk Category	LDL-C goal	Initiate TLC	Consider RX
Very high risk*	< 70	> 70	≥ 70
CHD or risk equivalent	< 100	> 100	≥ 130; 100–129, drug optional
2+ risk factors, 10-year risk 10%–20%**	< 130	≥ 130	≥ 130
2+ risk factors, 10-year risk < 10%**	< 130	≥ 130	≥ 160
0–1 risk factor	< 160	≥ 160	≥ 190; 160–189, drug optional

Note. *Established CHD who also have multiple risk factors, including diabetes, metabolic syndrome, or severe or poorly controlled risk factors.
**Percentage risk based on Framingham Risk Score Calculation (National Cholesterol Education Panel, 2001)

Adapted from *Third report on detection, evaluation and treatment of high blood cholesterol in adults (Adult Treatment Panel III)*, by National Cholesterol Education Panel (NIH Publication 01-3670), 2001, Bethesda, MD: NHLBI Health Information Center.

- Other medications may be given instead of or in addition to statins to modify cholesterol levels (see Table 11–7).

Table 11–7. Prescription Drug Therapy for Lipids

Drug Class	Medications	Primary Effect(s)	Nursing Considerations
Statins	Lovastatin (Mevacor) Fluvastatin (Lescol) Pravastatin (Pravachol) Simvastatin (Zocor) Atorvastatin (Lipitor) Rosuvastatin (Crestor) Pitavastatin (Livalo)	Lowers LDL Raises HDL +/– Lowers TG	Monitor for • Myalgias • Dark urine • Liver function tests

Fibrates	Gemfibrozil (Lopid) Fenofibrate (Triplix®, Lofibra®, Fenoglide®, Tricor®, Antara®)	Lowers TG Raises HDL	Contraindicated in severe hepatic and renal disease Monitor for: • Gallstones • GI upset • Myopathy
Nicotinic acid	Niacin (OTC) Niaspan®	Raises HDL Lowers TG Lowers LDL	Initial few doses cause severe flushing; aspirin taken 30 min before diminishes Monitor for: • Myopathy • GI upset • GI bleeding • Liver function • Hyperglycemia • Hyperuricemia/gout symptoms
Cholesterol absorption inhibitor	Ezetimibe (Zetia®)	Lowers LDL Lowers TG	Monitor for: • Diarrhea • Other GI symptoms
Bile acid resins	Colestipol WelChol™	Lowers LDL	Monitor for: • Constipation • Elevated TG
Fish oil	Lovaza®	Lowers TG	Monitor for: • Eructation • Taste perversion • GI upset

INTERVENTIONAL TREATMENT
- Percutaneous coronary intervention (PCI): used for treatment of single or multivessel disease; placement of intracoronary stents greatly reduces the likelihood of restenosis.
- Coronary artery bypass grafting (CABG): most efficacious for patients with > 50% stenosis of the left main coronary artery or triple-vessel disease who have a reduced ejection fraction (35% to 50%); also yields better long-term outcomes than PCI in people with diabetes.

Special Considerations
- As stated previously, women, persons with diabetes, and older persons tend to have more atypical/vague presentations of ischemic heart disease.
- Studies show that women who have an MI are less likely than men to receive treatments known to improve survival.
- Patients should be educated on the action, importance, and possible side effects of each medication that they take. It should be emphasized that coronary ischemia is a chronic condition with a high mortality rate. Optimal therapy requires strict adherence to both medication and lifestyle therapies.
- Anemia can exacerbate coronary ischemia, especially when hemoglobin is < 7 g/dL.

Follow-up

EXPECTED OUTCOMES
- Patient will have sufficient exercise tolerance to engage in activities of daily living without angina.
- Patient will verbalize understanding of steps to take when angina occurs, and differentiate between stable and unstable angina (which might be from acute coronary syndrome.)
- Patient will have minimal or at least tolerable side effects from his or her medication regimen.
- Patient will verbalize understanding that treatment of ischemic heart disease either by lifestyle modifications or pharmacologic interventions is a lifelong requirement to prevent complications and reduce the risk of death.

COMPLICATIONS
- Congestive heart failure is the most common complication of ischemic heart disease, resulting from damage to the myocardium that impairs pumping and cardiac output.
- Coronary ischemia also can precipitate sudden cardiac death.

VALVULAR HEART DISEASE

Description
- The four cardiac valves maintain unidirectional blood flow through the heart.
- Valves that are stiff and don't open well are called "stenotic" and valves that don't close well and allow for backward flow of blood are called "incompetent," "insufficient," or "regurgitant."
- Stenotic valves lead to myocardial hypertrophy as the heart pumps against increased resistance.
- Incompetent valves contribute additional blood to a cardiac chamber that is full or filling, thus causing volume overload and chamber dilation.
- Acquired valvular disease most commonly affects the aortic and mitral valves, which will be the focus of this section.

Etiology
- Rheumatic fever in childhood (5% to 15% of cases: greatly decreased over the past few decades)
- Valve degeneration or calcification with age
- Myocardial infarction, which can damage papillary muscles and lead to valve dysfunction
- Systemic disease such as lupus and scleroderma
- Infective endocarditis
- Marfan syndrome, caused by a genetic defect that leads to excessive growth of long bones of the body and connective tissue problems affecting the cardiovascular system, eyes, and skin

Incidence and Demographics
- Calcific aortic stenosis affects 2% to 4% of persons over age 65.
- Bicuspid aortic valve is found in 1% to 2% of the population, mostly men.
- Women have mitral stenosis 4 to 5 times more often than men.

Risk Factors
- Age
- Rheumatic heart disease
- Ischemic heart disease
- IV drug use
- Periodontal disease

Prevention and Screening
- Age-related valvular calcification is not preventable.
- Prevention of ischemic heart disease, discussed in the previous section, in turn protects valvular function.
- Routine screening for valvular dysfunction is not cost-effective.
- Evaluation by echocardiography is performed as indicated based on symptoms of valve dysfunction or presence of a murmur noted on physical exam.

Assessment

HISTORY
- Subjective symptoms will vary based on which valve is affected and whether it is stenotic or insufficient, and also whether the condition developed slowly or suddenly (such as acute rupture of a cord causing a flail valve).
  - Valvular insufficiency will produce symptoms of chamber overload, such as dyspnea at rest or on exertion, orthopnea, paroxysmal nocturnal dyspnea, cough, fatigue, weakness, edema, and possibly chest pain.
  - Valvular stenosis impedes forward flow of blood and causes chamber hypertrophy. Symptoms of reduced cardiac output are present, such as syncope, angina and dyspnea, and fatigue.
- History of ischemic heart disease or rheumatic fever
- Prior or current IV drug use

PHYSICAL EXAM
- Mitral insufficiency
  - Holosystolic murmur heard at the apex that radiates to the left axilla; S4 gallop with acute cause; PMI displaced laterally
  - Cardiac rhythm may be irregular due to atrial fibrillation or frequent atrial ectopic beats.
  - Blood pressure normal to low; pulse pressure narrow due to decreased stroke volume
  - Lung auscultation may reveal crackles or no sounds due to pleural effusion.
- Aortic insufficiency
  - Diastolic murmur is a high-pitched, "blowing" sound heard at the aortic area or left sternal border; more severe regurgitation will produce a longer murmur (holodiastolic); PMI displaced laterally
  - Elevated systolic pressure and low diastolic pressure (wide pulse pressure)
  - Chronic aortic insufficiency can cause other signs:
    - Waterhammer pulse: sharp upstroke then abrupt fall
    - de Musset sign: bobbing of head with each pulse
    - Traube's sign: "pistol shot" sound heard over the femoral arteries
- Aortic stenosis

- Systolic ejection murmur heard in the aortic area that radiates across the precordium to the apex as the condition worsens; the duration of the murmur increases and gets louder, eventually obliterating the S2 heart sound; S4 gallop is common
- Blood pressure is normal to high.
- Diminished carotid and peripheral pulses due to reduced ejection of blood

DIAGNOSTIC STUDIES
- CXR and ECG
- 2-D echocardiography
- Transesophageal echocardiography (better views of mitral valve)
- Right heart catheterization: measure pulmonary artery pressure
- Left heart catheterization

Nursing Management
- Mitral regurgitation
  - Medical: aimed at reducing afterload to promote forward flow of blood with medications such as ACEIs, nitrates, and hydralazine; reducing volume with diuretics; antibiotic prophylaxis before dental and surgical procedures
  - Referral to a cardiologist is needed in patients who are symptomatic with fatigue, heart failure, or arrhythmias.
  - Surgical: valve repair or replacement (mechanical or tissue)
- Aortic insufficiency
  - Medical: antibiotic prophylaxis with dental, endoscopic, or surgical procedures; vasodilating drugs to reduce backward flow of blood: ACEIs, nifedipine, hydralazine
  - Follow-up: twice yearly history, physical, and CXR; annual ECG and echocardiogram
  - Surgical: Valve replacement is warranted in all symptomatic patients and is best performed before LV dysfunction develops; operative mortality is 3% to 10%, but for successful cases, 77% of persons are alive at 10 years.
- Aortic stenosis
  - Medical: antibiotic prophylaxis to prevent endocarditis; avoidance of extreme exertion with moderate to severe disease; periodic echocardiograms are performed to track disease progression (frequency depends on severity of stenosis)
  - Surgical: Valve replacement is indicated in symptomatic patients and those with severe stenosis and LV dysfunction; balloon valvuloplasty is an alternative palliative therapy to relieve symptoms in patients whose surgical mortality risk is too high.

Special Considerations
- All patients who receive a prosthetic valve require anticoagulation for 6 to 12 weeks. The highest risk for thromboembolism occurs in the first days to months after surgery. Once the valve has endothelialized, the risk of thrombus formation is less, and persons with tissue valves are maintained on aspirin.
- Patients who receive a mechanical valve will require lifelong anticoagulation with warfarin due to a continued risk of clotting. International normalized ratio (INR) should be maintained between 2.5 and 3.5.
- Red blood cell destruction occurs with mechanical valves so these patients should be monitored for anemia.

Follow-up

EXPECTED OUTCOMES
- Patient with valvular disease will ensure antibiotic prophylaxis prior to any invasive or dental procedure to prevent endocarditis.
- Patient with mitral or aortic insufficiency will adhere to the chronic medication regimen needed to reduce afterload and alleviate symptoms.
- Patient with a valvular disorder will understand and report symptoms of congestive failure or reduced cardiac output immediately.
- Patient with a mechanical prosthetic valve will keep frequent (usually monthly or more often) follow-up appointments to monitor level of anticoagulation.

COMPLICATIONS
- Congestive heart failure is the most common complication of valvular heart disease. Once symptoms develop and left ventricular dysfunction occurs, prognosis worsens for valve replacement surgery.
- Coronary heart disease often occurs concurrently in patients with valvular disease, which worsens prognosis and increases chances of sudden cardiac death.

CONGESTIVE HEART FAILURE (CHF)

Description
- A syndrome whereby blood output by the heart is insufficient to meet metabolic demands of the tissues.
- Reduced renal blood flow leads to activation of the rennin-angiotensin-aldosterone system (RAAS). Angiotensinogen is made in the liver and is converted by rennin in the kidney to angiotensin I. Angiotensin I is then converted to angiotensin II by angiotensin-converting enzyme (ACE). Angiotensin II is a potent vasoconstrictor and binds to the AT1 receptor, producing harmful cardiac effects, and also to the A2 receptor, which has beneficial cardiac effects. Angiotensin II also stimulates the release of aldosterone, which leads to sodium and water retention in the kidney. In addition to RAAS activation, the sympathetic nervous system also is stimulated through baroreceptor activation in the left ventricle, aortic arch, and carotid sinus. This leads to catecholamine release, resulting in an increase in heart rate and vasoconstriction. Initially, these compensatory mechanisms improve cardiac output, but ultimately lead to a more dysfunctional myocardial state.
- There are two types of heart failure:
  - Systolic heart failure occurs when the ventricle is too weak to pump blood. Most common cause is myocardial infarction.
  - Diastolic heart failure occurs when the ventricle is too stiff and noncompliant to fill with an adequate volume of blood to provide sufficient stroke volume. Most common cause is longstanding hypertension.

Etiology
- Causes of heart failure
  - Ischemic disease/MI
  - Valvular disease
  - Cardiomyopathy: irreversible primary disease of the heart muscle that results in severe dysfunction. There are three types:

- Dilated: caused by alcohol or cocaine consumption, viral infection, or idiopathic
- Hypertrophic: due to myocardial hypertrophy that most commonly affects the intraventricular septum; most common cause of sudden death in young athletes
- Restrictive: least common, characterized by impaired diastolic relaxation in absence of ventricular hypertrophy
- Hypertension
- Myocarditis: inflammation of the myocardium, which may be caused by viral, fungal, parasitic, or bacterial infections; peripartum condition; cocaine use; chest radiation; or other causes; often leads to dilated cardiomyopathy
- Pulmonary hypertension
- Exacerbating factors
  - Noncompliance with medications/diet
  - Infection (pneumonia, urinary tract infection)
  - Anemia
  - Stress
  - Arrhythmias (particularly tachycardia or atrial fibrillation)
  - Excessive salt intake
  - Digoxin toxicity
  - Thyroid disease
  - Pulmonary emboli
  - New medications that can cause volume overload or interfere with action of chronic medications: nonsteroidal anti-inflammatory drugs (NSAIDs), thiazolidinediones (TZDs for treating diabetes mellitus)

Incidence and Demographics
- About 5 million Americans have a diagnosis of CHF.
- Prevalence increases with age and is about 9% in persons over age 80.
- Approximately 400,000 new cases are diagnosed annually.
- CHF is the most costly Medicare diagnosis-related group (DRG).

Risk Factors
- Ischemic heart disease
- Hypertension
- Any risk factors for the above disease processes

Prevention and Screening
- Prevention of CHF involves preventing the underlying disease processes that lead to poor myocardial function.
- There is no "screening" for CHF. Since it is a known complication of hypertension and ischemic heart disease, persons with these conditions should be carefully followed for any change in symptoms or exam results that might suggest development of CHF.
- Assessment

  HISTORY
  - Subjective data: decreased exercise tolerance, dyspnea, orthopnea, paroxysmal nocturnal dyspnea (PND), cough or wheezing, fatigue, leg or abdominal swelling
  - History of HTN, diabetes, hyperlipidemia, coronary or valvular disease, peripheral vascular disease, rheumatic fever, exposure to cardiotoxic agents (antineoplastics)
  - Social history: illicit drug use, tobacco use, alcohol consumption
  - Family history: premature CAD, cardiomyopathy, sudden death

PHYSICAL EXAM
- Blood pressure may be elevated or low
- Weight gain
- Neck: jugular venous distention
- Lungs: basilar crackles or diminished sounds with effusion, wheezing
- Heart: S3 or S4 gallop, displaced PMI, tachycardia, weak pulses
- Abdomen: hepatomegaly, positive hepatojugular reflex
- Genitourinary (GU): decreased urine output
- Skin: cyanosis, pallor
- Neurologic: altered mental status

DIAGNOSTIC STUDIES
- Complete blood count (CBC)
- Urinalysis
- Blood chemistries and magnesium
- B-type natriuretic peptide (BNP)
  - Produced in the ventricles in response to stress (elevated pressure)
  - Low level rules out HF
- Renal and hepatic function tests
- Thyroid function tests
- Chest x-ray
  - Shows increased interstitial markings, vascular engorgement, cardiomegaly, or pleural effusions
- 12-lead ECG
- Two-dimensional echocardiogram
  - This test measures ejection fraction (EF), which is used to differentiate systolic versus diastolic failure and evaluate wall motion. In systolic failure, the EF is reduced (< 50%); in diastolic failure EF is high (> 50%) (see Box 11–1).

Box 11–1. Left Ventricular Ejection Fraction

Normal LVEF	High LVEF	Low LVEF
EDV = 100 mL	EDV = 60 mL	EDV = 120 mL
SV = 60 mL	SV = 50 mL	SV = 25 mL
EF = 60%	EF = 85%	EF = 20%
HR = 70	HR = 70	HR = 70
CO = 4.2 L/min	CO = 3.5 L/min	CO = 1.7 L/min

EDV: end diastolic volume, amount of blood filling ventricle at end diastole
SV: stroke volume, amount of blood ejected with each ventricular contraction
EF: ejection fraction, percentage of blood ejected with each contraction
HR: heart rate
CO: cardiac output, amount of blood pumped in 1 minute; HR × SV

CLASSIFICATION

- Two classification systems are used for heart failure. The New York Heart Association (NYHA) classification focuses on functional capacity and the American College of Cardiology/American Heart Association (ACC/AHA) Stages of Heart Failure combines functional capacity and structural changes to guide treatment and reduce morbidity and mortality.
  - NYHA Classification
    - Class I: Early, no symptoms
    - Class II: Mild symptoms with ordinary activity
    - Class III: Advanced; comfortable only at rest
    - Class IV: Severe; symptoms at rest
  - ACC/AHA Stages of Heart Failure
    - Stage A: All patients with cardiac risk factors
    - Stage B: Patients with structural heart disease but no symptoms
    - Stage C: Patients who have current or prior symptoms of HF; includes NYHA Class I, II, and III
    - Stage D: Patients with advanced structural heart disease and marked symptoms at rest; includes NYHA Class IV

Differential Diagnosis

- Pneumonia
- Chronic obstructive pulmonary disease (COPD) exacerbation
- Asthma
- Pulmonary embolus
- Renal disease
- Liver disease

Nursing Management

NONPHARMACOLOGIC TREATMENT

- Heart-healthy diet (low fat/cholesterol, low sodium, high fiber)
- Regular exercise (unless decompensated)
- Smoking cessation
- Limit alcohol
- No illicit drugs
- Influenza and pneumococcal vaccines
- Monitor daily weights (plan of action if weight increases by 2 to 3 lbs)
- Focus on control of risk factors for other underlying/aggravating diseases (such as diabetes, ischemic heart disease)
  - Nursing interventions
    - Place patient in semi-Fowler's position to decrease preload (volume return to the heart)
    - Organize activities to provide adequate rest for patients who are decompensated

PHARMACOLOGIC TREATMENT

- Angiotensin-converting enzyme inhibitor (ACEI): alleviate symptoms and block the neurohormonal cascade that ensues with HF; hypotension possible with initiation; must follow creatinine and potassium.

- Beta blockers (BB): must be started slowly in patients with compensated HF or may worsen symptoms; permit up-regulation of beta receptors and improve cardiac function over time; monitor for bradycardia, heart block, fatigue, hypotension (first 24 to 48 hours); often necessary to separate the doses of ACEI and BB.
- Loop diuretics: used to control volume overload; most rapid symptom relief.
- Digoxin: may be used in patients with atrial fibrillation or those with systolic dysfunction.
- Aldosterone antagonists: usually added in patients with persistent symptoms after treatment with the above medications; monitor for hyperkalemia and gynecomastia.
- Angiotensin receptor blockers (ARBs): sometimes used in persons who cannot tolerate ACEIs.
- Hydralazine and nitrates: older therapy for HF that is often used in patients who cannot tolerate ACEIs because of renal dysfunction, or as add-on medications to lower BP.
- Warfarin: indicated for patients with atrial fibrillation and some patients at high risk of embolization due to severely dilated left ventricles.

Special Considerations

- Treatment in patients with diastolic dysfunction (normal EF) varies slightly.
  - Sodium restriction is more critical: very volume-sensitive.
  - Avoid over-diuresis.
  - Verapamil and diltiazem often are used to enhance "relaxation" of the ventricle; these medications have negative inotropic effects and are never used in patients with systolic dysfunction.
  - Maintenance of sinus rhythm is important; atrial fibrillation further compromises ventricular filling.
  - Focus on decreasing left ventricular hypertrophy (strict BP control).
- Younger patients with Stage IV heart failure may be candidates for heart transplantation or left ventricular assist devices as a bridge to transplant.
- 30% to 50% of patients with CHF die suddenly of cardiac arrhythmias; implantable pacemaker-defibrillators reduce this risk by 36% (COMPANION trial).
- Biventricular pacing or "cardiac resynchronization therapy" has been shown to improve symptoms and reduce morbidity and mortality in patients with severe symptoms despite optimal medical management.
- Advance directives are important for all patients with chronic, terminal illness.
- Hospice care may be appropriate for patients with end-stage CHF.

Follow-up

EXPECTED OUTCOMES
- Patient will verbalize knowledge of action and dosage for each medication.
- Patient will weigh self daily.
- Patient will verbalize understanding that compliance with medications is paramount to prevent hospitalization, improve quality of life, and minimize morbidity and mortality.
- Patient will recognize signs and symptoms of worsening heart failure and notify a healthcare provider immediately or implement predefined plan of action (such as extra diuretic dosage).
- Patient will have optimal exercise tolerance to complete activities of daily living.
- Patient will verbalize an action plan for lifestyle modifications to improve outcomes in HF.

COMPLICATIONS
- Sudden cardiac death is the most serious complication of CHF.
- Class IV heart failure patients have a mortality of 50% at 6 months.
- Most common reasons for hospital readmission are lack of adherence to medication and diet therapy, inadequate control of BP and ischemia, and underuse of ACEIs.

ARRHYTHMIAS

Description
- Result from abnormal conduction or automaticity of the heart that changes the rate and rhythm. Rhythm disturbances range in severity from benign to life-threatening.

Etiology
- Myocardial ischemia or infarction
- Organic heart disease
- Drug effects
- Electrolyte abnormalities
- Degenerative changes in the conduction system

Incidence and Demographics
- Most common in persons with ischemic or structural heart disease
- Increased incidence with age

Risk Factors
- Same as risk for ischemic heart disease and hypertension

Prevention and Screening
- Preventive efforts are aimed at prevention of ischemic disease and hypertension.
- Routine screening is not performed. Ambulatory monitors or event recorders are used in patients experiencing symptoms of arrhythmias.

Assessment

HISTORY
- Subjective: palpitations, near-syncope or syncope, falls, shortness of breath, chest pain, fatigue, weakness, dizziness
- Family history of arrhythmia or sudden cardiac death
- Social history: use of alcohol, illicit drugs, caffeine, tobacco
- Medication review (including herbal/natural preparations)

PHYSICAL EXAM
- Blood pressure may be elevated or decreased
- Neck: abnormal carotid pulsations
- Heart: irregular rhythm, abnormal rate
- Lungs: increased respiratory rate; normal auscultation unless patient has pulmonary congestion secondary to the arrhythmia
- GU: reduced urine output
- Extremities: pallor, cold, clammy
- Neuro: altered mental status if cerebral perfusion is compromised

DIAGNOSTIC STUDIES
- 12-lead ECG
- Exercise ECG
- Ambulatory ECG (24- to 48-hour Holter monitor)
- Event monitor: useful for infrequent arrhythmias that are symptomatic; on some models, patient must activate the "record" button when experiencing symptoms; usually worn 30 days or until an event is recorded
- Serum electrolytes and magnesium to rule out imbalance

Nursing Management
- Goal is to restore normal sinus rhythm when possible.

NONPHARMACOLOGIC TREATMENT
- Carotid sinus massage
- Valsalva maneuver

PHARMACOLOGIC TREATMENT
- Quinidine
- Flecainide
- Propranolol
- Amiodarone
- Sotalol
- Verapamil
- Diltiazem

INTERVENTIONAL TREATMENT
- Pacemaker
- Implantable cardioverter-defibrillator (ICD)
- Cardioversion
- Electrophysiologic study with catheter ablation

Special Considerations
- Atrial fibrillation (AF)
  - Results from multiple impulses fired by the atria at a rate > 300 beats per minute (bpm); impulses are randomly conducted by the AV node at a rate usually 100 to 180 bpm.
  - Atria lose organized contractile activity and just "quiver," which allows for stagnation of blood and thrombus formation.
  - High prevalence in older patients and those with structural heart disease.
  - Rhythm compromises cardiac output by reducing the ventricular filling (loss of atrial kick) and thereby reducing stroke volume.
  - Goals of treatment: restoration of sinus rhythm (when possible), ventricular rate control, prevention of thromboembolus.
  - Warfarin therapy is initiated to maintain an INR between 2.0 and 3.0.
  - Pradaxa (dabigatran) is a direct thrombin inhibitor recently approved for anticoagulation in AF. It is dosed b.i.d. and doesn't require monitoring, but costs about $8/day.

Follow-up

EXPECTED OUTCOMES
- Patient will maintain normal BP and evidence of adequate tissue perfusion.

- Patient will verbalize understanding of medication regimen needed to minimize risk of cardiac arrhythmias.
- Patients requiring anticoagulation will demonstrate understanding of medication regimen, dietary restrictions, and how to identify abnormal bleeding.

COMPLICATIONS
- Syncope
- Hip fracture
- Fall with other injury
- Sudden cardiac death
- Seizure
- Cerebrovascular accident
- Arterial embolization (with AF)

CAROTID ATHEROSCLEROSIS

Description
- Atherosclerosis is a ubiquitous disease (not localized). When plaque accumulates in carotid arteries, it can dislodge and embolize to the brain.

Etiology
- 90% of all extracranial carotid lesions are due to atherosclerosis.
- Carotid occlusion may be implicated in cerebrovascular accident (CVA), but is not the only cause.

Incidence and Demographics
- Stroke is the third leading cause of death in the United States and is the leading cause of disability.

Risk Factors
- Age
- Diabetes
- HTN
- Dyslipidemia
- Smoking
- Other risk factors of atherosclerosis

Prevention and Screening
- Prevention of atherosclerosis is the same for disease in any area of the body. (See Ischemic Heart Disease above.)
- There are no recommendations for screening of asymptomatic persons with a normal physical exam.
- Screening for carotid occlusion is accomplished by carotid ultrasound (Doppler) to quantify the severity of the lesion when a carotid bruit is heard on physical exam.
- Patients also may be "screened" after experiencing symptoms that suggest carotid occlusion, such as amaurosis fugax or symptoms of transient cerebral ischemia.

Assessment

HISTORY
- Subjective symptoms: transient neurologic symptoms, such as unilateral numbness or weakness, problems with speech or understanding, problems with walking or balance, or transient blindness; elevated BP; headache
- Social history: smoking
- Family history: atherosclerotic cardiovascular disease, stroke

PHYSICAL EXAM
- BP may be high or low
- Eyes: visual field exam
- Neck: carotid bruits
- Heart: rate/rhythm, murmurs
- Abdomen: bruits
- Neurologic: focal sensory or motor dysfunction, speech, gait

DIAGNOSTIC STUDIES
- Carotid ultrasound
- Computed tomography (CT) angiogram
- Magnetic resonance angiography (MRA)

Nursing Management

NONPHARMACOLOGIC TREATMENT
- Lifestyle modifications for atherosclerosis, discussed above under Ischemic Heart Disease.

PHARMACOLOGIC TREATMENT
- Antiplatelet therapy
  - Aspirin 81 to 325 mg/day
  - Plavix (clopidogrel) 75 mg/day
  - Aggrenox (aspirin/dipyridamole) 25/200 mg b.i.d.
  - Lipid-lowering therapy
  - Antihypertensive therapy

INTERVENTIONAL TREATMENT
- Carotid endarterectomy (CEA)
  - Patients with TIA symptoms with ipsilateral severe carotid stenosis (70% or greater)
  - Symptomatic patients with moderate stenosis (50% to 69%)
  - Asymptomatic patients with > 60% stenosis
- Carotid angioplasty and stenting (CAS)
  - Patients who are not candidates for surgery because of severe heart or lung disease, prior head/neck surgery or radiation, or prior CEA

Special Considerations
- Asymptomatic persons with carotid bruits have a 1.5% chance of stroke at 1 year and 7.5% at 10 years. Trial data show no benefit for surgery in these patients.

EXPECTED OUTCOMES
- Patients with asymptomatic carotid disease will verbalize need for regular follow-up with healthcare provider and need for continued medication and lifestyle therapy to prevent progression of atherosclerosis.
- Patient will maintain normal vital signs in the postoperative period.
- Post-CEA patient will have adequate ventilation and be free of excessive swelling in the neck (from hematoma formation).

COMPLICATIONS
- Risk of untreated severe carotid stenosis (> 70%) is stroke (26% in 2 years).
- Possible risks of CEA are stroke, bleeding, infection, MI, or seizures. These risks are very low with an experienced surgeon and institution.

ABDOMINAL AORTIC ANEURYSM (AAA)

Description
- Abnormal dilation in the arterial wall, usually occurring below the renal arteries and above the bifurcation of the iliac arteries.

Etiology
- Develops when degeneration occurs in the media of the artery, causing weakening of the arterial walls.
- Elevated blood pressure furthers weakens the arterial walls and enlarges the aneurysm.
- 90% result from atherosclerosis.

Incidence and Demographics
- AAA occurs predominantly in White men between the ages of 65 and 75 who have smoked tobacco.
- Incidence is 2% to 4% in the general population.
- Ruptured AAA accounts for 15,000 deaths annually.

Risk Factors
- Age
- Male sex
- White race
- Cigarette smoking
- Atherosclerosis
- Family history of AAA in first-degree relative

Prevention and Screening
- U.S. Preventive Services Task Force (USPSTF) recommends one-time screening for AAA by ultrasound in men between ages 65 and 75 who have ever smoked.
- Most AAAs are found incidentally on an imaging study or physical exam.
- Eliminating risk factors for atherosclerosis and controlling blood pressure are the most important aspects of prevention.

Assessment

HISTORY
- Symptoms of leak or rupture include severe, sudden low back, flank, or groin pain; syncope.

PHYSICAL EXAM
- Physical findings may be subtle
- BP in both arms
- Tachycardia
- Neck and other arteries for bruits
- Cyanosis and mottling
- Pulsatile abdominal mass (present in less than half of cases)
- Abdominal bruit or lateral propagation of the aortic pulsation

DIAGNOSTIC STUDIES
- Ultrasound: diagnostic accuracy approaches 100%
- Can often be visualized on a plain radiograph of the abdomen
- CT or MRI for special circumstances

Differential Diagnosis
- Renal colic

Nursing Management

NONPHARMACOLOGIC TREATMENT
- Smoking cessation
- Control of other atherosclerotic risk factors
- "Watchful waiting": Surveillance by ultrasound every 6 to 12 months is employed to assess size and rate of expansion. Risk of rupture is highest in AAA larger than 5.5 cm or with a rate of expansion that exceeds 0.5 cm in 6 months.

PHARMACOLOGIC TREATMENT
- BP reduction with beta blockers to reduce the rate of expansion

INTERVENTIONAL TREATMENT
- In persons with a life expectancy of 2 years or more, intervention should be offered when the AAA is 4.5 cm, because risk of rupture increases precipitously from this point.
- AAA repair with graft
  - Potential complications: renal failure, amputation, graft infection, ischemic colitis, paraplegia from spinal cord ischemia, and aortoenteric fistula.
- Endovascular stent-grafting
  - Not a good option for patients with a life expectancy greater than 3 years because 3 years is the average life of the stent-graft; then it must be replaced.
  - "Endoleak," in which blood fills the AAA via the anastomotic site or collateral vessels, is the most common complication.

Special Considerations
- AAAs are largely asymptomatic until they are sufficient size to press on surrounding tissues.
- Older men who smoke are at highest risk and thus should be screened by ultrasound.

Follow-up

EXPECTED OUTCOMES
- Patient will verbalize symptoms of possible leak and remain under close medical follow-up.

COMPLICATIONS
- 50% of untreated AAA patients die of rupture within 2 years of diagnosis.
- More than 85% die within 5 years.

CHRONIC LOWER EXTREMITY ARTERIAL OCCLUSIVE DISEASE (PAOD OR PAD)

Description
- Insufficient arterial circulation from the aorta into the legs; process usually spares the upper extremities.

Etiology
- Caused by atherosclerosis.
- Lesions are most prone to develop at major bifurcations.
- Because the process occurs slowly, development of collateral vessels is common.

Incidence and Demographics
- Affects 12% to 20% of adults 65 and older.
- PAD is a marker of systemic atherosclerosis.
- Blacks are affected most.

Risk factors
- Age
- Diabetes
- Black
- Smoking
- Other risk factors of atherosclerosis
- Elevated plasma homocysteine

Prevention and Screening
- In the general population, only 10% of persons with PAD have classic symptoms (intermittent claudication).
- Must have a high index of suspicion with a person who has leg symptoms of any kind and risk factors for atherosclerosis.
- Prevention involves eliminating risk factors for atherosclerosis, particularly smoking cessation and controlling diabetes.
- Regular exercise.
- Maintain a healthy body weight and low-fat, low-cholesterol diet.

Assessment

HISTORY

- Classic presentation involves pain in the legs or buttocks with walking; pain is relieved by rest.
  - Location of pain
  - Distance person can walk before onset
- 40% have no leg pain.
- 50% have leg symptoms that are different from claudication.
- Acute arterial occlusion presents with the 6 "Ps."
  - Pain: sudden and severe
  - Pallor
  - Pulselessness
  - Paresthesia
  - Poikilothermia or "polar": referring to a cold extremity
  - Paralysis
- Social history: smoking
- Family history: atherosclerotic cardiovascular disease of any type
- Review of systems: exertional chest pain, erectile dysfunction, pain at night relieved by hanging leg over side of bed, sores on feet/legs

PHYSICAL EXAM

- SBP in the arm and leg (used to calculate ABI, see Box 11–2)
- Skin/hair/nails: brittle nails, absent hair on toes and lower legs, thin skin that is shiny and pale with elevation
- Dependent rubor: Extremity is pale on elevation, then becomes mottled or dark red when lowered
- Neck: carotid bruits
- Heart: rate/rhythm, peripheral pulses, femoral bruits
- Abdomen: bruits (aorta and iliacs)
- Neurologic: neurosensory exam of legs

DIAGNOSTIC STUDIES

- Ankle-brachial index (ABI; see Box 11–2)
- Doppler ultrasound: noninvasive test that shows decreased flow distal to the occlusion
- Angiography

Differential Diagnoses

- Diabetic neuropathy
- Spinal stenosis
- Lumbar disc disease

Nursing Management

NONPHARMACOLOGIC TREATMENT

- Walking program: patients are encouraged to walk to the point of claudication, then rest until pain is relieved. This action is repeated, aiming for 5 to 10 minutes total at first. Duration is gradually lengthened to about 50 minutes (35 minutes walking/15 minutes resting). This activity improves collateral circulation, but must be continued

indefinitely to maintain benefits. *Note:* Best results are achieved in a supervised exercise setting, much like cardiac rehabilitation.
- Smoking cessation
- Lipid management
- Control of diabetes mellitus
- Control of HTN
- Counseling regarding proper foot care
  - Check feet daily
  - Keep clean and moisturized
  - Nail care may need to be done by podiatrist
  - Protect feet from injury: shoes, socks, no temperature extremes

PHARMACOLOGIC TREATMENT
- Homocysteine is lowered by B vitamins and folic acid, though no studies have demonstrated that lowering levels improves outcomes
- Antiplatelet therapy
  - Aspirin 81 to 325 mg/day
  - Plavix (clopidogrel) 75 mg/day
- Lipid-lowering therapy
- Improve functional status (reduce claudication)
  - Cilostazol (Pletal): improves ability to exercise; contraindicated in CHF
  - Pentoxifylline (Trental): less effective, but side effects are rare

INTERVENTIONAL TREATMENT
- Angioplasty with or without stent
- Bypass surgery
- Thrombolytic therapy for acute occlusion
- Amputation for incurable infection or gangrene

Special Considerations
- Persons with PAD have a fourfold to fivefold greater risk of dying from a cardiovascular event than those without disease.
- Very high prevalence of disease has been noted in patients who also have chronic renal insufficiency.

EXPECTED OUTCOMES
- Patient will incorporate lifestyle changes for risk factor reduction.
- Postintervention patients will maintain distal pulses, warm skin temperature, and absence of pain.
- Patient will participate in a regular progressive walking program to maximize exercise capability.

COMPLICATIONS
- Disease is asymptomatic in up to 40% of persons, meaning that they have an increased risk of mortality and no symptoms.
- Peripheral arterial insufficiency can lead to many complications from immobility and nonhealing wounds.

Box 11-2. Measuring Ankle-Brachial Index (ABI)

1. Place the patient in the supine position.
2. Measure systolic blood pressure using a Doppler probe in both arms.
3. Select the higher of these two values as the brachial reading.
4. Measure the systolic BP in both legs at the dorsalis pedis (DP) and posterior tibial (PT) arteries.
5. Select the higher of the pressures in each ankle.
6. Values are determined by dividing the higher ankle pressure in each leg by the higher arm pressure.
7. Interpret that values as follows:
   a. 1.0–1.1   Normal
   b. 0.9   Minimal disease
   c. 0.5–0.8   Moderate disease; often have exercise claudication
   d. < 0.5   Severe disease; often have pain at rest

VENOUS THROMBOEMBOLISM (VTE)

Description
- Formation of a blood clot in the deep venous system of the lower extremity

Etiology
- Virchow's triad
  - Venous stasis
  - Injury of the vascular intima
  - Altered coagulability

Incidence and Demographics
- About 1 million cases per year in the United States
- Nearly two-thirds result from hospitalization
- 300,000 persons die each year

Risk Factors
- Hereditary disorders of coagulation
- Acquired hypercoagulability
- Surgery
- Major medical illness
- Immobility
- Air travel
- Cancer and some cancer treatments
- Central lines
- Pregnancy, oral contraceptives, or hormone replacement therapy
- Obesity (BMI > 30)

Prevention and Screening
- Prevention of VTE focuses on elimination of risk factors, for example avoiding long periods of immobility.

- Risk during air travel can be reduced by adequate hydration, seated leg exercises, and walking as much as possible during the flight.
- Guidelines from the American College of Chest Physicians recommend the following for hospitalized patients:
  - Use of aspirin alone is not recommended.
  - Mechanical thromboprophylaxis (intermittent pneumatic compression or other) should only be used for persons at high risk for bleeding or as an adjunct to anticoagulation therapy.
  - Patients with medical illness, major trauma, or spinal cord injury and patients undergoing major surgery (stratified by type of surgery) are recommended to receive either low–molecular weight heparin (LMWH), low-dose unfractionated heparin (LDUH), or fondaparinux (Arixtra).

Assessment

HISTORY
- Pain, tenderness, warmth, or swelling of extremity
- Risk factors for VTE (recent surgery or major illness, pregnancy, prolonged inactivity, use of oral contraceptives or hormone replacement therapy, leg trauma)

PHYSICAL EXAM
- Warmth, edema, erythema along the site
- Dilated veins (collaterals) may be seen
- Observe for Homans' sign. (Note: This test has poor positive and negative predictive value and thus is not really useful clinically; however, it is still a standard of care to check for it.)

DIAGNOSTIC STUDIES
- D-dimer: measures level of fibrin degradation products; test has good negative predictive value (99%), but often is elevated in absence of VTE; elevation may be caused by malignancy, active bleeding, trauma, infection, or recent surgery.
- Duplex ultrasonography: procedure of choice for diagnosis.
- Contrast venography: gold standard for diagnosis, but requires contrast dye injection and has thus lost favor to ultrasonography.
- Spiral CT of the chest or ventilation/perfusion (V/Q) scanning is appropriate when pulmonary embolus is suspected; both are discussed further in that section.

Differential Diagnosis
- Cellulitis
- Popliteal (Baker's) cyst
- Trauma
- Muscle/tendon damage
- Venous insufficiency with stasis dermatitis
- CHF or renal failure (usually cause bilateral swelling)

Nursing Management

NONPHARMACOLOGIC TREATMENT
- Use of compression stockings at 30 to 40 mm Hg pressure is recommended for 1 to 2 years after acute DVT to prevent postthrombotic syndrome (PTS).

- Education regarding anticoagulation therapy with warfarin.
  - Frequent follow-up with blood monitoring will be needed to minimize risk of bleeding.
  - Dietary intake of Vitamin K should remain consistent over the course of a week; it is no longer recommended to avoid foods that are high in vitamin K.
  - Warfarin should be taken in the evening (preferably), roughly at the same time each day.
  - Use an electric razor and avoid aspirin, products containing aspirin, and herbal products unless otherwise instructed by a healthcare provider.

PHARMACOLOGIC TREATMENT
- Unfractionated heparin (UFH) to maintain aPTT (activated partial thromboplastin time) 1.5 to 2.5 times higher than control aPTT.
- Low-molecular weight heparin (LMWH) subcutaneously; no monitoring is required except in patients who are obese, pregnant, or have renal insufficiency.
- Fondaparinux (Arixtra) is given in combination with a vitamin K antagonist (VKA) such as warfarin.
- Warfarin therapy also is started and overlapped for a minimum of 5 days or until the INR is between 2.0 and 3.0 for at least 24 hours.
- Thrombolytic therapy may be used in certain cases.
- Treatment duration depends on the likelihood of recurrence.
  - 3 months with VKA for patients with a first DVT due to a transient cause; goal for INR is 2.0 to 3.0.
  - Patients who have DVT without an identified cause and who request less frequent blood testing can be maintained at an INR of 1.5 to 1.9 after the initial 3 months of therapy; this is preferred over stopping warfarin.
  - Patients with active malignancy, certain coagulopathies, or multiple unexplained recurrent DVTs require long-term anticoagulation.

Special Considerations
- Proximal thromboembolism (popliteal vein or above) has a risk of 50% for pulmonary embolism if not treated.
- Approximately 25% of calf vein thromboses, if not treated, will propagate to the popliteal vein or higher.

Follow-up

EXPECTED OUTCOMES
- Patient will verbalize importance of regular medical follow-up to manage anticoagulation.
- Patient will show evidence of resolving VTE on therapy, e.g., decreased edema, pain.
- Patient will verbalize understanding of bleeding precautions.

COMPLICATIONS
- Pulmonary embolus is the most serious complication of untreated VTE.
- One-third of patients with acute DVT will develop postthrombotic syndrome, which can lead to venous stasis ulcers and their associated problems.
- 300,000 Americans have a pulmonary embolism each year and 25% of those present with sudden death or die within 30 days of symptom presentation (usually because of incorrect diagnosis). The mortality rate for patients who are properly treated is only 2% to 8%.

CHRONIC VENOUS INSUFFICIENCY/ POSTTHROMBOTIC SYNDROME

Description
- Chronic dependent swelling of the lower extremities that can lead to dermatitis, cellulitis, or ulceration.

Etiology
- Condition occurs due to destruction or incompetence of the valves in the deep venous system of the legs. Can be a complication of VTE or can occur in patients without a diagnosis of prior VTE.

Incidence and Demographics
- 6 to 7 million persons in the United States have evidence of venous stasis.
- Affects about 40% of the population to some degree.

Risk Factors
- Age
- Obesity
- History of DVT or phlebitis
- Leg trauma
- More common in women, but may be due to relative longevity
- Varicose veins
- Inactivity
- Family history

Prevention and Screening
- Prevention of advanced disease associated with skin discoloration and chronic ulceration can be prevented by early use of graduated compression stockings.

Assessment

HISTORY
- Lower extremity swelling, may be asymmetric or unilateral, that usually improves with elevation and worsens with prolonged standing or sitting
- Skin discoloration and itching
- Visible veins or varicosities
- Leg fullness, aching, or heaviness, usually worse on standing
- Nocturnal leg cramps

PHYSICAL EXAM
- Lower extremity edema, which may be unilateral or bilateral
- Hyperpigmentation of the skin affected, due to hemosiderin deposits in the subcutaneous tissues; most common on the medial ankle and medial portion of the lower leg
- Ulceration, often occurring on the medial ankle region

DIAGNOSTIC STUDIES
- Venous insufficiency is basically a diagnosis of exclusion that is supported by history and physical exam.
- Duplex ultrasound can be used to identify venous reflux and also to exclude a diagnosis of DVT.

Differential Diagnosis
- DVT
- Congestive heart failure
- Renal failure
- Liver failure/hypoalbuminemia
- Lymphatic obstruction
- Drug effects

Nursing Management

NONPHARMACOLOGIC TREATMENT
- Avoid prolonged sitting or standing.
- Walking, bicycling or swimming as an exercise program for persons with mild to moderate disease can improve long-term symptoms.
- Graded compression stockings are the mainstay of therapy. Properly fitted stockings should apply 30 to 40 mm Hg compression at the ankle and gradually decrease toward the proximal leg. (Note: Compression stockings are avoided in patients with concomitant arterial insufficiency.)
- Nongradient stockings or compression with elastic bandage wraps may cause a tourniquet effect and should not be used.

PHARMACOLOGIC TREATMENT
- No oral medications are effective.
  - Diuretics can cause intravascular volume depletion and associated complications of dizziness, falls, etc.
  - Avoidance of medications known to cause swelling (e.g., calcium channel blockers, pioglitazone) as a side effect can be helpful.
- Antibiotics are rarely useful for treating venous ulcers.

INTERVENTIONAL TREATMENT
- All methods of venoablation are effective. Symptoms resolve and ulcers heal once the volume of venous reflux is reduced below a critical level.
- Available therapies include:
  - Valvuloplasty
  - Endovenous laser therapy (EVT)
  - Radiofrequency ablation (RFA)
  - Sclerotherapy
  - Vein stripping with ligation

Special Considerations
- Patients can have a varicosity that ruptures, requiring hospitalization to control bleeding.
- Patients with concomitant arterial insufficiency are very difficult to manage.

- Chronic ulcers are difficult to heal without reduction in edema (venous reflux). These wounds often require application of compression dressings or a zinc gelatin boot (Unna's boot).
- Large ulcers may require excision and skin grafting, but this treatment is rarely effective unless venous reflux is corrected.

Follow-up

EXPECTED OUTCOMES
- Patient will comply with daily use of graduated compression stockings, the most successful treatment for venous insufficiency.
- Patient will have minimal leg discomfort and maximal exercise tolerance.

COMPLICATIONS
- Untreated venous insufficiency can lead to:
  - Recruitment and malfunction of additional veins
  - Chronic pain
  - Recurrent cellulitis
  - Chronic nonhealing ulcers
  - DVT
  - Pulmonary embolus
  - Secondary lymphedema

Pulmonary System

GENERAL APPROACH

- The pulmonary system is responsible for ventilation and oxygenation, and in conjunction with the cardiovascular system, supports the function of all organ systems through the delivery of oxygenated blood.
- Ventilation is the process of moving air in and out of the alveoli.
- Perfusion refers to the delivery of blood through the pulmonary vasculature that surrounds the alveoli.
- In a healthy lung, inhaled oxygen diffuses from the alveoli into the blood and carbon dioxide, which is a byproduct of cellular metabolism, diffuses from the blood into the alveoli to be exhaled.
- Respiration is under neural and chemical control.
  - Chemoreceptors in the medulla oblongata and in the carotid bodies respond to changes in hydrogen ion concentration and arterial oxygen levels.
  - Chemoreceptors send signals to the respiratory center in the medulla oblongata.
  - Nerve impulses are then transmitted to the pons, which regulates respiratory muscles.
  - Excess levels of carbon dioxide stimulate the rate and depth of ventilation.
- Most diseases of the lung affect either ventilation or perfusion, producing a mismatch, thus altering oxygen or carbon dioxide delivery.
- Lung anatomy dictates that breath sounds must be auscultated in the anterior and lateral fields to properly assess the upper lobes and right middle lobe; and posterior fields must be auscultated to assess the lower lobes.

- Chronic lower respiratory disease is the 4th leading cause of death in the United States, behind heart disease, cancer, and stroke.
- Lung disease cost $42.6 billion in healthcare costs and lost productivity in 2007.
- Most lung disease in this country results from tobacco abuse, making this healthcare problem largely preventable.

RED FLAGS

- Clubbing of the nails is rare in emphysema and chronic bronchitis and suggests another cause, such as bronchiectasis or bronchogenic carcinoma.
- Any person with chronic unexplained symptoms—especially fever, sweats, weight loss, anorexia, or cough—should be evaluated for tuberculosis.

Common Disorders of the Pulmonary System

CHRONIC OBSTRUCTIVE PULMONARY/LUNG DISEASE (COPD, COLD)

Description
- An umbrella term used to refer to emphysema and chronic bronchitis, two diseases that often occur in the same patient and result in narrowed airways and air trapping.

Etiology
- Caused by an inflammatory reaction in the lungs, most commonly triggered by cigarette smoking.
- In emphysema, the inflammation leads to destruction of the alveolar airspaces, thereby reducing the surface area for gas exchange.
- In the larger airways, inflammation causes stimulation and hypertrophy of mucous glands, leading to the daily productive cough of chronic bronchitis.

Incidence and Demographics
- 13.5 million Americans, or about 5% of the population, have COPD.
- 15 million Americans are estimated to be undiagnosed or in the early stages.
- Number of deaths in women is slightly higher.

Risk Factors
- Cigarette smoking
- Age
- Genetic factors
- Air pollution
- Occupational dust exposure
- Respiratory infections
- Asthma

Prevention and Screening

- Prevention of COPD is best accomplished by avoidance of primary or secondary inhalation of cigarette smoke.
- According to the Global Obstructive Lung Disease (GOLD) guidelines, persons over the age of 40 with any of the following indicators should be screened with spirometry:
  - Dyspnea that is progressive, persistent, or worse with exercise
  - Chronic cough with or without sputum
  - Chronic sputum production
  - Exposure to tobacco smoke, occupational dust, or chemicals, or smoke from home cooking or heating fuels

Assessment

HISTORY

- Exposure to risk factors
- Tobacco history including age at onset of smoking, average number of packs smoked per day, and number and duration of quit attempts
- Past medical history:
  - Asthma
  - Allergies
  - Sinusitis
  - Other respiratory illnesses
- Presence of comorbidities:
  - Heart disease
  - Musculoskeletal disease
  - Osteoporosis
  - Malignancies
- Family history of COPD or chronic respiratory disease
- Respiratory symptoms, such as cough, sputum, dyspnea
- Impact of disease on patient's life

PHYSICAL EXAM

- Although certain characteristic physical findings may be seen in patients with COPD (usually with advanced disease), these are not diagnostic.
  - Posture: often leaning forward with hands resting on thighs
  - Chest
    - Increased anterior-posterior diameter (1:1) = barrel chest
    - Decreased movement of the rib cage on inspiration and increased movement of the abdominal wall
  - Pulmonary
    - Pursed-lip breathing with prolonged expiratory time
    - Increased resonance on chest percussion
    - Diminished transmission of breath sounds
    - Early inspiratory crackles
  - Heart
    - Medial displacement of the point of maximum impulse (PMI)
    - Often a pronounced cardiac impulse in the epigastrium due to pulmonary hypertension

- Note: Development of right heart failure or cor pulmonale may cause neck vein distention, peripheral edema, hepatomegaly, and a systolic murmur from tricuspid regurgitation (over the epigastrium).
- Extremities
  - Tobacco-stained fingers
  - Clubbing of nails is rare and suggests bronchiectasis or bronchogenic carcinoma.

DIAGNOSTIC STUDIES
- Chest x-ray: abnormal only with advanced disease; findings include flattening of diaphragm, hyperinflation, narrowed cardiac silhouette, and increased retrosternal airspace on the lateral view
- Spirometry: used for diagnosis and assessment of severity (see Box 11–3)
- High-resolution CT of the chest may be helpful in some cases.
- Arterial blood gas measurement can determine hypoxemia and hypercapnia; useful in later stages
- Other testing for special circumstances
  - Carbon monoxide diffusing capacity: helpful for distinguishing emphysema from asthma
  - CBC, Gram stain and culture of sputum, or Purified Protein Derivative (PPD) test may be needed if infection is suspected.
  - Serum protein electrophoresis to evaluate for a-1 antitrypsin deficiency in young patients with severe disease that is disproportionate to smoking history
  - Electrocardiogram in severe disease when cor pulmonale is suspected; in COPD, ECG will show a vertical or indeterminate heart axis and low voltage; in cor pulmonale, expect a right-axis deviation and enlarged P waves

Box 11–3. Spirometry Measurements*

FVC = total amount of air that can be forcefully exhaled after deep inhalation
FEV_1 = amount of air that can be forcefully exhaled in 1 second
FEV_1/ FVC or FEV_1 % = percentage of total air leaving the lung in 1 second

*Many other measurements can be obtained, but these are considered the most useful.

Differential Diagnosis
- Asthma
- Congestive heart failure
- Acute bronchitis
- Bronchiectasis

Nursing Management
- Management of COPD is based on the stage of severity (GOLD criteria; see Table 11–8).

Table 11–8. COPD Severity

Stage	Severity	% Predicted FEV_1
I	Mild	$\geq 80\%$
II	Moderate	$\geq 50\%$ but $< 80\%$
III	Severe	$\geq 30\%$ but $< 50\%$
IV	Very Severe	$< 30\%$

Adapted from COPD diagnosis and management at-a-glance desk reference by the Global Initiative for Chronic Obstructive Lung Disease, 2011, retrieved from http://www.goldcopd.org/Guidelines/guidelines-resources.html

NONPHARMACOLOGIC TREATMENT
- Smoking cessation is the single most important lifestyle intervention (all stages).
- Elimination of environmental irritants; limit outdoor activities at times of poor air quality.
- Avoid potentially harmful drugs: beta blockers, sedatives, antihistamines, narcotics.
- Consider a pulmonary rehabilitation program if one is available (Stage II).

PHARMACOLOGIC TREATMENT (SEE BOX 11–4)
- Prevention of infection
  - Yearly influenza vaccinations
- Early treatment of recurrent or chronic infections as indicated by a change in the quantity, color, or character of sputum
  - Doxycycline, erythromycin, amoxicillin, or Bactrim DS
  - Frequent or more severe exacerbations may require Augmentin, second-generation macrolide, or quinolone.
- Short-acting bronchodilator when needed (Stage I)
- Add one or more long-acting bronchodilators (Stage II)
- Add inhaled corticosteroids if repeated exacerbations (Stage III)
- Add long-term oxygen with chronic respiratory failure (Stage IV)
  - Supplemental oxygen has been shown to prolong life and improve quality of life in hypoxemic patients.
  - Indications
    - $PaO_2 \leq 55$ mm Hg or $SaO_2 \leq 88\%$ breathing room air
    - PaO_2 56–59 mm Hg or SaO_2 89% with concurrent cor pulmonale or polycythemia
    - $PaO_2 \geq 60$ mm Hg or $SaO_2 \geq 90\%$ with significant exercise-induced or sleep-induced hypoxemia

Box 11–4. COPD Treatments

β_2 Agonists

These medications stimulate $beta_2$ receptors in the lung, causing bronchodilation. The short-acting β_2 agonists are the most important "rescue" medications for acute shortness of breath in both COPD and asthma. These drugs include albuterol (Proventil® HFA), levalbuterol (Xopenex®), and pirbuterol (Maxair®). They are administered by metered-dose inhaler (MDI) or by nebulizer. β_2 agonists are also available in sustained release or long-acting forms:

salmeterol (Serevent®) and formoterol (Foradil®). Older adults with ischemic heart disease can develop angina from the tachycardia caused by these medications.

Education regarding proper use of inhaled medications is critical. Patients should be required to return demonstration of new delivery devices as well as those that they have been using. Use of a spacer device on the standard MDI can improve the delivery of medication to the lungs. Many persons do not receive full benefit from inhaled medications because of improper technique.

Anticholinergics

Inhaled anticholinergics inhibit vagal stimulation and prevent contraction of smooth muscle in the airway as well as decreasing mucus production. Ipratropium bromide (Atrovent®) is a short-acting medication that requires dosing four times daily. Tiotropium bromide (Spiriva®) may be dosed once daily.

Inhaled Corticosteroids

These medications are indicated in patients who achieve improvement in FEV_1 after a 6- to 12-week trial or who have frequent exacerbations. Examples are budesonide (Pulmicort®), and fluticasone (Flovent®). Oral corticosteroids are beneficial during acute exacerbations to improve symptoms and decrease hospital length of stay.

Theophylline

This medication may be added to other therapies during times of exacerbation or for persons with severe disease. Theophylline has bronchodilating effects and also improves respiratory muscle function. The major drawback is the potential for toxicity due to multiple drug interactions and reduced clearance in the elderly.

Antibiotics

Broad-spectrum antibiotics often are prescribed for treatment of acute exacerbations believed to be secondary to bacterial infection. Because presence of a bacterial pathogen is difficult to prove (by sputum culture) in patients who are not intubated, clinical therapy usually covers this possibility.

INTERVENTIONAL TREATMENT
- Lung volume reduction surgery (Stage IV)
- Lung transplantation

Special Considerations
- 5-year survival decreases with FEV_1 reduction.
- Smoking cessation reduces the rate of decline in lung function.
- Oral corticosteroids at doses of 30 mg to 60 mg prednisone daily for 7 to 14 days will shorten the duration of symptoms for patients with exacerbations.
- Chronic hypoxemia leads to pulmonary hypertension and cor pulmonale, which is associated with poor survival.
- People who are underweight can improve their symptoms by increasing caloric intake, primarily protein and fat calories (rather than carbohydrates, which increase carbon dioxide production).

Follow-up

EXPECTED OUTCOMES
- Patient will have adequate ventilation.
- Patient will learn techniques for energy conservation in order to complete activities of daily living.
- Patient will recognize symptoms of exacerbation and notify the healthcare provider immediately.

COMPLICATIONS
- Recurrent infections (exacerbations) as previously mentioned.
- Patients with large bullae can have a bullous rupture, causing pneumothorax (see Box 11–5) and further compromising breathing status.
- Factors associated with a poor prognosis:
  - Very low FEV_1 = severe airflow obstruction
  - Poor exercise capacity
  - Shortness of breath
  - Continued smoking
  - Frequent exacerbations
  - Extremes of body weight
  - Respiratory failure or cor pulmonale

Box 11–5. Pneumothorax

Pneumothorax is a collection of air or gas in the pleural cavity between the chest wall and the lung. Pneumothoraces may be small and asymptomatic or large, causing shortness of breath and hypoxemia. A tension pneumothorax occurs when air continues to leak and is trapped during expiration, causing increased pressure on the lung. Tension pneumo can lead to hypotension and cardiac arrest. Causes of pneumothorax include spontaneous rupture of a congenital bleb, bullous emphysema, chest trauma, blast injury, or a complication of medical treatment (such as insertion of a central IV line).

ASTHMA

Description
- Chronic inflammatory disease of the airway with episodic, variable airflow limitation and bronchospasm, often triggered by an environmental exposure, causing cough, wheezing, chest tightness, and shortness of breath

Etiology
- Increased tendency to have bronchospasm is also called "airway reactivity" or "bronchial hyperresponsiveness."
- Bronchospasm usually occurs after exposure to an allergen or irritant (such as odors or cold, dry air).
- Mechanisms causing airway reactivity are not completely understood.
- Airway inflammation is at the heart of the problem, with submucosal infiltration with white blood cells and mast cells, edema, and vascular engorgement.
- Inflammation leads to chronic changes in airway morphology and fixed obstructive changes in lung function.

Incidence and Demographics

- 300 million persons affected worldwide.
- 14 to 15 million Americans, including almost 5 million children.
- Increasing prevalence since the 1970s.

Risk Factors

- Caused by environmental and genetic factors that are not completely understood.
- History of atopic disease (eczema, hay fever, multiple allergies).
- Obesity.
- GERD (found in 80% of persons with asthma).
- Maternal tobacco use during pregnancy and after delivery.
- Poor air quality.

Prevention and Screening

- Avoidance of known irritants is one of the cornerstones of asthma control in persons with airway reactivity (see Box 11–6).
- No screening is recommended in asymptomatic patients.

Box 11–6. Common Asthma Triggers

Allergens
- Dust mites
- Pollen
- Molds
- Animal dander

Environmental changes
- Heat
- Cold

Smoke
- Tobacco
- Wood

Strong odors or fumes
- Perfumes
- Paint
- Hair spray

Respiratory infections

Assessment

HISTORY
- Duration, frequency, and severity of attacks
- Specific triggers of symptoms
- Cough that is worse at night or in early morning
- Seasonal variations and other allergy symptoms
- Tobacco use or secondhand exposure
- Respiratory medications and adherence
- Other medications that may aggravate symptoms: beta blockers, ACE inhibitors (ACEIs)

- Other conditions or irritants
  - Home condition: dust mites, cockroaches, mold
  - Gastroesophageal reflux disease (GERD)
  - Sulfites found in wines, seafood, dried fruits, and other processed foods
  - Obesity

PHYSICAL EXAM
- Acute asthma attack
  - Frightened appearance
  - Respiratory pattern
    - Initial: deep, slow with prolonged expiration
    - Late: rapid, shallow with expiratory grunting
  - Use of accessory muscles
  - Hyperinflation (expansion) of lungs with decreased respiratory excursion
  - Ineffective cough
  - Tachycardia
  - Pulsus paradoxus (decrease in systolic BP > 15 mm Hg during inspiration) seen with severe exacerbation
  - Diffuse expiratory wheezes or silence during severe attacks
- Chronic asthma
  - Nasal signs of allergic rhinitis: pale mucosa, clear drainage, swollen turbinates
  - Chest exam is often normal
  - May elicit expiratory wheezing with forced expiration

DIAGNOSTIC STUDIES
- Spirometry: used to define baseline lung function
- Peak flow measurement: performed at home to monitor the severity of airflow obstruction
  - Values vary with height, age, and gender
  - Values are compared to patient's "personal best"
    - 80% to 100% of personal best = good control
    - 50% to 80% = acute exacerbation
    - < 50% = severe exacerbation; emergency treatment indicated
- Chest x-ray: usually normal during asymptomatic phases
- CBC: eosinophils are commonly seen in the peripheral blood smear
- Skin testing: may be needed to identify specific allergens or triggers
- RASTs: blood testing for allergen-specific IgE used instead of skin testing
- Methacholine challenge: test used when the diagnosis of asthma is not clear

Differential Diagnoses
- Vocal cord dysfunction
- Upper airway obstruction
- Tumor
- Congestive heart failure
- Pulmonary embolus
- Cough due to other cause such as ACEIs or GERD
- COPD

Nursing Management

NONPHARMACOLOGIC TREATMENT
- Avoidance of environmental triggers and aggravating factors such as tobacco smoke, poor air quality, other known allergens, beta blockers, foods containing sulfites
- Some patients have sensitivity to aspirin and nonsteroidal anti-inflammatory drugs
- Increased fluids
- Humidification

PHARMACOLOGIC TREATMENT
- Annual influenza vaccination
- The NIH Expert Panel on Asthma Treatment recommends a stepwise approach to pharmacologic therapy (see Table 11–9).
- Many medications used for asthma are also used in COPD (see Box 11–4).
- Leukotriene Receptor Antagonists (LTRA) are indicated for asthma and control of allergic rhinitis (see Box 11–7).

Table 11–9. Classification and Treatment of Asthma

Step	Symptoms	Night-time Symptoms	Lung Function	Treatment
Step 6 Severe Persistent	Symptoms through-out day, most days SABA (short-acting beta$_2$-agonist) several times a day Limited activity	Most nights	$FEV_1 < 60\%$ predicted FEV_1/FVC reduced > 5%	High-dose inhaled corticosteroid (ICS) + long-acting beta$_2$ agonist (LABA) and oral corticosteroid *and* Consider omalizumab for patients who have allergies
Step 5 Severe Persistent	Symptoms through-out day, most days SABA several times a day Limited activity	Most nights	$FEV_1 < 60\%$ predicted FEV_1/FVC reduced > 5%	High-dose ICS + LABA *and* Consider omalizumab for patients who have allergies
Step 4 Severe Persistent	Symptoms through-out day, most days SABA several times a day Limited activity	Most nights	$FEV_1 > 60\%$ predicted FEV_1/FVC reduced > 5%	Medium-dose ICS + LABA Alternative: Medium-dose ICS + leukotriene receptor antagonist (LTRA), theophylline, or zileuton

cont.

Table 11–9. Classification and Treatment of Asthma (cont.)

Step 3 Moderate Persistent	Daily symptoms Daily use of inhaled SABA Some limitation in activity	> 1 time a week	FEV_1 > 60% to < 80% predicted FEV_1/FVC reduced 5%	Low-dose ICS +LABA or Medium-dose ICS Alternative: Low-dose ICS + LTRA, theophylline or zileuton
Step 2 Mild Persistent	Symptoms > 2 times a week but not daily Minor limitation in activity	3 to 4 times a month	FEV_1 > 80% predicted FEV_1/FVC normal	Low-dose ICS Alternatives: Cromolyn, LTRA, nedocromil, or the-ophylline
Step 1 Intermit-tent	Symptoms < 2 times/week No activity limita-tion	< 2 times a month	Normal FEV_1 between exacerbations FEV_1 > 80% predicted FEV_1/FVC normal	SABA as needed

*The presence of one of the features of severity is sufficient to place a patient in that category. An individual should be assigned to the most severe grade in which any feature occurs. The characteristics noted in the figure are general and may average because asthma is highly variable. Normal FEV_1/FVC for 60- to 70-year-olds is 70%.

Note. Reprinted from Expert Panel Report 3: *Guidelines for the diagnosis and management of asthma*, 2007, by the National Asthma Education and Prevention Program, Washington, DC: U.S. Department of Health and Human Services.

Box 11–7. Leukotriene Receptor Antagonists

Montelukast (Singulair®)
Zafirlukast (Accolate®)
Zileuton (Zyflo®)

Block the action of leukotrienes, inflammatory mediators that cause asthma symptoms

- Management of acute exacerbations: therapy depends on severity of symptoms, but may include any of the following:
  - More frequent use of short-acting beta agonist (inhaled or nebulized)
  - Course of oral corticosteroids
  - Office visit or emergency care

Special Considerations
- Symptoms usually develop in childhood, but can begin in adulthood
- There is a broad range of symptom severity in patients with asthma, from a few episodes of wheezing during their lifetime to severe daily symptoms that affect lifestyle and function.

- Systemic corticosteroids can have a number of adverse effects, including hypertension, elevated blood glucose, cataracts, osteoporosis, and confusion and agitation, especially in patients with underlying cognitive impairment.

Follow-up

EXPECTED OUTCOMES
- Patient will regain normal ABGs and FEV_1 that is more than 80% of personal best.
- Patient will demonstrate proper use of inhaled medications and verbalize understanding of purpose and use of each.
- Patient will avoid environmental triggers that might precipitate an asthma attack.
- Patient will monitor peak flow with a home meter to identify exacerbations early and seek appropriate treatment.

COMPLICATIONS
- Underdiagnosis and ineffective therapy contribute heavily to morbidity and mortality.
- Status asthmaticus is an acute asthma attack that does not respond to usual therapy of bronchodilators and steroids. Without emergency intervention, this condition can lead to respiratory and cardiac arrest.

PULMONARY EMBOLISM (PE)

Description
- Blockage of a main artery in the lung or one of its branches by a substance that has traveled through the bloodstream.

Etiology
- PEs are usually due to blood clots, but can also be caused by air, fat, or amniotic fluid.
- This section will address PE that is secondary to venous thromboembolism (VTE).

Incidence and Demographics
- 650,000 pulmonary emboli are diagnosed yearly in the United States.
- Occurrence rate is about 1 case per minute.

Risk Factors
- COPD
- Congestive heart failure
- Hypercoagulable states
- Hypertension (HTN)
- Heavy cigarette smoking
- Age
- Black (50% higher incidence than among Whites)
- Surgery
- Major medical illness
- Immobility
- Air travel
- Cancer and some cancer treatments
- Central lines
- Pregnancy, oral contraceptives, or hormone replacement therapy
- Obesity (BMI > 30)

Prevention and Screening

- Prevention of PE mirrors prevention of VTE.
- Elimination of risk factors; for example, avoiding long periods of immobility.
- Risk during air travel can be reduced by adequate hydration, seated leg exercises, and walking as much as possible during the flight.
- Guidelines from the American College of Chest Physicians recommend the following prophylaxis for VTE in hospitalized patients:
  - Use of aspirin alone is not recommended,
  - Mechanical thromboprophylaxis (intermittent pneumatic compression or other) should only be used for persons at high risk for bleeding or as an adjunct to anticoagulation therapy.
- Patients with medical illness, major trauma, or spinal cord injury and patients undergoing major surgery (stratified by type of surgery) are recommended to receive either low molecular weight heparin (LMWH), low-dose unfractionated heparin (LDUH), or fondaparinux (Arixtra).

Assessment

HISTORY
- Previous history of VTE
- Surgery within past 4 weeks
- Current estrogen use
- Active cancer
- Family history of VTE
- Immobilization
- Shortness of breath, cough, hemoptysis
- Pleuritic chest pain
- Apprehension
- Syncope

PHYSICAL EXAM
- Low-grade fever, tachycardia, tachypnea, and elevated work of breathing
- Elevated jugular venous pressure
- Reduced oxygen saturation (< 95%)
- S3 or S4 gallop heart sound
- Lung crackles or pleural friction rub

DIAGNOSTIC STUDIES
- Chest x-ray: often normal in persons with PE; findings are nonspecific if present; may be useful to rule out mimic diseases.
- D-dimer assay: negative test rules out PE in patients with low probability of disease; a positive test isn't helpful because it can be elevated for other reasons.
- Ventilation-perfusion scanning (V/Q): used when CT not available or dye load is contraindicated.
- Contrast-enhanced spiral CT.
- Pulmonary angiography: previous "gold standard," but losing favor due to dye requirement, pain, and invasive nature of the test.

Differential Diagnoses

- Chest trauma
- Pneumonia
- Pericarditis
- Cardiac tamponade
- Dissecting aortic aneurysm
- Pneumothorax
- Myocardial infarction
- Primary pulmonary hypertension
- Pulmonary edema
- Congestive heart failure

Nursing Management

NONPHARMACOLOGIC TREATMENT
- Education regarding anticoagulation therapy with warfarin.
  - Frequent follow-up with blood monitoring will be needed to minimize risk of bleeding.
  - Dietary intake of vitamin K should remain consistent over of time; it is no longer recommended to avoid foods that are high in vitamin K.
  - Warfarin should be taken in the evening (preferably), roughly at the same time each day.
  - Use an electric razor and avoid aspirin or products containing aspirin and herbal products unless instructed by a healthcare provider.

PHARMACOLOGIC TREATMENT
- Oxygen, even with normal PaO_2.
- Unfractionated heparin (UFH) to maintain activated partial thromboplastin time (aPTT) 1.5 to 2.5 times higher than control aPTT.
- Low molecular weight heparin (LMWH) subcutaneously; no monitoring is required except in patients who are obese or pregnant, or have renal insufficiency.
- Warfarin therapy is also started and overlapped for a minimum of 5 days or until the international normalized ratio (INR) is between 2.0 and 3.0 for at least 24 hours.
- Fibrinolytic therapy may be indicated with massive PE and hemodynamic instability.
- Treatment duration depends on the likelihood of recurrence.
  - Average length of therapy is 3 to 6 months.
  - Patients with active malignancy, certain coagulopathies, or multiple unexplained recurrent PEs require long-term anticoagulation.

INTERVENTIONAL TREATMENT
- Vena cava filter may be inserted if:
  - Major contraindications to anticoagulation
  - Bleeding complications from anticoagulation
  - Recurrent VTE despite adequate therapy

Special Considerations

- Approximately 25% of calf vein thromboses, if not treated, will propagate to the popliteal vein or higher, where they are at greater risk of embolization.

Follow-up

EXPECTED OUTCOMES
- Patient will maintain hemodynamic stability and cardiopulmonary tissue perfusion.
- Patient will maintain adequate ventilation and oxygenation.
- Patient will verbalize understanding of bleeding precautions.

COMPLICATIONS
- If the embolus obstructs arterial blood supply, pulmonary infarction can occur.
- Massive PE can cause right heart failure, shock, and adult respiratory distress syndrome (ARDS).
- Twenty-five percent of patients with PE present with sudden death or die within 30 days of diagnosis (usually because of incorrect diagnosis). The mortality rate for patients who are properly treated is only 2% to 8%.

PNEUMONIA

Description
- Pneumonia is an inflammatory illness of the lung resulting in alveolar fluid accumulation.
- There are two broad types of pneumonia based on the location of acquisition: hospital- or community-acquired.
- Community-acquired pneumonia (CAP) is infection that occurs in an outpatient setting or in a patient with no history of hospitalization or long-term care residence for 14 days or longer before symptom onset.
- Hospital-acquired pneumonia (HAP), also called nosocomial pneumonia, occurs 48 hours or longer after admission to a hospital or long-term care facility.

Etiology
- Usually caused by microaspiration of pathogens that colonize the oropharynx (see Table 11–10).
- Bacterial pathogens are most common, but infection can also be caused by viruses, fungi, or parasites.
- Hygiene issues and poor dentition can increase oral colonization.

Table 11–10. Causative Organism in Pneumonia

Community-Acquired Pneumonia	Hospital-Acquired Pneumonia
Strep pneumoniae	S. aureus (MRSA)
Haemophilus influenzae	Strep pneumoniae (drug-resistant)
Legionella sp. or atypical pathogens	Gram-negative enterics
Influenza, other viruses	Anaerobes
S. aureus (following influenza)	

Incidence and Demographics
- Leading cause of infectious death in the United States
- More than 3 million cases annually in the United States

- Accounts for over 600,000 hospitalizations
- Combined with influenza, ranks as the seventh leading cause of death
- Ninety percent of mortality is in the elderly

Risk Factors
- Advanced age
- Alcoholism
- Altered mental status
- Smoking
- Chronic lung disease
- Poor dental hygiene
- Upper respiratory infection
- Neurological deficits (history of CVA, Parkinson's disease, dementia)
- Feeding tubes

Prevention
- Annual influenza vaccination
- Pneumococcal vaccination
- Feeding precautions for patients with feeding tubes, neuromuscular weakness, or confusion
- Proper dental hygiene
- Prompt treatment of upper-respiratory illness in high-risk persons

Assessment
- The clinical presentation of pneumonia can vary based on the age of the patient. Healthy, relatively young persons have "typical symptoms," while older persons and those with more comorbid illness have a more subtle presentation (see Table 11–11).

Table 11–11. Clinical Presentation of Pneumonia

Typical Presentation	Presentation in the Elderly
Fever	Confusion
Cough	Falls
Shortness of breath	Anorexia
Leukocytosis	Decreased functional ability
Tachycardia	Dehydration
	Tachypnea
	Exacerbation of other illness (DM, CAD)

HISTORY
- Presence and duration of the following symptoms:
  - Fever, chills, sweats
  - Cough (productive or nonproductive); appearance of sputum
  - Shortness of breath
  - Fatigue, muscle aches, anorexia, chest pain, headache
  - History of chronic lung disease or asthma
  - Tobacco use

PHYSICAL EXAM
- General appearance may range from no distress to critically ill
- Fever (normal temperature or hypothermia common in elders)
- Tachypnea, tachycardia
- Reduced oxygen saturation
- Lung exam: abnormal lung sounds, crackles, "A to E" changes, dullness on percussion, and increased tactile fremitus over consolidated areas
- Abdominal exam: tenderness
- Mental status: alert versus altered

DIAGNOSTIC STUDIES
- Chest x-ray: presence of infiltrate on CXR is diagnostic in presence of clinical symptoms; also identifies multilobar involvement or pleural effusion, which indicates severe disease.
- Sputum Gram stain and culture: (if properly collected) may be helpful to guide treatment.
- CBC.
- Electrolytes, renal and liver function tests: can help determine need for hospitalization.
- Hospitalized patients may also have the following tests:
  - Arterial blood gases
  - Two sets of blood cultures
  - Serologic testing for HIV (human immunodeficiency virus; if at risk)
  - Acid-fast stain and culture for cough of longer than 1 month duration with weight loss
  - Urinary antigen assay for *Legionella* (very ill, immunocompromised, unresponsive to B-lactam antibiotics

Differential Diagnoses
- COPD
- Lung abscess
- Pulmonary embolism
- Congestive heart failure
- Neoplasm
- Tuberculosis
- Atelectasis

Nursing Management

NONPHARMACOLOGIC TREATMENT
- Rest
- Increased fluid intake
- Humidification
- Avoidance of tobacco smoke
- Avoidance of cough suppressants

PHARMACOLOGIC TREATMENT
- Treatment is based on Gram stain and culture when available
- Guidelines for CAP (see Table 11–12).
  - Antibiotic therapy, usually 7 to 14 days
  - Hospitalized patients usually have 2 days of IV antibiotics followed by 12 days of oral.

Table 11–12. Empiric Treatment of Community-Acquired Pneumonia

Patient Variable	Treatment Options
Previously healthy No risk factors No recent antibiotic therapy	Macrolide (erythromycin, clarithromycin, azithromycin) *or* doxycycline
Recent antibiotic therapy (last 3 months) Comorbid illnesses: COPD, diabetes, renal failure, CHF, malignancy, or immunosuppression	Respiratory fluoroquinolone (levofloxacin, moxifloxacin) *or* Macrolide *plus* Beta-lactam
In regions with high rates (> 25%) of macrolide-resistant *S. pneumoniae*, without morbidities	Respiratory fluoroquinolone (levofloxacin, moxifloxacin) *or* Macrolide *plus* Beta-lactam

Adapted from L. A. Mandell, R. G. Underink, A. Anzueto, et al., 2007, Infectious Diseases Society of America / American Thoracic Society consensus guidelines on the management of community acquired pneumonia in adults, *Clinical Infections Diseases*, 44(S2), 27–72.

INTERVENTIONAL TREATMENT
- Diagnostic thoracentesis for patients with pleural effusion

Special Considerations
- Older adults have an increased risk of aspiration (especially with altered cognition or level of consciousness), reduced ability to clear the airway, and decreased immune function.
- Patients who receive empiric antibiotic therapy early have better outcomes than those whose treatment is delayed.

Follow-up
- Smokers and patients over 40 should have a CXR 4 to 8 weeks after treatment to rule out bronchogenic carcinoma that might have been obscured by the pneumonia.

EXPECTED OUTCOMES
- Patient will regain and maintain normal blood gas values.
- Patient will complete antibiotic regimen as prescribed.
- Patient will maintain adequate nutrition and hydration during course of illness.

COMPLICATIONS
- Empyema
- Septic shock
- Respiratory failure
- Meningitis
- Endocarditis

ADULT RESPIRATORY DISTRESS SYNDROME

Description
- A form of pulmonary edema that follows acute lung injury from trauma, sepsis, pneumonia, aspiration, drug/alcohol abuse, or burns and can quickly lead to respiratory failure and death.

Etiology
- Inflammation of the lung parenchyma leads to diffuse alveolar damage and the release of cytokines and other inflammatory mediators.
- Increased alveolar-capillary membrane permeability leads to fluid accumulation in the interstitial spaces and small airways.
- Reduced surfactant production causes stiffening of the lung tissues and further impairs gas exchange.
- The end result is respiratory failure and severe hypoxemia.

Incidence and Demographics
- About 190,000 persons are affected annually.
- Mortality rate is about 30%, which is down from 50% to 70% 20 years ago.

Risk Factors
- Pneumonia
- Sepsis
- Trauma
- Aspiration
- Burns
- Acute pancreatitis
- Any acute illness

Prevention and Screening
- No prevention known.
- Early medical treatment is imperative for best outcomes.

Assessment

HISTORY
- Acute onset of shortness of breath and sometimes confusion within 48 hours of any precipitating illness or event

PHYSICAL EXAM
- Tachypnea, tachycardia
- Increased work of breathing
- Lung exam abnormal: crackles, wheezes, consolidation
- Remainder of exam will vary based on the underlying cause of the respiratory insult

DIAGNOSTIC STUDIES
- Arterial blood gas
  - If $PaO_2:FiO_2$ is < 300 mm Hg, acute lung injury (ALI) is present.
  - If $PaO_2:FiO_2$ is < 200 mm Hg, ARDS is present.
- Chest x-ray: bilateral infiltrates that spare the costophrenic angles

- Pulmonary artery wedge pressure < 18 mm Hg or absence of clinical signs of left ventricular failure

Differential Diagnoses
- Cardiogenic pulmonary edema
- Diffuse pulmonary hemorrhage
- Pneumonia
- Pulmonary vasculitis

Nursing Management

NONPHARMACOLOGIC TREATMENT
- Mechanical ventilation with positive end-expiratory pressure (PEEP).
- High-frequency jet ventilation is sometimes used.
- Prone positioning of patient has been shown to improve atelectasis and thus improve oxygenation, but not improve survival.
- Fluid restriction or diuresis: improved outcomes in clinical trials.

PHARMACOLOGIC TREATMENT
- Moderate-dose corticosteroids: no large-scale trial has shown benefit.
- Antibiotic therapy is given based on sputum culture and sensitivity. More than 60% of ARDS patients have a nosocomial infection.
- Sedatives, narcotics, and neuromuscular blocking agents to assist with ventilation and patient comfort.

INTERVENTIONAL TREATMENT
- Extracorporeal membrane oxygenation (ECMO) is sometimes used to support patients with refractory hypoxemia.

Special Considerations
- Death may result from complications of underlying disease or from complications of mechanical ventilation.
- Survivors usually regain near-normal lung function.

Follow-up

EXPECTED OUTCOMES
- Patient will regain spontaneous ventilatory function and normal arterial blood gases with treatment.

COMPLICATIONS
- Lung barotrauma
- Pulmonary embolism
- Cardiac arrhythmias
- Acute renal failure
- Disseminated intravascular coagulation (DIC)
- Pneumothorax
- Tracheal injury/stenosis
- Malnutrition
- Death

LUNG MALIGNANCY

Description
- Bronchogenic carcinoma is divided into two cell types:
  - Small-cell (also called oat cell; SCLC) tends to be detected at more advanced stages; grows rapidly and metastasizes early.
  - Non-small-cell (NSCLC) includes squamous cell, adenocarcinoma, and large-cell carcinoma (75% to 80% of lung cancers).

Etiology
- Tobacco exposure
- Ionizing radiation
- Asbestos exposure
- Heavy metals

Incidence and Demographics
- Most common type of cancer
- Leading cause of cancer death in both men and women
- Rare in persons younger than 40
- Peak incidence is age 70 to 74 in women and age 75 to 79 in men
- Women are more likely than men to have lung cancer that is not related to smoking

Risk Factors
- Cigarette smoking (90% of lung cancers due to tobacco)
- Exposure to radon
- Chronic exposure to talc
- Exposure to heavy metals such as arsenic, nickel, petroleum products
- Exposure to asbestos
- Genetic factors play a role

Prevention and Screening
- Avoid tobacco exposure (both direct and secondhand).
- Chest x-rays and cytology as screening measures have not improved survival.
- Currently no recommended screening tests.

Assessment

HISTORY
- Persistent cough, hemoptysis
- Hoarseness or dysphagia
- Recurrent pneumonia or bronchitis
- Anorexia, weight loss, fatigue

PHYSICAL EXAM
- No characteristic physical exam findings

DIAGNOSTIC STUDIES
- Chest x-ray
- CBC

- CT of chest
- Arterial blood gas measurement
- Pulmonary function tests
- ECG
- Sputum cytology
- Bronchoscopy
- Transthoracic needle aspiration
- If metastasis is suspected:
  - MRI brain
  - Total body bone scan

Differential Diagnoses

- Pneumonia
- Sarcoidosis
- Tuberculosis
- COPD
- Pulmonary embolism

Nursing Management

NONPHARMACOLOGIC TREATMENT
- Smoking cessation
- Removing other harmful exposures
- Nutritional support

PHARMACOLOGIC TREATMENT
- Treatment is based on staging of the cancer (see Table 11–13).

Table 11–13. Staging of Non-Small-Cell Lung Cancers

Stage	Criteria	Treatment
I	Non-small-cell lung cancer	Surgery
II	Non-small-cell lung cancer with lymph node or chest wall invasion	Surgery Curative XRT or XRT then curative surgery + adjuvant chemotherapy
III-A	Non-small-cell lung cancer with lymph node and chest wall invasion that requires resection of the lung and ribs	Surgery Chemotherapy Surgery + post-operative XRT
III-B	Non-small-cell lung cancer with more invasion than in stage III-A that requires a wider, more invasive excision	XRT Chemotherapy Chemotherapy + XRT XRT then surgical resection
IV	Non-small-cell lung cancer with distant metastasis	Palliation of symptoms; therapies only used to curtail quality compromising effects of tumor

Adapted from *Treatment of lung cancer* by the National Cancer Institute, n.d., retrieved from http://www.cancer.gov/cancertopics/treatment/lung

INTERVENTIONAL TREATMENT
- Surgical resection of NSCLC is often curative.
- SCLC is rarely operable.

Special Considerations
- Risk of lung cancer gradually declines for 15 years after a person stops smoking, at which point the risk becomes similar to a nonsmoker's.
- Side effects of treatment may be worse than the course of the disease, particularly in elderly patients.
- Smoking cessation campaigns have decreased the number of men who smoke, but have not had an impact on teenage or women smokers.
- Weight loss is a marker of poor prognosis.

Follow-up

EXPECTED OUTCOMES
- Patient will regain lost weight and maintain adequate nutritional status.
- Patient will verbalize precautions to prevent infection in their immunocompromised state.

COMPLICATIONS
- Most complications result from treatment with immunosuppressive therapies.
- Fracture is a complication of bone metastasis.
- Seizures could result from brain metastasis.
- Head or neck swelling can result from tumor compression of the superior vena cava.

TUBERCULOSIS (TB)

Description
- TB is an infectious disease caused by *Mycobacterium tuberculosis*, often seen where people live in close proximity.
- TB mostly affects the lungs, but in 15% of cases disease can be seen elsewhere in the body such as kidneys, bones, skin, or reproductive and urinary systems.

Etiology
- Bacilli are transmitted by droplet particles that are aerosolized from the cough or sneeze of an infected person.
- Several hundred bacilli must be inhaled to infect an immunocompetent person, but only a few are needed to infect a compromised host.
- Incubation period from infection to positive skin test is 2 to 10 weeks.
- Two types of disease exist:
  - Latent tuberculosis infection (LTBI)
    - After exposure, person develops local illness in upper lobes of lungs, but the immune system "walls off" the infection.
    - No symptoms occur and person is not contagious.
    - Disease can remain inactive for decades.
  - Active disease
    - Exposed person develops acute illness
    - Bacillus causes inflammation and necrosis of lung parenchyma

Incidence and Demographics
- According to the World Health Organization (WHO), more than one-third of the world's population is currently infected with the TB bacillus.
- About 5% to 10% of persons infected will become ill or contagious at some point in their lives.
- In 2009, about 11,5000 cases were reported in the United States.
- Rate of death from TB in the United States is declining.
- Worldwide, TB accounts for 2 million deaths annually and is increasing, mostly due to the HIV epidemic.
- In the United States, racial minorities are disproportionately affected.

Risk Factors
- Age (risk factor for reactivation)
- HIV
- AIDS
- Chemotherapy
- Organ transplantation
- IV drug use
- Chronic renal failure
- Diabetes mellitus
- Chronic lung disease
- Poor nutritional status
- Leukemia, lymphoma, or any malignancy

Prevention and Screening
- Screening with TB skin test (PPD) is required for many professionals who have contact with the public (health care, cosmetology, etc.).
- Recent converters or persons with known exposure should be considered for chemoprophylaxis with Isoniazid (INH) for 6 to 12 months.

Assessment

HISTORY
- Night sweats
- Fever
- Weight loss and anorexia
- Cough, hemoptysis
- Any chronic, unexplained symptoms
- Prior skin test results or chest x-rays
- Country of origin and foreign travel
- Contact with known infected person

PHYSICAL EXAM
- May be entirely normal
- Fever, weight loss
- Crackles heard in the upper posterior chest
- Evidence of pleural effusion
- Lymphadenopathy

DIAGNOSTIC STUDIES
- Tuberculin skin test (TST or Mantoux)
  - Only way to identify infection before it has progressed to disease.
  - Anergy testing for persons with a compromised immune response is no longer recommended.
  - Two-step test is recommended in older adults and persons who will require serial testing (such as healthcare workers).
    - Some persons infected with M. *tuberculosis* have a negative response to TST if infection occurred a number of years ago.
    - Repeating the TST 1 to 3 weeks after the initial negative test may "awaken" the immune system and allow a positive response to the test (booster phenomenon).
    - A second positive test indicates infection and need for evaluation and treatment (see Table 11–14).

Table 11–14. Classification of Tuberculin Skin Test Reactions

Induration Measurement	Considered Positive In
≥ 5 mm	HIV-infected persons Recent contacts of person with infectious TB Persons with CXR suggestive of prior TB Organ transplant recipients Persons who are immunosuppressed (on prednisone or TNF-α antagonists)
≥ 10 mm	Recent immigrants (within 5 years) from high-prevalence countries Injection drug users Persons with pre-existing medical conditions: malnutrition, diabetes, chronic renal failure, cancer, gastrectomy, jejunoileal bypass Residents or employees of high-risk congregate settings (prisons, LTC facilities, homeless shelters, hospitals) Mycobacteriology lab personnel Children younger than 4 years of age
≥ 15 mm	All persons

Adapted from *Latent tuberculosis infection: A guide for primary healthcare providers* by the Centers for Disease Control and Prevention, 2010, retrieved from http://www.cdc.gov/tb/publications/LTBI/diagnosis.htm#1

- Interferon-gamma release assays (IGRAs)
  - Measure a person's immune reactivity to specific mycobacterial antigens
  - Advantages of this test over TST:
    - Requires a single test
    - Does not cause booster phenomenon
    - Less subject to reader bias
    - Unaffected by BCG vaccine and most environmental mycobacteria
- Chest x-ray: ordered in persons with a positive TST or IGRA result or persons with known contact with an infected individual

- CBC
- Liver function tests and electrolytes
- Erythrocyte sedimentation rate (ESR)
- Urinalysis (looking for sterile pyuria)
- Sputum test for acid-fast bacillus

Differential Diagnoses
- Malignancy
- COPD
- Asthma
- Pneumonia
- Bronchiectasis
- Silicosis

Nursing Management

NONPHARMACOLOGIC TREATMENT
- Isolation for new, confirmed cases
- Must be reported to the CDC

PHARMACOLOGIC TREATMENT
- LTBI is treated with isoniazid (INH) or rifampin.
  - Liver toxicity is the major risk of INH.
- Multiple drugs are given in the initial treatment of active TB and may include:
  - First-line: INH, rifampin, rifapentine, pyrazinamide, ethambutol
  - Second-line medications for drug-resistant disease: cycloserine, ethionamide, fluoroquinolones, p-aminosalicylic acid, streptomycin, and others

Special Considerations
- If patient is high-risk (HIV-infected, young child, TB contact), directly observed therapy (DOT) is recommended.

Follow-up
- Patients should visit a healthcare provider monthly while receiving treatment to assess for signs of hepatitis, check adherence, and review possible drug interactions.

EXPECTED OUTCOMES
- Patient with active TB will regain normal ventilation and oxygenation.
- Patient will verbalize importance of adherence to prescribed drug therapy.
- Patient will promptly report signs and symptoms of organ dysfunction in other systems.

COMPLICATIONS
- Disseminated disease is most common in the elderly, HIV-infected persons, and persons on immunosuppressive medications. TB can affect virtually any body system.
- Drug-resistant TB can develop when medications are misused or mismanaged:
  - Patient doesn't complete full course of treatment.
  - Healthcare providers prescribe the wrong drugs, dose, or length of treatment.
  - Drugs are of poor quality.
  - Multidrug-resistant TB is resistant to INH and rifampin.

- Extensively drug-resistant TB is a rare type of disease that is also resistant to two of the second-line therapies.
- Bronchopleural fistulas can lead to pneumothorax.
- Liver toxicity is the most serious risk of treatment.

REFERENCES

American Lung Association. (n.d.). *Acute respiratory distress syndrome (ARDS)*. Retrieved from http://www.lungusa.org/lung-disease/acute-respiratory-distress-syndrome/

American Lung Association. (n.d.). *Understanding Lung Cancer*. Retrieved from http://www.lungusa.org/lung-disease/lung-cancer/about-lung-cancer/understanding-lung-cancer.html

Centers for Disease Control and Prevention. (2010). *Chronic obstructive pulmonary disease.* Retrieved from http://www.cdc.gov/copd/

Centers for Disease Control and Prevention. (2010). *Latent tuberculosis infection: A guide for primary healthcare providers.* Retrieved from http://www.cdc.gov/tb/publications/LTBI/diagnosis.htm#1

Ferebee, L. (2006). Respiratory function. In S. E. Meiner & A. G. Lueckenotte (Eds.), *Gerontological nursing* (pp. 504–534). St. Louis, MO: Mosby-Elsevier.

Fiebach, N. H., Kern, D. E., Thomas, P. A., & Ziegelstein, R. C. (Eds.). (2007). *Barker, Burton and Zieve's principles of ambulatory medicine* (7th ed.). Philadelphia: Lippincott Williams & Wilkins.

Geerts, W. H., Berggvist, D., Pinero, G. F., Heit, J. A., Samama, C. M., Lassen, M. R., & Colwell, C. W. (2008). Prevention of venous thromboembolism: American College of Chest Physicians Evidence-Based Clinical Practice Guidelines (8th Edition). *Chest, 133*(6 Suppl), 381s–453s.

Granton, J. T., & Grossman, R. F. (1993). Community-acquired pneumonia in the elderly patient: Clinical features, epidemiology, and treatment. *Clinical Chest Medicine, 14*, 537–553.

Kim, E. S. H., & Bartholomew, J. R. (2010). *Venous thromboembolism.* Retrieved from http://www.clevelandclinicmeded.com/medicalpubs/diseasemanagement/cardiology/venous-thromboembolism/

Mandell, L. A., Wunderink, R. G., Anzueto, A., Bartlett, J. G., Campbell, G. D., Dean, N.C., ... American Thoracic Society (2007). Infectious Diseases Society of America/American Thoracic Society consensus guidelines on the management of community acquired pneumonia in adults. *Clinical Infectious Diseases, 44*(S2), 27–72.

Mills, E. J. (Ed.). (2005). *Handbook of medical-surgical nursing* (4th ed.). Philadelphia: Lippincott Williams & Wilkins.

Mimio, A. M., & Smith, B. L. (2001). Deaths: Preliminary data for 2000. *National Vital Statistics Reports, 49*(12), 5.

National Cancer Institute. (n.d.). *Treatment of lung cancer.* Retrieved from http://www.cancer.gov/cancertopics/treatment/lung

National Cholesterol Education Panel. (2001). *Third report on detection, evaluation and treatment of high blood cholesterol in adults (Adult Treatment Panel III)* (NIH Publication 01–3670). Bethesda, MD: NHLBI Health Information Center.

National Cholesterol Education Program. (2001). Risk assessment tool for estimating 10-year risk of developing hard CHD. *Third Report of the Expert Panel on Detection, Evaluation, and Treatment of High Blood Cholesterol in Adults (Adult Treatment Panel III).* Bethesda, MD: NHLBI Health Information Center. Retrieved from http://hp2010.nhlbihin.net/atpiii/calculator.asp?usertype=prof

O'Connor, R. E. (2010). *Abdominal aneurysm.* Retrieved from http://emedicine.medscape.com/article/756735-overview

Singh, N. (2010). *Atherosclerotic disease of the carotid artery.* Retrieved from http://emedicine.medscape.com/article/463147-overview

Steele, L. L., & Steele, J. R. [2006]. Cancer. In S. E. Meiner & A. G. Lueckenotte (Eds.), *Gerontological nursing* (pp. 382–410). St. Louis, MO: Mosby-Elsevier.

Sutherland, S. F. (2010). *Pulmonary embolism.* Retrieved from http://emedicine.medscape.com/article/759765-overview

Weiss, R. (2009). *Venous insufficiency.* Retrieved from http://emedicine.medscape.com/article/1085412-overview

Woods, S. L., Froelicher, E. S., Motzer, S. A., & Bridges, E. J. (2004). *Cardiac nursing* (5th ed.). Philadelphia: Lippincott Williams & Wilkins.

Gastrointestinal System

Jo Nell Wells, PhD, RN-BC, OCN

Common Gastrointestinal Disorders

GENERAL APPROACH

Gastrointestinal (GI) conditions are generally categorized into lower or upper GI disorders or liver, pancreas, and biliary tract problems. GI conditions make up many of the most common medical-surgical conditions nurses see. Treatment plans can include preventive health practices, medications, surgical therapies, or all of these approaches. Some disorders are easily managed and others can be life-threatening. Careful GI assessment is the foundation for care for all GI conditions.

GASTROESOPHAGEAL REFLUX DISEASE (GERD)

Description
- GERD is not a disease but a syndrome.
- GERD is any clinically significant symptomatic condition or histopathologic alteration secondary to reflux of gastric contents into the lower esophagus.
- Many people experience few symptoms while others develop inflammatory esophagitis as a result of exposure to gastric juices.
- GERD is a chronic condition.

Etiology

- No single cause.
- It results when the lower esophagus defenses are overcome by the reflux of acidic gastric contents into the esophagus.
- Predisposing factors include hiatal hernia, incompetent lower esophageal sphincter (LES) and impaired esophageal motility, and delayed gastric emptying.

Incidence and Demographics

- GERD is the most common upper GI problem seen in adults.
- Approximately 14% to 20% of the U.S. population experiences GERD symptoms at least once a week.

Risk Factors

- LES pressure can be reduced by certain foods such as caffeine and chocolate, drugs such as anticholinergics, obesity, pregnancy, cigarette and cigar smoking, and hiatal hernia.

Prevention and Screening

- Lifestyle modification to avoid aggravating factors (see above).
- Diet can aggravate but does not cause GERD. Teach patient to eat small frequent meals, avoid late evening meals and snacking, take fluids between rather than with meals to reduce gastric distention, and reduce intra-abdominal pressure with weight management.

Assessment

HISTORY
- Assess for heartburn after meals or when bending over or reclining; intolerance of spicy, acidic, or fatty foods; dyspepsia; hypersalivation; and reports of noncardiac chest pain.
- Gastric symptoms include early satiety, postmeal bloating, nausea, and vomiting.

PHYSICAL EXAM
- Assess for respiratory symptoms, including wheezing, coughing, dyspnea, nocturnal coughing resulting in disturbed sleep patterns; hoarseness; sore throat; lump in the throat and choking; belching of hot, bitter, or sour liquid into the throat or mouth.
- Assess for respiratory complications of GERD asthma, chronic bronchitis, and pneumonia.
- Assess for dental erosion, especially in the posterior teeth.

DIAGNOSTIC STUDIES
- Diagnostic studies performed to determine the cause of the GERD include:
  - Barium swallow
  - Endoscopy to assess the LES competence and degree of inflammation if present, potential scarring, and strictures
  - Biopsy and cytologic specimens to differentiate stomach or esophageal carcinoma from Barrett esophagus
  - Radionuclide tests to detect reflux of gastric contents and the rate of esophageal clearance
  - Motility studies (manometry)
  - 24-hour ambulatory pH monitoring

- For this test, a small tube with a pH electrode is inserted through the nose into the esophagus. The electrode is attached to a small box worn on the belt that records the data, later analyzed via computer.
- Endoscopic procedures allow visualization of the esophageal, gastric, and duodenal mucosa through a lighted endoscope (gastroscope). The procedure can be used to evaluate esophageal and gastric motility and to collect secretions and tissue specimens for further analysis.
  - In esophagogastroduodenoscopy (EGD), the gastroenterologist views the GI tract through a viewing lens and can take still photographs or video through the scope to document findings. Endoscopic retrograde cholangiopancreatography (ERCP) is an endoscopic procedure to provide radiographic visualization of the biliary and pancreatic ducts.

Nursing Implications for Diagnostic Study: Upper Endoscopy (EGD) and ERCP

BEFORE PROCEDURE
- Explain the procedure. Teach the patient that no discomfort is associated with the dye injection but that minimal gagging may occur during the initial introduction of the scope into the oral pharynx. Inform the patient that breathing will not be compromised by the insertion of the endoscope.
- Obtain informed consent.
- Keep patient NPO (nothing by mouth) for 4 to 8 hours prior to the test.
- Assess baseline vital signs; assess for any allergies to iodine, seafood, or contrast media; remove dentures; establish IV access; administer antibiotic prophylaxis as ordered.
- Administer appropriate premedication as ordered. Assure patient safety. Maintain bedrest after premedication.

DURING PROCEDURE
- Assist the patient to the supine or left side position. The patient is sedated with a narcotic and a sedative/hypnotic.
- Assist the physician to spray the patient's pharynx with a local anesthetic (lidocaine [Xylocaine]) to reduce the gag reflex and lessen the discomfort caused by the scope passage.
- Provide safety precautions for the patient; stand at the patient's side; monitor changes in heart rate, breathing, and blood pressure.

POSTPROCEDURE
- Monitor vital signs. Do not allow the patient to eat or drink until the gag reflex returns. Check for gag reflex by applying gentle pressure on a tongue depressor placed on the back of the tongue.
- Observe for and report abdominal distention and signs of perforation, GI bleeding, or possible pancreatitis, including chills, fever, pain, vomiting, and tachycardia. Notify the physician immediately. This may indicate the onset of ERCP-induced pancreatitis.
- Observe safety precautions until the effects of the sedative have worn off.
- Monitor the patient for signs of respiratory depression. Medication (e.g., naloxone [Narcan]) should be available to counteract serious respiratory depression. Resuscitative equipment also should be present.

- Inform the patient that he or she may be hoarse and have a sore throat for several days. Drinking cool fluids and gargling will help relieve some of this soreness.

HOME CARE RESPONSIBILITIES
- A sore throat is expected. Gargling with a soothing mouthwash may help.
- Notify the physician immediately if increasing abdominal pain, nausea, fever, shaking chills, or vomiting occurs. These may be the early signs of cholangitis.
- Encourage the patient to eat lightly for the next 12 to 24 hours.

Nursing Management

- GERD is a chronic, lifelong condition best managed by the patient. Teach patients and family GERD risk factors; medication side effects; to keep head of bed elevated 4 to 6 inches; and to not lie down for 2 to 3 hours after eating. Instruct to see HCP if symptoms persist.
- Surgery may be used for patients who do not respond to pharmacologic and lifestyle management.
  - Surgical therapy (antireflux surgery)
  - Fundoplication
  - Hill gastropexy
- Postoperative care focus: Prevent respiratory complications, maintain fluid and electrolyte balance, prevent infections.
  - Assess respiratory rate and rhythm, pulse rate and rhythm, and signs of pneumothorax (e.g., dyspnea, chest pain, cyanosis). Deep breathing is essential.
  - Administer medications to prevent postoperative nausea and vomiting and to control pain.
- Diet: Add solids gradually so that stomach is not over-distended. Record intake and output (I&O). Avoid gas-forming foods and gastric distention.

NONPHARMACOLOGIC TREATMENT
- Elevate head of bed on 4- to 6-inch blocks.
- High-protein, low-fat diet with avoidance of foods that decrease LES pressure or irritate acid-sensitive esophagus.
- Endoscopic care: intraluminal valvuloplasty, radiofrequency therapy, injection or implantation of foreign material.

PHARMACOLOGIC TREATMENT
- Antacids: Gelusil, Maalox, Mylanta
- Antisecretory agents
  - H2-receptor blockers (e.g., cimetidine, famotidine, nizatidine, ranitidine)
  - Proton pump inhibitors (PPIs; e.g., esomeprazole, lansoprazole, omeprazole, pantoprazole, rabeprazole)
- Prokinetic therapy (e.g., metoclopramide [Reglan])
- Cholinergic drugs to increase LES pressure (e.g., bethanechol)
- Cytoprotective agents (e.g., alginic acid-antacid [Gaviscon] and sucralfate [Carafate])

See Table 12–1 for major nursing implications for selected GI medications.

Special Considerations
- See below.

Follow-up

EXPECTED OUTCOMES
- Surgical repair should decrease symptoms. Symptom recurrence rate ranges from 10% to 30% over a 20-year period. Patients should avoid nonsteroidal anti-inflammatory drugs (NSAIDs) for 10 days minimum after surgery and other treatment procedures.

COMPLICATIONS
- If untreated, GERD can result in esophagitis, esophageal scarring, stricture, dysphagia, Barrett esophagus (esophageal metaplasia).
- Respiratory complications include cough, bronchospasm, laryngospasm and cricopharyngeal spasm, chronic bronchitis, aspiration pneumonia, and dental erosion.

Table 12-1. Medication Administration: Drugs Used to Treat GERD, Gastritis, and Peptic Ulcer Disease

Medication	GI Treatment Purpose	Nursing Implications
Antibiotics		
Amoxicillin (Amoxil)	Antibiotic that assists with eradicating H. pylori bacteria in the gastric mucosa	May cause diarrhea Do not use in patients with penicillin allergy
Clarithromycin (Biaxin)	Same as above	GI upsets; altered taste Do not give with warfarin (Coumadin)
Metronidazole (Flagyl)	Useful as an antibacterial and antiprotozoal agent to eradicate H. pylori; administered with other antibiotics and proton pump inhibitors	Administer with meals to decrease GI upset risk May cause anorexia and metallic taste Avoid with alcohol Flagyl increases anticoagulation effects of warfarin (Coumadin)
Tetracycline (Achromycin V, Tetracyn, Sumycin)	Bacteriostatic effect assists to eradicate H. pylori	May cause photosensitivity reaction; warn patient to wear sunscreen May cause GI upset Must be used with caution in patients with renal or hepatic impairment Avoid milk or dairy products to achieve maximum effect
Antidiarrheal		
Pepto-Bismol (bismuth subsalicylate)	Suppresses H. pylori bacteria in the gastric mucosa and assists with healing of mucosal ulcers	Take on an empty stomach Given concurrently with antibiotics to treat PUD

cont.

Table 12–1. Medication Administration (cont.)

Histamine-2 (H2) receptor antagonists	To treat PUD: relieve pain, promote healing, prevent ulcer recurrence, and prevent complications. Decrease amount of HCl produced by stomach by blocking action of histamine on histamine receptors of parietal cells in the stomach	Use these meds with caution in patients with renal or hepatic dysfunction Follow prescriber's orders for administration around meal times
Cimetidine (Tagamet)		Least expensive of meds in this category; available over the counter (OTC) May cause confusion, agitation, or coma in the elderly or those with renal or hepatic insufficiency Long-term use may cause diarrhea, dizziness, gynecomastia Can increase levels of other meds (e.g., amiodarone, amitriptyline, benzodiazepines, metoprolol, nifedipine, phenytoin, warfarin [Coumadin])
Famotidine (Pepcid)	Same as cimetidine	May cause diarrhea Do not administer to patients with penicillin allergy
Nizatidine (Axid)	Same as cimetidine	May cause GI upset, headache, altered taste Assess for possible drug interactions with many drugs (e.g., lovastatin, warfarin [Coumadin])
Ranitidine (Zantac)	Same as cimetidine	Administer with meals to decrease GI upset; may cause anorexia and metallic taste Patient should avoid alcohol
Proton pump inhibitors of gastric acid (PPIs)		
Esomeprazole (Nexium) Lansoprazole (Prevacid) Omeprazole (Prilosec) Rabeprazole (AcipHex) Pantoprazole (Protonix)	Primarily used to treat PUD, relieve pain, promote healing, prevent ulcer recurrence, and prevent complications Decrease gastric acid section by slowing the hydrogen-potassium-adenosine triphosphatase (H+, K+-ATPase) pump on the surface of the parietal cells of the stomach	PPIs are generally very safe, but are contraindicated in cases of hypersensitivity to the drug itself or to a component of the formulation; oral pill forms should be taken whole/intact Nexium should be taken at least 1 hour before a meal Prilosec and Prevacid should be taken just before eating Protonix and AcipHex may be taken without regard to food When Protonix is given IV, an in-line filter must be used to remove any precipitate

Prostaglandin E1 analogs		
Misoprostol (Cytotec)	Synthetic prostaglandins; protect the gastric mucosa from agents that cause ulcers; also increase mucus production and bicarbonate levels	Should be taken on an empty stomach Works in combination with antibiotics for ulcer treatment
Sucralfate (Carafate)	Form a viscous substance in the presence of gastric acid to provide a protective barrier, binding to the surface of the ulcer, and prevent digestion by pepsin	Least expensive of meds in this category; available OTC May cause confusion, agitation, or coma in the elderly or those with renal or hepatic insufficiency Long-term use may cause diarrhea, dizziness, gynecomastia Exerts many drug-drug interactions (e.g., amiodarone, amitriptyline, benzodiazepines, metoprolol, nifedipine, phenytoin, warfarin [Coumadin])
Prokinetic agents		
Metoclopramide (Reglan)	Increase resting tone of esophageal sphincter, and tone and amplitude of upper GI contraction to promote gastric emptying and intestinal transit	Used to treat symptoms of GERD Give 30 minutes before meals and at bedtime Available for IV infusion; protect IV bag from light during infusion by using protective cover provided by the company Can cause sedation, fatigue, restlessness, agitation, headache, insomnia, confusion, GI upsets, dry mouth, urticaria or rash, periorbital edema, and extra pyramidal symptoms Immediately report restlessness and involuntary movements, facial grimacing, rigidity, or tremors Presents interactions with other central nervous system (CNS) depressants
Antacids	The primary use for antacids is PUD; these meds work to neutralize gastric acid and promote healing and pain relief; antacids should be taken regularly (e.g., 7 times a day: 1 and 3 hours after each mean and at mealtime)	

cont.

Table 12–1. Medication Administration (cont.)

Magnesium compounds (Magnesium hydroxide [milk of magnesium]; magnesium oxide)	Same as above	May cause diarrhea Can cause magnesium toxicity (CNS depression) in patients with renal impairment
Aluminum compounds (Amphojel, Basaljel)	Same as above	Can cause constipation and hypophosphatemia
Calcium compounds (Tums, Titralac)	Same as above	Can cause constipation, acid rebound, or milk-alkali syndrome Releases CO_2
Sodium compounds (sodium bicarbonate)	Same as above	Does not cause constipation or diarrhea Does increase systemic pH so not used routinely to treat ulcers Used to treat acidosis and to alkalinize urine high risk of sodium-loading Releases CO_2.
Other (e.g., Magaldrate [complex of magnesium/ aluminum compounds])		

HIATAL HERNIA (HH)

Description
- Protrusion of a portion of the stomach into the esophagus through an opening, or hiatus, in the diaphragm.
- Types
  - Sliding: The junction of the stomach and esophagus is above the hiatus of the diaphragm and a part of the stomach slides through the opening.
  - Paraesophageal or rolling: The esophagogastric junction remains in the normal position, but the fundus and greater curvature of the stomach roll up through the diaphragm, forming a pocket alongside the esophagus.

Etiology
- Unknown

Incidence and Demographics
- Incidence is difficult to determine; but HH is the most common abnormality found on UGI x-ray examination. Common in older adults and occurs more often in women than men.

Risk Factors
- Diaphragm muscle weakening
- Increase in intra-abdominal pressure (obesity, pregnancy, ascites, tumors, tight girdles, intense physical exertions, and heavy lifting on a continual basis)
- Increasing age
- Trauma
- Poor nutrition
- Forced recumbent position (prolonged illness)
- Congenital weakness

Prevention and Screening
- Avoid or eliminate risk factors.

Assessment

HISTORY
- Persons with HH may be asymptomatic or have signs and symptoms similar to those described for GERD (i.e., belching, indigestion, heartburn after eating or lying supine).

PHYSICAL EXAM
- Patients may experience severe burning pain when bending over, which is relieved by sitting or standing. Sometimes symptoms are similar to gallbladder disease, peptic ulcer disease, and angina.

DIAGNOSTIC STUDIES
- Barium swallow and/or endoscopic visualization

Nursing Management
- See GERD.

NONPHARMACOLOGIC TREATMENT
- Surgical therapy goal: Reduce the hernia, provide an acceptable LES pressure, and prevent movement of the gastroesophageal junction. Standard technique includes Nissan laparoscopic procedure, for example, herniotomy (excision of the hernia sac), herniorrhaphy (closure of the hiatal defect, an antireflux procedure), and gastropexy (attachment of the stomach subdiaphragmatically to prevent reherniation).

PHARMACOLOGIC TREATMENT
- See GERD.

Special Considerations
- Increased incidence with aging. Medications commonly taken by older patients can decrease lower esophageal pressure (LES; e.g., nitrates, calcium channel blockers, antidepressants).
- Some older adults are asymptomatic or have less severe symptoms. Assess for bleeding or respiratory complications.
- An older adult with cardiovascular and pulmonary problems may not be a good candidate for surgical intervention.
- Additionally, lifestyle modifications may be more difficult in this age group.

Follow-up

EXPECTED OUTCOMES
- Surgical risks are reduced with laparoscopic procedures. See gerontological considerations above.

COMPLICATIONS
- Esophagitis, esophageal bleeding, respiratory complication (e.g., aspiration pneumonia). Esophageal bleeding is a medical emergency and during an episode of bleeding, management of airway and prevention of aspiration of blood are critical factors.

PEPTIC ULCER DISEASE (PUD)

Description
- Peptic ulcer disease is a condition characterized by erosion of the GI mucosa resulting from the digestive action of hydrochloric acid and pepsin. Any portion of the GI tract that comes into contact with gastric secretions is susceptible to PUD, including the lower esophagus, stomach, and duodenum. Peptic ulcer may be chronic, with spontaneous remissions and exacerbations. Exacerbations may be associated with trauma, infection, or other physical or psychologic stressors.

Etiology
- Various factors can disrupt the gastric mucosa and allow pathophysiologic acid back-diffusion into mucosa. This prompts destruction of mucosal cells and histamine release, which increases acid and pepsin release, causing further mucosal erosion. Resulting destruction of blood vessels and bleeding results in ulceration.
- H. pylori alters gastric secretion and produces tissue damage leading to PUD in many individuals.
- Zollinger-Ellison syndrome is PUD caused by a gastrinoma, or gastrin-secreting tumor of the pancreas, stomach, or intestines. Gastrinomas may be benign, although 50% to 70% are malignant tumors. Characteristic ulcer-like pain is common, and steatorrhea (excess fecal fat), bleeding, and persistent diarrhea may occur.

Incidence and Demographics
- There are approximately 500,000 new cases of ulcers diagnosed and more than 4 million recurrences of PUD each year. The incidence of PUD in patients over 60 years of age is increasing, probably related to the increased use of aspirin and other NSAIDs.

Risk Factors
- A variety of agents are known to destroy the mucosal barrier. These include ulcerogenic drugs, NSAIDs such as aspirin, and corticosteroids.
- Other risk factors include low socioeconomic status, living conditions such as crowded and unsanitary surroundings, and unclean food or water.
- Additionally, risk increases with cigarette smoking, family history of PUD, personal history of ulcer, and advanced age.

Prevention and Screening

- Peptic ulcer disease is difficult to predict; however, nurses can promote health by advising patients to avoid risk factors such as excessive aspirin or NSAID use and cigarette smoking.
- When GI irritating or ulcerogenic medications must be taken, enteric-coated preparation or coadministration with a proton pump inhibitor (PPI) or misoprostol (Cytotec) should be considered.
- Screening: upper GI endoscopy with biopsy; *H. pylori* testing of breath, urine, blood, tissue; UGI barium contrast study; complete blood count; urinalysis; liver enzymes; serum electrolytes.
- See *Nursing Implications for Diagnostic Study: Upper Endoscopy (EGD) and ERCP* under GERD above.

Assessment

HISTORY

- The person with PUD may have no pain or other symptoms because the gastric and duodenal mucosa are not rich in sensory pain fibers. Silent PUD is more likely to occur in older adults and those taking NSAIDs.
- Family history of PUD, chronic alcohol abuse, smoking, caffeine use.
- History of chronic kidney disease, pancreatic disease, chronic obstructive pulmonary disease, serious illness or trauma, hyperparathyroidism, cirrhosis of the liver, Zollinger-Ellison syndrome.
- Use of aspirin, other nonsteroidal anti-inflammatory drugs (NSAIDS, corticosteroids).
- Prolonged surgeries, sustained severe burns or trauma.

PHYSICAL EXAM

- When pain does occur, gastric ulcer pain is located high in the epigastrium, occurs about 1 to 2 hours after meals, and is described as "burning" or "gaseous." Pain can occur when the stomach is empty or when food has been ingested. If the ulcer has eroded through the gastric mucosa, food tends to aggravate rather than alleviate the pain. For some patients the earliest symptoms will be due to a serious complication such as perforation.
- Duodenal ulcer pain may be described as "burning" or "cramplike." Pain is located in the midepigastric area behind the sternum or as back pain. Pain usually occurs 2 to 4 hours after meals. It can also be seasonal in nature.
- Anemia

DIAGNOSTIC STUDIES

- See above.
- Abnormal upper gastrointestinal endoscopic and barium studies.
  - Lab tests, including CBC, urinalysis, serum electrolytes; guaiac-positive stools; positive blood, urine, breath, or stool tests for *H. pylori*.
  - Liver enzyme studies help determine any liver problems, such as cirrhosis, that may complicate PUD treatment.
  - Stools are routinely tested for the presence of blood.
  - A serum amylase determination is done to determine pancreatic function when posterior duodenal ulcer penetration of the pancreas is suspected.

Nursing Management

- See above.
  - Assess for weight loss; anorexia; nausea and vomiting; hematemesis; dyspepsia; heartburn; belching; black and tarry stools; and epigastric tenderness.
  - Teach patient and family about diet modifications, rationale for avoiding cigarettes, alcohol, OTC drugs unless approved by the healthcare provider, the need to take all medications prescribed to avoid relapse. Explain the importance of reporting increased nausea and/or vomiting, epigastric pain, and bloody emesis or tarry stools.
  - Encourage the patient and family to discuss needed lifestyle changes and living with a chronic illness.
  - See Special Considerations below for the patient who has a gastrostomy or jejunostomy tube placement.

NONPHARMACOLOGIC TREATMENT

- No longer necessary are bland or restricted diets. Patients are encouraged to maintain good nutrition, avoid foods that cause GI upset for them, and consume balanced meals at regular intervals. Mild alcohol intake is not harmful but smoking should cease because smoking slows the rate of healing and increases the rate of relapses.

PHARMACOLOGIC TREATMENT

- See Table 12–1
  - Antisecretory agents
    - H2-receptor blockers: cimetidine (Tagamet); famotidine (Pepcid), Nizatidine (Axid), ranitidine (Zantac)
    - Proton pump inhibitors (PPIs): esomeprazole (Nexium), lansoprazole (Prevacid), omeprazole (Prilosec), pantoprazole (Protonix), rabeprazole (AcipHex).
  - Antibiotics for *H. pylori*: amoxicillin, metronidazole (Flagyl), tetracycline, clarithromycin (Biaxin)
  - Antacids: many varieties
    - Single substance (Basaljel, Riopan, Rolaids, Phosphaljel)
    - Mixtures of aluminum hydroxide and magnesium salts (Gaviscon, Gelusil, Maalox, Mylanta)
    - Mixtures of calcium carbonate and aluminum and magnesium hydroxides (Camalox)
  - Mixtures of calcium carbonate, magnesium carbonate, and magnesium oxide (Alkets)
  - Side effects of antacid therapy include:
    - Aluminum hydroxide gels: constipation, phosphorus depletion with chronic use
    - Calcium carbonate: constipation or diarrhea, hypercalcemia, milk-alkali syndrome, renal calculi
    - Magnesium preparations: diarrhea, hypermagnesemia
    - Sodium preparations: milk-alkali syndrome when used with large amounts of calcium; use with caution with patients on sodium restrictions
  - Anticholinergic: used occasionally to decrease cholinergic/vagal stimulation of hydrochloric acid
  - Cytoprotectives: sucralfate (Carafate)
  - Other medications: tricyclic antidepressants (e.g., imipramine [Tofranil] and doxepin [Sinequan]) and SSRIs contribute to pain relief and reduced acid secretion

Special Considerations

NURSING CARE OF THE PATIENT WITH A GASTROSTOMY OR JEJUNOSTOMY TUBE
- Patients who have had extensive gastric surgery or who require long-term enteral feedings to maintain nutrition may have a gastrostomy or jejunostomy tube inserted. Special care of the ostomy insertion site should include:
  - Tube placement assessment: Aspirate stomach contents and check the gastric aspirate. Intestinal aspirate generally presents a pH of 7 or higher while a gastric aspirate presents as a pH of 5 or less. (Auscultation is ineffective in determining feeding tube placement.)
  - Tube insertion site cleansing: Clean around tube with prescribed cleansing solution every shift and as needed. Report changes in the insertion site, drainage, or lack of healing.
  - Abdominal assessment: Assess for distention, bowel sounds, and tenderness to evaluation functioning of the GI tract.
  - Tube site care: Use sterile technique until healing is complete. Clean technique is appropriate after the site heals because the GI tract is not a sterile environment. Clean technique includes removal of old dressing, site cleansing with soap and water and thorough rinsing; apply skin barrier as needed to prevent peristomal skin excoriation and tape tube to skin or skin barrier with hypoallergenic tape. If using gauze pads to redress the site, do not cut them because threads may enter the wound, causing irritation and increasing the risk of inflammation.
  - Irrigate the tube with 30 to 50 mL of water, and clean the tube inside and out as ordered. Soft gastric tubes may require cleaning of the inner lumen with a special brush to maintain patency.
  - Provide patient mouth care or teach patient to perform self-care to stimulate saliva production and lubrication to mucous membranes.
  - Teach patient and family the long-term care of the tube. Refer to a home health agency or visiting nurse for support and reinforcement of learning.

Follow-up

EXPECTED OUTCOMES
- PUD can recur even after surgery. If the patient is willing to make required lifestyle adjustments, a successful rehabilitation is more likely.

COMPLICATIONS
- Acute exacerbation with bleeding, increased pain and discomfort, nausea, and vomiting
- Gastric outlet obstruction
- Perforation of GI mucosa with life-threatening bleeding and peritonitis.
- Surgery for PUD is uncommon due to currently available antisecretory medications. Surgical procedures include the Billroth I procedure (subtotal gastric resection with gastroduodenostomy anastomosis) or the Billroth II procedure (subtotal gastric resection with gastrojejunostomy anastomosis), vagotomy (partial or complete severing of the vagus nerve), or pyloroplasty (surgical enlargement of the pyloric sphincter to facilitate the easy passage of contents from the stomach). After surgery the gastric aspirate is observed for color, amount, and odor. The color is expected to be bright red

with a gradual darkening with the first 24 hours and changes to yellow-green within 36 to 48 hours. If the nasogastric (NG) tube becomes clogged during this time, the healthcare provider may order periodic gentle irrigations with normal saline solution. It is essential that the NG suction is working and the tube remains patent to avoid strain on the anastomosis. This can lead to stomach distention and result in rupture of the sutures, leakage of gastric contents into the peritoneal cavity, hemorrhage, and possible abscess formation. If the tube must be replaced or repositioned, the surgeon will do so, not the nurse.

- The nurse assesses bowel sounds for decreased peristalsis and lower abdominal discomfort that may indicate intestinal obstruction. Accurate intake and output records must be kept. Vital signs are monitored and recorded every 4 hours. The patient should be kept comfortable and free of pain with prescribed drugs and frequent position changes. If open surgery was performed, the incision is relatively high in the epigastrium and may interfere with deep breathing and coughing measures. The nurse should encourage splinting the area with a pillow to promote coughing, deep breathing, and protection of the suture line.
- Observe the dressing for signs of bleeding or odor and drainage indicative of infection. Encourage early ambulation. Maintain NG suction and IV therapy. When fluids are well tolerated, the tube is removed and fluids are increased with a slow progression to regular foods.
- Pernicious anemia may be a long-term complication of gastrectomy due to the loss of intrinsic factors produced by the parietal cells. The patient my require cobalamin (vitamin B12) replacement therapy.

COMMON POST-OP GI SURGERY COMPLICATIONS

- Dumping syndrome: Approximately one-third to one-half of patients experience dumping syndrome after PUD surgery because removal of a large portion of the stomach and the pyloric sphincter results in a large bolus of hypertonic fluid entering the intestine and fluid being drawn into the bowel lumen. This creates a decrease in plasma volume along with distention of the bowel lumen and rapid intestinal transit. Symptoms occur at the end of a meal or within 15 to 30 minutes after eating. The patient reports overall weakness, sweating, palpitations, and dizziness. Also, the patient reports abdominal cramps, borborygmi (loud bowel sounds produced by hyperactive intestinal peristalsis), and the urge to defecate. These indicators usually last for no longer than an hour after meals.
- Dumping syndrome therapy: The patient should be advised not to overload the stomach, eat six small meals a day, reduce drinking to no more than 4 ounces of fluids with a meal, wait at least 30 minutes after a meal to drink additional fluids, and eat low-carbohydrate meals with moderate protein and fat content. The amount of time these restrictions should be followed varies according to the patient's clinical condition and progress.

GASTRITIS

Description

- Gastritis is an inflammation of the gastric mucosa. It may be acute or chronic and may be diffused or localized. Gastritis results from a breakdown in the normal gastric mucosal barrier, which normally protects the stomach tissue from autodigestion by hydrochloric acid (HCl) and the enzyme pepsin. When the barrier is broken, HCl diffuses back into the mucosa. The acid back-diffusion results in tissue edema, disruption of capillary walls with plasma lost into the gastric lumen, and possible hemorrhage.

Etiology

- Causes of gastritis are drugs, diet, microorganisms, pathophysiologic conditions, environmental and other factors. For example:
  - Drugs: aspirin, corticosteroids, NSAIDs
  - Diet: alcohol; spicy, irritating food
  - Microorganisms: *H. pylori,* Salmonella, Staphylococcus
  - Pathophysiologic conditions: burns, large hiatal hernia, physiologic stress, reflux of bile and pancreatic secretions, renal failure (uremia), sepsis, shock
  - Environmental factors: radiation, smoking
  - Other: endoscopic procedures, nasogastric suction, psychologic stress
- Autoimmune atrophic gastritis is a form of chronic gastritis that affects both the fundus and the body of the stomach and is associated with an increased risk of gastric cancer.

Incidence and Demographics

- Gastritis is one of the most common problems affecting the GI tract.

Risk Factors

- See Etiology above.

Prevention and Screening

- Eliminating the cause and preventing or avoiding it in the future is generally all that is needed to treat acute gastritis.

Assessment

HISTORY
- Assess ingestion or presence of risk factors.

PHYSICAL EXAM
- Perform a thorough GI assessment and history. Clinical manifestations include anorexia, nausea and vomiting, epigastric tenderness, and a feeling of fullness. Hemorrhage is commonly associated with alcohol abuse and at times may be the only symptom.
- Chronic gastritis manifestations are similar to those of acute gastritis. See below.

DIAGNOSTIC STUDIES
- Diagnosis of acute gastritis is most often based on a history of drug and alcohol use. The diagnosis of chronic gastritis may be delayed or completely missed because symptoms are nonspecific.

- Endoscopic examination with biopsy to obtain a definitive diagnosis.
- Breath, urine, serum stool, or gastric tissue biopsy and analysis for *H. pylori*.
- Complete blood count (CBC) to assess for anemia from blood loss or lack of intrinsic factor.
- Stools tested for occult blood.
- Gastric analysis to determine achlorhydria associated with sever atrophic gastritis.
- Serum test for antibodies to parietal cells and intrinsic factor (IF).

Nursing Management

- The plan of care is supportive and similar to care needed for nausea and vomiting.
- Clear liquids are resumed when acute symptoms have subsided, with gradual reintroduction of solid, bland foods.

NONPHARMACOLOGIC TREATMENT

- During the acute phase of gastritis, bed rest and nothing by mouth (NPO) status is implemented; in severe cases, a nasogastric (NG) tube may be used, either for lavage of the precipitating agent from the stomach or with suctioning to keep the stomach empty and free of noxious stimuli.

PHARMACOLOGIC TREATEMENT

- IV fluids may be prescribed to replace fluids and electrolytes lost through vomiting and occasional diarrhea.
- Antiemetics often are given for nausea and vomiting.
- Antacids are used for relief of abdominal discomfort, and H2-histamine receptor (H2R) blockers (e.g., ranitidine [Zantac], cimetidine [Tagamet]) or proton pump inhibitors (PPIs; e.g., omeprazole [Prilosec], lansoprazole [Prevacid]) will reduce gastric acid (HCl) secretion.

Special Considerations

- Treatment of chronic gastritis focuses on evaluation and elimination of the specific cause. To eradicate *H. pylori* infection, antibiotics are used. For the patient with pernicious anemia, lifelong injections of cobalamin are needed. Some patients have no symptoms directly associated with the gastric lesion.
- When the acid-secreting cells are lost or do not function as a result of atrophy, the source of intrinsic factor is lost and cobalamin (vitamin B12) cannot be absorbed in the ileum, resulting in pernicious anemia.

Follow-up

EXPECTED OUTCOMES

- Acute gastritis is self-limiting, lasting from a few hours to a few days, with complete healing of mucosa expected.
- The patient with chronic gastritis may have to adapt to lifestyle changes and strictly adhere to medication regimens.

COMPLICATIONS

- An interdisciplinary team approach in which the physician, nurse, dietitian, and pharmacist provide consistent information and support may increase patient success in making needed lifestyle changes to control chronic gastritis.

IRRITABLE BOWEL SYNDROME (IBS)

Description
- IBS is a chronic functional disorder characterized by intermittent and recurrent abdominal pain and stool pattern irregularities. It is classified as IBS with diarrhea, IBS with constipation, or IBS with mixed diarrhea and constipation.

Etiology
- Unknown. Stimulation of visceral afferent fibers by the presence of stool or gas in the GI tract, resulting in perception of discomfort or pain.

Incidence and Demographics
- IBS is a common problem occurring in approximately 10% to 15% of the Western population. In the United States, approximately 2 to 2.5 times as many women as men seek health care for IBS.

Risk Factors
- Stress, psychological factors, prior gastroenteritis, and specific food intolerances.

Prevention and Screening
- For some patients, psychologic factors such as depression, anxiety, and posttraumatic stress disorder play a role in the pathophysiology of IBS.
- Encourage the patient to verbalize concerns to a trusted healthcare provider.

Assessment

HISTORY
- Abdominal pain, distention, excessive flatulence, bloating, a continual defecation urge, urgency, and sensation of incomplete evacuation.

PHYSICAL EXAM
- No specific physical exam findings. Extraintestinal findings in women include migraine headache, insomnia, fibromyalgia. Men are less likely to admit symptoms or seek help for symptoms.

DIAGNOSTIC STUDIES
- Diagnosis is made based on history of the above symptoms, past health history of psychosocial factors such as physical or sexual abuse, family history, and drug and diet history. Diagnostic tests are selectively used to rule out more serious disorders with similar symptoms such as colorectal cancer, peptic ulcer disease, inflammatory bowel disease, and malabsorption disorder (e.g., celiac disease).
- Standardized criteria for IBS (Rome criteria) include:
  - Abdominal discomfort or pain for at least 12 weeks within 12 months that has at least two of the following characteristics: 1) relieved with defecation, 2) change in stool frequency, and 3) change in stool appearance.

Nursing Management

- Establish a trusting relationship and encourage patient to verbalize concerns and anxiety.
- Encourage patient to keep diary of symptoms, diet, and episodes of stress to help identify factors that seem to trigger the IBS symptoms.
- Teach about diet high in fiber and elimination of gas-producing foods (e.g., broccoli, cabbage) and to substitute yogurt for milk products to help determine whether lactose intolerance is causing symptoms.
- Instruct patient that high fiber ingestion can increase IBS symptoms of bloating and gas pain, at least initially.

  NONPHARMACOLOGIC TREATMENT
  - Diet containing at least 20 g per day of dietary fiber or bulking agent such as Metamucil
  - Other therapies: cognitive-behavioral therapy, relaxation and stress management techniques, acupuncture, hypnosis

  PHARMACOLOGIC TREATMENT
  - Bulk-forming laxatives, antispasmodic agents (e.g., dicyclomine [Bentyl]) before meals to decrease pain associated with food ingestion. However, this drug has anticholinergic side effects which may limit its use.
  - For diarrhea, loperamide (Imodium), a synthetic opioid to decrease GI transit time and enhance GI water absorption and sphincter tone.
  - For IBS-related constipation: lubiprostone (Amitza).

Special Considerations

- For women with severe IBS and diarrhea who have not responded to other IBS therapies: alosetron (Lotronex), an antidiarrheal only available through physicians registered with the manufacturer.

Follow-up

EXPECTED OUTCOMES
- No single therapy has been found to be effective for all patients with IBS.

COMPLICATIONS
- Patients may experience severe constipation and ischemic colitis. Report immediately the occurrence of abdominal pain and blood in stool.

LARGE INTESTINE POLYPS AND COLORECTAL CANCER

Description

- Polyps arise from the mucosal surface of the colon and project into the lumen; all are considered abnormal and should be removed. Some are flat and broad-based while others are pedunculated or stalk-like. Most are asymptomatic but may present as rectal bleeding and with occult blood in the stool.

- Familial adenomatous polyposis (FAP), a rare genetic disorder, presents as multiple (thousands) of polyps and presents an 80% lifetime risk of developing colorectal cancer. These patients also develop cancer at younger than 40 years of age. Children of patients with FAP should be screened at puberty and then annually. Total colectomy with ileostomy is the treatment of choice.
- Colorectal cancer: Adenocarcinoma is the most common type and begins as a polyp arising from the colon and rectum mucosal lining. As it grows, it becomes invasive and penetrates the muscularis mucosae; tumor cells gain access to the regional lymph nodes and vascular system and can spread to distant sites.

Etiology
- See above.

Incidence and Demographics
- Colorectal cancer is the third most common form of cancer and the second leading cause of cancer-related deaths in the United States. It has a slow onset and symptoms do not appear until the disease is quite advanced; it is more common in men than women. Mortality rates are highest among Black men and women. About 90% of new cases are detected in persons over age 50 and about 25% occur in patients with a family history. Hereditary diseases, such as FAP, account for only about 5% to 10% of cases. Hereditary nonpolyposis colorectal cancer (HNPCC) syndrome (also known as Lynch syndrome) is the most common inherited form of hereditary colorectal cancer.

Risk Factors
- Increasing age
- Family history in a first-degree relative or personal history
- Colorectal polyps
- Inflammatory bowel disease (IBD) for more than 10 years
- FAP or HNPCC
- Obesity (BMI over 30 kg/m^2)
- Diet high in animal fat (e.g., more than 7 servings per week of red meat)
- Cigarette use
- Alcohol (over 4 drinks/wk)

Prevention and Screening
- Changes in stool consistency unrelated to dietary changes should be assessed for colon polyps/cancer.
  - Colonoscopy every 10 years starting at age 50. Colonoscopy is the gold standard for screening of the entire colon, during which biopsies can be obtained and polyps can be immediately removed and sent to the lab for histologic examination. Screening for high-risk patients should begin before age 50.
  - Digital rectal exam (DRE) and fecal occult blood test (FOBT) with annual exam. All positive tests are followed up with a colonoscopy.
  - Modify relevant risk factors. Physical exercise and a diet with large amounts of fruits, vegetables, and grains may decrease risk. NSAIDs (e.g., aspirin) may decrease risk.

Assessment

HISTORY

- Family or personal history of breast or ovarian cancer, FAP, villous adenoma, adenomatous polyps, IBD
- Use of medications affecting bowel function (e.g., cathartics, antidiarrheal drugs)
- Weakness or fatigue
- Diet patterns: high-calorie, high-fat, low-fiber diet, anorexia, weight loss, nausea and vomiting
- Elimination pattern: any change in bowel habits; alternating diarrhea and constipation; defecation urgency; rectal bleeding; mucoid stools; black, tarry stools; increased flatus; decrease in stool caliber; feeling of incomplete evacuation; abdominal or low back pain; tenesmus

PHYSICAL EXAM

- Clinical manifestations are usually non-specific or do not appear until the disease is advanced.
- General head-to-toe assessment for pallor (anemia), cachexia, lymphadenopathy (later signs).
- GI: Assess for palpable abdominal mass, distention, ascites, hepatomegaly, rectal bleeding, alternating constipation and diarrhea, change in stool caliber (narrow, ribbonlike).

DIAGNOSTIC STUDIES

- Digital rectal exam (DRE) and fecal occult blood test (FOBT)
- Barium enema
- Sigmoidoscopy
- Colonoscopy
  - Once colonoscopy and tissue biopsies confirm colorectal cancer, additional lab studies are done:
    - CBC (to assess for anemia)
    - Liver function tests (may or may not verify metastasis)
    - MRI, CT scan of abdomen, and/or ultrasound to detect extent of disease and metastasis
    - Carcinoembryonic antigen (CEA) test (helpful to assess recurrence after surgery or chemotherapy)

Nursing Management

- In the hospitalized patient, the nurse will assist in precolonoscopy preparation such as bowel cleansing with 24 hours of clear liquids only and using one of the oral preparations such as polyethylene glycol (PEG) lavage solutions (e.g., GoLYTELY) or sodium phosphate liquid or pills. Patients may find the GoLYTELY preps challenging to drink all the required amounts, experience nausea and bloating. With the sodium phosphate pills, risks exist for fluid and electrolyte imbalance in patients with heart, kidney, and/or liver disease.
- Advise the patient with diabetes to consult with his or her physician about medication adjustment to prevent hyperglycemia or hypoglycemia resulting from the dietary modification required in preparing for the colonoscopy.
- Instruct all patients, especially the elderly, to maintain adequate fluid, electrolyte, and caloric intake while undergoing bowel cleansing.

- Special precautions must be taken for some patients. Implantable defibrillators and pacemakers are at high risk of malfunction if electrosurgical procedures (i.e., polypectomy) are performed in conjunction with colonoscopy. A cardiologist should be consulted before the test is performed and the defibrillator should be turned off. Careful patient monitoring during the procedure is required.
- Nursing diagnoses related to colorectal cancer include:
  - Diarrhea or constipation related to altered bowel elimination patterns
  - Acute pain related to difficulty in passing stools because of partial or complete obstruction
  - Fear related to diagnosis of cancer and accompanying therapies, and possible terminal disease
  - Ineffective coping related to cancer diagnosis and treatment side effects

Pre-op care priorities
- Provide information about prognosis and future screening and support in dealing with the diagnosis.
- Prepare patients for ostomy care. All nurses working with patients who have ostomies should advocate for the patient to receive information about and to discuss a) sexual dysfunction if this is a complication of the patient's surgery; b) practical stoma care techniques; and c) issues surrounding social interaction, employment, body image, and sexuality. When an enterostomal therapist (ET nurse) is available, work together to address all these discussion areas.
- If an abdominal perineal resection is planned, provide intense emotional support to cope with prognosis and extreme change in body appearance and function. Also teach side-to-side positioning and proper sitting for taking a sitz bath. Sitting on a toilet is discouraged until the perineal wound is well healed.

Post-op care priorities
- See colostomy care under Special Considerations below.
- Wound care: After abdominal perineal resection, alert all care personnel to avoid rectal temperatures, suppository use, or other procedure that could damage sutures.
- Assess and provide meticulous care for the patient who has open and packed wounds. Examine the wound regularly and record bleeding, excessive drainage, and unusual odor. The perineal wound is usually irrigated with normal saline when the dressing is changed several times a day. Aseptic technique is always used. Reinforce abdominal dressing and change frequently to keep it clean and dry. Assess all drainage for amount, color, and consistency. The drainage is usually serosanguineous. The packing generally stays in place for 2 to 3 days; longer times may result in sepsis and cavity rigidity and deter healing.
- Assess skin at drain sites and the suture line for inflammation and keep it clean and dry. Report fever and elevated WBC counts. For an unclosed perineal wound, patient care may include warm sitz baths at 100.4° F to 106° F for 10 to 20 minutes three to four times a day to assist in tissue debridement, provide comfort, and increase circulation to the area.
- Assess for phantom pain and be very careful to differentiate phantom sensations from perineal abscess pain. For pain and itching around the wound, administer antipruritic agents as ordered.

NONPHARMACOLOGIC TREATMENT

Invasive procedures:

- Surgical therapy for polyps: Laser photocoagulation can be performed endoscopically to destroy small tumors, provide palliation for advanced tumors to remove obstruction, and is useful for patients who cannot tolerate major surgery.
- Colorectal cancer surgery: Location of the rectal lesion determines the surgical procedure. The optimal procedure is bowel resection with reanastomosis of the remaining segment.
- Abdominal-perineal resection is performed when the cancer is located within 5 cm of the anus and results in two wounds and a stoma. This procedure is very extensive and involves an abdominal incision through which the proximal sigmoid is brought through the abdominal wall to form a permanent colostomy. The distal sigmoid, rectum and anus are removed through a perineal incision which may be closed around a drain or left open with packing to allow healing by granulation. Complication risk is high and can include delayed wound healing, hemorrhage, persistent perineal sinus tracts, infections, and urinary tract and sexual dysfunction.
- Radiation therapy: May be used postoperatively as an adjuvant to surgery and chemotherapy or as a palliative measure for patients with metastatic cancer. The purpose of radiation is to reduce tumor size and provide symptomatic relief.

PHARMACOLOGIC TREATMENT

- Chemotherapy: When a patient has positive lymph nodes or metastatic disease, chemotherapy is used as an adjuvant therapy following colon resection and a primary treatment for nonresectable colorectal cancer. First-line agents are 5-fluorouracil (5-FU) plus leucovorin and irinotecan (Camptosar).
- Biologic and targeted therapy: Monoclonal antibodies cetuximab (Erbitux) and panitumumab (Vectibix) target epidermal growth factor receptor. Another drug, bevacizumab (Avastin), prevents the formation of new blood vessels (angiogenesis).

Special Considerations

- Colostomy care: Ostomies are described according to location and type and include the ileostomy, transverse, and sigmoid. The stool consistency from the bowel through the stoma will depend on the location of the ostomy and can range from liquid, to semiliquid in the ascending colon, to formed if passing from the sigmoid area.
- An ileostomy will drain continually and a bag must be worn at all times to collect drainage. A sigmoid ostomy drainage will resemble normal formed stool and some patients are able to regulate emptying time so they do not need to wear a collection bag.
- The major types of ostomies are end stoma, loop ostomy, and double-barreled:
  - An end stoma is constructed by dividing the bowel and bringing out the proximal end as a single stoma. If the remaining (distal) end is left in place, it is oversewn (Hartmann's pouch) and at times is reanastomosed and the stoma closed (takedown).
  - A loop stoma is usually temporary and is constructed by bringing a bowel loop to the abdominal surface and then point the anterior loop wall to allow for fecal passage. There is one stoma with a proximal and distal opening and intact posterior wall that separates the two openings. The bowel loop generally is held in place with a plastic rod for 7 to 10 days to prevent slippage back into the abdominal cavity.
  - A double-barreled stoma presents with two separate stomas. The distal colon is not removed but bypassed, and the proximal stoma is functional and diverts feces to the abdominal wall. The distal stoma, also called the mucous fistula, expels mucus from the distal colon.

GUIDELINES FOR IRRIGATING A COLOSTOMY

- Purpose: To empty the colon of feces, gas, or mucus, cleanse the lower intestinal tract, and establish a regular pattern of bowel elimination so that normal life activities may be pursued.
- Time of day: Select time for irrigation to match the patient's post-hospital pattern of elimination. Most often this is after a meal.
- Assemble needed supplies to include irrigating sleeve and belt. Irrigation container with 500 mL to 1500 mL of lukewarm tap water to hang 18 to 20 inches above the stoma (shoulder height). Assist patient to be seated on the toilet. Remove the dressing or pouch, apply an irrigating sleeve to the stoma. Place the end of the sheath in the commode. Continue with the following basic steps:
    1. Prime the irrigating catheter. Lubricate the catheter/cone and gently insert it into the stoma no more than 3 inches. Hold the shield/cone gently but firmly against the stoma to prevent backflow of water. Never force the catheter.
    2. Allow the lukewarm water to slowly enter the colon. If cramping occurs, clamp off the tubing and allow the patient to rest before continuing. Irrigation should continue over a 5- to 10-minute period.
    3. Hold the cone/shield in place 10 seconds after the water has been instilled, then gently remove it.
    4. Allow 10 to 15 minutes for most of the return; then dry the bottom of the sleeve/sheath and attach it to the top, or apply the appropriate clamp to the bottom of the sleeve.
    5. Leave the sheath in place for 30 to 45 minutes while the patient gets up and moves around.
    6. Cleanse the area with a mild soap and water; pat the area dry.
    7. Replace the colostomy dressing or appliance.
    8. Instruct patient to burp the bag when gas accumulates and to empty the bag when it becomes no more than half full.
- Include a close family member in the teaching for the patient's care when possible. Other patient teaching aspects of colostomy care include:
    - Provide a supportive environment and caring attitude to promote the patient's adaptation to the changes brought about by the surgery. Explore community resources such as home health nursing to assist in the transition to home care. Many patients need a home health care referral and the telephone number of the local chapter of the American Cancer Society.
    - Provide very specific directions about when to call the physician. Patients need to know which complications require prompt attention (i.e., bleeding from the colostomy wound, abdominal distention and rigidity, diarrhea, fever, wound drainage, disruption of suture line).
    - Explain if radiation therapy is planned, the possible side effects of anorexia, vomiting, diarrhea, and exhaustion.
    - Address patient concerns about odor or leakage from the pouch. Teach gas-forming foods to avoid.
    - Encourage the patient to discuss feelings about body image, sexuality, and sexual function.
    - Assist the patient in connecting with community resources to obtain needed ostomy supplies when discharge is planned.

Follow-up

EXPECTED OUTCOMES

- Prognosis and treatment correlate with pathologic staging. The preferred classification system is the tumor, node, metastasis (TNM) staging system of the American Joint Committee on Cancer. Prognosis worsens with greater size and depth of tumor, lymph node involvement, and metastasis.
- Polypectomy during colonoscopy can be curative if the cancer is contained within the polyps. If the cancer is localized, meaning there is no lymphatic or blood vessel involvement, colon resection with remaining cancer-free ends sewn back together can be curative. Radiation or chemotherapy is used if the cancer has spread to lymph nodes or into nearby tissue. Once the cancer has spread to distant sites, surgery is palliative.

COMPLICATIONS

- Colorectal cancer most commonly spreads to regional lymph nodes, liver, lungs, and peritoneum. From the liver, the cancer spreads to the lungs, bones, and brain. The growing tumor can obstruct the bowel. Other complications include bleeding, perforation, peritonitis, and fistula formation.

INFLAMMATORY BOWEL DISEASE (IBD)

Description

- Crohn's disease and ulcerative colitis are immunologically related disorders that are referred to as inflammatory bowel disease (IBD). Both diseases present with chronic inflammation of the intestine with periods of remission and exacerbation. Both diseases have much in common and in about one-third of the cases, a clear differentiation cannot be made between the two.

Etiology

- The cause is unknown and there is no cure. IBD is an autoimmune disorder believed to have a genetic influence. The normal inflammatory response is altered in patients with IBD.

Incidence and Demographics

- Both ulcerative colitis and Crohn's disease commonly occur during the teenage years and early adulthood, with a second peak around age 60 years. IBD is about four times more common among Whites compared with other racial groups and has the highest incidence among the Ashkenazi Jewish people and those of middle European origin.

Risk Factors

- Family history, altered immune response history, and lifestyle factors such as smoking.

Prevention and Screening

- Both ulcerative colitis and Crohn's disease present with many of the same symptoms; diarrhea, bloody stools, weight loss, abdominal pain, fever, and fatigue. However, the pattern of inflammation is different for the two diseases. In Crohn's disease, the inflammation involves all layers of the bowel wall and can occur anywhere in the GI tract from the mouth to the anus, but most commonly affects the terminal ileum and colon. Segments of normal bowel can be seen between diseased portions, the so-called skip lesions. The inflammation goes through the entire wall. Ulcerative colitis usually starts in the rectum and moves in a continual fashion toward the cecum and is considered a disease of the colon and rectum. Ulcerative colitis spreads in a continuous pattern; ulcerations occur in the mucosal layer, the innermost layer of the bowel wall.

Assessment

HISTORY
- Family history of ulcerative colitis, fatigue, malaise, infection, autoimmune disorders
- Medications used: antidiarrheals; see Prevention and Screening above

PHYSICAL EXAM
- GI system: nausea, vomiting, anorexia, weight loss, abdominal distention, hyperactive bowel sounds, abdominal cramps
- Elimination: observe stools for obvious and occult blood; report grossly bloody stools (hematochezia) may indicate hemorrhage and require emergency surgery; diarrhea, mucus, or pus in stools
- Other: intermittent fever, emaciated appearance, fatigue, pale skin with poor turgor, dry mucous membranes, skin lesions, anorectal irritation, skin tags, cutaneous fistulas
- Cardiovascular: tachycardia, hypotension
- Possible lab findings: anemia; leukocytosis; electrolyte imbalance; hypoalbuminemia; vitamin and trace metal deficiencies; guaiac-positive stool; abnormal sigmoidoscopic, colonoscopic, and/or barium enema findings

DIAGNOSTIC STUDIES
- CBC, erythrocyte sedimentation rate, genetic studies, serum chemistries, testing of stool for occult blood and infection, capsule endoscopy, barium contrast radiologic studies, sigmoidoscopy and colonoscopy with biopsy. Serum albumin may be decreased because of malabsorption, malnutrition, protein lost through intestinal lesions, and chronic inflammation. Folic acid and serum levels of most vitamins, including A, B complex, C, and the fat-soluble vitamins, often are decreased due to malabsorption.

Nursing Management
- Assess subjective and objective data acquired through history, physical exam, and diagnostic studies (above).
- Nursing goals for the IBD patient are that patient will
  - Experience a decrease in number and severity of acute exacerbations.
  - Maintain normal fluid and electrolyte balance.
  - Be free from pain or discomfort.
  - Comply with medical regimens.
  - Maintain nutritional balance.
  - Have improved quality of life.

SELECTED IMPLEMENTATIONS
- Maintain accurate intake and output records, noting number and appearance of stools.
- Support diarrhea control by performing actions to rest the bowel; encourage frequent, small feedings, adding bulk gradually to prevent bowel irritation. Teach to eliminate gas-forming and spicy foods and to eat low-fiber, high-protein, high-calorie diet to meet nutritional needs. Keep the patient clean, dry, and free of odor. Provide a deodorizer

in the room and ready access to a toilet. Meticulous perianal skin care using plain water (no harsh soap) is necessary to treat and prevent skin breakdown. Advocate for soothing compresses or prescribed ointment and sitz baths to reduce irritation and relieve anal discomfort.

- Teach stress management strategies. Encourage smokers to quit because smoking exacerbates Crohn's disease.
- Advocate for patient to receive psychotherapy if experiencing emotional problems. Inadequate coping mechanisms are sometimes due to early onset of the disease.
- Support sufficient rest periods to relieve and prevent fatigue. Plan activities around rest periods.

NONPHARMACOLOGIC
- High-calorie, high-vitamin, high-protein, low-residue, lactose-free diet (if lactase-deficient)

PHARMACOLOGIC
- Aminosalicylates (local anti-inflammation effect)
- Antimicrobials (prevent or treat infection; e.g., metronidazole [Flagyl], *ciprofloxacin* [Cipro], clarithromycin [Biaxin])
- Corticosteroids (anti-inflammation effect) p.o., or topical as suppository, foam, or enema and/or IV in severe cases
- Immunosuppressants (to suppress immune response; e.g., azathioprine [Imuran], cyclosporine)
- Biologic therapy (immunomodulator to suppress the cytokine tumor necrosis factor [TNF]; e.g., infliximab [Remicade])
- Antidiarrheals (decrease GI motility; e.g., diphenoxylate and atropine [Lomotil], loperamide [Imodium]); caution: When giving antidiarrheal medications to a patient with IBD, closely observe for manifestations of toxic megacolon: fever, tachycardia, hypotension, dehydration, abdominal pain and cramping, and an abrupt relief of diarrhea
- Hematinics and vitamins (e.g., ferrous sulfate, ferrous gluconate, iron dextran injection [Imferon cobalamin], zinc, folate) correct iron deficiency anemia and promote healing

Special Considerations
- About 75% of patients with Crohn's disease will require surgery to induce remissions, but recurrence rates are high. Approximately 25% to 40% of patients with ulcerative colitis will need surgery. Indications for surgical therapy for IBD include drainage of abdominal abscess, failure to respond to conservative therapy, fistulas, inability to decrease corticosteroids, intestinal obstruction, massive hemorrhage, perforation, severe anorectal disease, and suspicion of carcinoma. Surgery is reserved for emergency situations such as bleeding, obstruction, peritonitis or when medical treatment has failed.
- Surgical procedures to treat chronic ulcerative colitis include:
  - Total colectomy with ileoanal reservoir: These two procedures are performed approximately 8 to 12 weeks apart and usually result in a decreased number of bowel movements over a 24-hour period. The patient is able to control defecation at the anal sphincter.
  - Total proctocolectomy with permanent ileostomy: This is a one-stage operation. The terminal ileum is brought out to form the stoma (ostomy), usually in the right lower quadrant below the belt line. Continence is not possible.

- Total proctocolectomy with continent ileostomy (Kock pouch): The pouch acts as reservoir and is drained at regular intervals by insertion of a catheter. This procedure is rarely used today due to valve failure, leakage, and pouchitis.

EXPECTED OUTCOMES
- This is a chronic illness and patients usually experience exacerbations and remission of symptoms. Excellent teaching resources are available from the Crohn's and Colitis Foundation of America.

COMPLICATIONS
- Local (confined to the GI tract): hemorrhage (leading to anemia), strictures, perforation with possible peritonitis, fistulas, perineal abscess, and colonic dilation (if > 5 cm is called toxic megacolon). Patients with toxic megacolon are at risk for perforation and may need an emergency colectomy. Additionally, fat malabsorption, small bowel cancer (with Crohn's) and colorectal cancer (with ulcerative colitis).
- Systemic (extraintestinal): fever, anorexia, malaise, thromboembolism, kidney stones, sclerosing cholangitis, gallstones, and osteoporosis.

DIVERTICULOSIS AND DIVERTICULITIS

Description
- Diverticulosis and diverticulitis conditions are generally treated at home.
- Diverticulosis is the presence of diverticula, dilated sacs or outpouchings of the mucosa through the circular smooth muscle of the intestinal wall. Multiple **non**inflamed diverticula are present in diverticulosis. Diverticula are most commonly found in the sigmoid colon.
- The condition is diverticulitis when the diverticula become inflamed. The inflammatory process can spread to the surrounding area in the intestine.

Etiology
- The etiology of diverticulosis of the ascending colon is unknown. Diverticula in the sigmoid colon are associated with high luminal pressures from a deficiency in dietary fiber intake combined with a loss of muscle mass and collagen with the aging process.

Incidence and Demographics
- Diverticular disease is common. It affects 5% of the U.S. population by age 40 years and 50% by age 80 years.
- Approximately 15% of patients with diverticulosis progress at some point to acute diverticulitis.
- The disease is most prevalent in Western, industrialized populations that consume diets low in fiber and high in refined carbohydrates.
- The incidence of diverticulosis rises with increasing age and is associated with obesity in people under age 40.
- Men and women are equally affected.

Risk Factors
- Lack of dietary fiber
- Stool retention
- Bacteria in the diverticulum

Prevention and Screening

- Asymptomatic diverticular disease is typically diagnosed on routine sigmoidoscopy or colonoscopy.
- Diverticulitis presents with localized pain over the involved area of the colon. Additionally, fever, leukocytosis and sometimes a palpable mass is found.
- Elderly patients with diverticulitis may be afebrile, with a normal WBC count and little abdominal tenderness.

Assessment

HISTORY
- Most cases are asymptomatic.
- If symptoms are present, typically the patient reports abdominal pain or cramping, and/or changes in bowel habits, but no symptoms of inflammation.

PHYSICAL EXAM
- Assess bowel sounds, presence and location of abdominal tenderness or masses.
- Assess stool for occult blood.

DIAGNOSTIC STUDIES
- Physical examination, CBC, urinalysis, flat and upright x-rays of the abdomen.
- These are followed by ultrasound and CT scan with contrast to confirm diagnosis and evaluate the disease severity.
- A barium enema is done to determine narrowing or obstruction of the colon lumen.
- A colonoscopy may be performed to rule out polyps or lesions.
- A patient with acute diverticulitis should not have a barium enema or colonoscopy because of the possibility of perforation and peritonitis.

Nursing Management

- Teach the patient about the condition to promote understanding of the disease process and encourage adherence to the prescribed regimen to decrease risk of complications.
- Observe for peritonitis.
- Observe WBC.
- If the patient requires surgery and a colostomy is performed, the nursing care is the same as for these procedures.

NONPHARMACOLOGIC TREATMENT
- High-fiber, high-residue diet, mainly from grains and cereals, fruits and vegetables, and decreased intake of fat and red meat.
- Promote daily activity, weight reduction if obese.
- With acute diverticulitis, the goal is to allow the colon to rest and the inflammation to subside. The patient is kept NPO, on bed rest, and given parenteral fluids.

PHARMACOLOGIC TREATMENT
- In acute diverticulitis, broad-spectrum antibiotics are required. Pentazocine (Talwin) may be prescribed for relief of pain associated with diverticulitis because it causes less increase in colonic pressure than morphine or meperidine (Demerol).
- A stool softener such as docusate sodium (Colace) may be prescribed; however, laxatives are avoided to avoid further increase in intraluminal pressure in the colon.

Special Considerations
- Bowel rest and antibiotic therapy are usually adequate.
- Surgery is reserved for patients with complications such as an abscess or obstruction that cannot be managed medically. The usual surgical procedures involve resection of the involved colon with a primary anastomosis with bowel cleansing or a temporary diverting colostomy, which is re-anastomosed after the colon heals.

Follow-up

EXPECTED OUTCOMES
- Usually managed in outpatient settings

COMPLICATIONS
- Rare with diverticula
- Diverticulitis perforation can occur and result in peritonitis, a life-threatening condition
- Other possibilities:
  - Abscess and fistula formation
  - Bowel obstruction
  - Ureteral obstruction
  - Bleeding
- Diverticulitis is the most common cause of lower GI hemorrhage; although bleeding may be significant, it usually stops spontaneously

INTESTINAL OBSTRUCTION

Description
- This disorder occurs when intestinal contents cannot pass through the GI tract and requires prompt treatment because it is a potentially life-threatening condition.
- Obstructions may be partial or complete and some may resolve without surgery.
- The most dangerous obstruction is a strangulated bowel with the blood supply cut off. Without emergency surgery, the bowel will become necrotic and rupture, leading to massive infection and death.

Etiology
- Mechanical obstruction most often occurs in the small intestine and surgical adhesion is the most common cause.
- Obstruction can occur within days of surgery or several years later.
- Carcinoma, volvulus (twisted bowel), and diverticular disease can cause large bowel obstruction.
- Hernias and tumors also can precipitate obstruction.
- Nonmechanical obstruction may stem from paralytic (adynamic) ileus, lack of intestinal peristalsis (detectable by the absence of bowel sounds), peritonitis, acute pancreatitis, acute appendicitis, electrolyte abnormalities (especially hypokalemia), or thoracic or lumbar spinal fractures.

Pathology

- Bacteria flourish when the small bowel is obstructed and stimulate intestinal secretion of fluids into the bowel, leading to distention and rising intraluminal bowel pressure.
- Electrolyte-rich fluids cannot be absorbed and are lost into the peritoneal cavity.
- If the obstruction is high (e.g., pylorus), metabolic alkalosis results from the loss of gastric hydrochloric acid (HCl) through vomiting or NG intubation.
- Small bowel obstruction leads to rapid dehydration.
- With a large bowel obstruction, most GI fluids are absorbed before reaching the obstruction and solid fecal material accumulates until symptoms of discomfort appear.

Incidence and Demographics

- None available.

Risk Factors

- See Etiology above.

Prevention and Screening

- Close assessment of bowel sounds and patient reports of abdominal pain, nausea, and vomiting.
- Encourage early post-op ambulation to stimulate GI peristalsis.

Assessment

HISTORY

- See Etiology above.

PHYSICAL EXAM

Clinical manifestations can vary depending on obstruction location.

- (See Pathology above.) Bowel sounds may present as high-pitched above the obstruction, or may be absent. The patient may report borborygmi (audible abdominal sounds due to GI hypermotility).
- The patient may have a slight low-grade temperature elevation unless strangulation or peritonitis has occurred, at which time the temperature will rise.
- Small intestine obstructions present with rapid onset of clinical manifestations: frequent and large-volume vomiting; colicky, cramplike, intermittent pain; bowel movements for a short time; and greatly distended abdomen. Metabolic alkalosis may occur with vomiting.
- Large intestine obstructions present with a gradual onset of clinical manifestations: vomiting is rare, pain is low-grade and cramping, bowel movements cease, and abdomen is moderately distended. Metabolic acidosis may occur with loss of HCl through vomiting.

DIAGNOSTIC STUDIES

- Thorough history and physical
- Abdominal x-rays to assess for gas and fluid presence in intestine versus intraperitoneal spaces
- Barium enemas to locate large intestinal obstruction **if** perforation is not suspected
- Sigmoidoscopy or colonoscopy
- CT scan

- Lab tests
- CBC
- Serum electrolytes
- Amylase
- BUN
- An elevated WBC may indicate perforation or strangulation
- Stool assessment for occult blood

Nursing Management

- Assessment: detailed patient history and physical examination
  - Inspect abdomen for scars, visible masses and distention; palpate for muscle guarding, tenderness, rigidity; pain location, duration, intensity, and frequency.
  - Nausea and vomiting onset, frequency, color, odor, and amount
  - Bowel sounds and function and passage of flatus
  - Fluid and electrolyte balance, skin turgor, I&O hourly via urinary catheter. Immediately report hourly output less than 0.5 mL/kg of body weight (approximately less than 30 mL per hour), which could indicate potential for acute renal failure. Rising serum creatinine and BUN level are also manifestations of acute renal failure.
- Key nursing diagnoses include:
  - Acute pain
  - Deficient fluid volume
  - Imbalanced nutrition
- Goals are:
  - Relief of obstruction and return to normal bowel function
  - Minimal to no discomfort
  - Normal fluid and electrolyte status

  ### NONPHARMACOLOGIC TREATMENT
  - Provide comfort measures to promote a restful environment; keep distraction and visitors to a minimum.
  - Provide excellent post-op care, NG tube to decompress the bowel.

  ### PHARMACOLOGICTREATMENT
  - Pain medications
  - IV fluids to restore fluid volume and electrolytes (e.g., normal saline or lactated Ringer's), with addition of potassium to IV fluids after renal function is verified
  - Antiemetics

Special Considerations

- NG tube care:
  - Assess every 4 hours for patency.
  - Assess nares for irritation; clean and dry daily and apply water-soluble lubricant.
  - Apply new tape daily and when needed.
- Mouth care:
  - Encourage and assist the patient to brush teeth frequently.
  - Provide easy access to mouthwash and water for rinsing the mouth and petroleum jelly or water-soluble lubricant for the lips.

Follow-up

EXPECTED OUTCOMES

- See Goals above (under Nursing Management). Surgery may result in partial or total colectomy, colostomy, or ileostomy. Parenteral nutrition may be necessary in some cases to correct nutritional deficits.

COMPLICATIONS

- Small bowel obstruction: Hypovolemia and hypovolemic shock with multiple organ dysfunction; can lead to death. Acute renal failure and impaired pulmonary ventilation may occur.
- Large bowel obstruction: Increasing pressure within the obstructed colon impairs circulation to the bowel wall, making gangrene and perforation potential complications. Infection and recurring adhesions can result.

VIRAL HEPATITIS

Description

- Hepatitis is inflammation of the liver and may be acute or chronic. When chronic it may increase the risk for liver cancer. Liver tissue inflammation alters metabolism of nutrients, drugs, alcohol, and toxins as well as bile elimination.
- With mild cases (e.g., hepatitis A), the liver is not significantly damaged, while hepatitis B and C can result in severe liver damage.
- Hepatitis A is sometimes referred to as "infectious hepatitis," has an abrupt onset but typically is benign and self-limiting with few long-term consequences.
- Hepatitis B can cause acute hepatitis, chronic hepatitis, rapidly progressive hepatitis (fulminant), or a carrier state. Chronic hepatitis may cause few symptoms but is the primary cause of liver damage leading to cirrhosis, liver cancer, and liver transplantation.
- Note: Toxic hepatitis is caused by many substances. Common causes include alcohol, acetaminophen, benzene, carbon tetrachloride, halothane, chloroform, and poisonous mushrooms.

Etiology

- At least 5 viruses are known to cause hepatitis. In the United States, cases are primarily caused by hepatitis A, hepatitis B, and hepatitis C. The viruses initiate an immune response that causes inflammation and necrosis of hepatocytes.
- Three primary effects of liver damage are decreased liver cell function, impaired bilirubin conversion and excretion leading to jaundice, and interrupted liver blood flow with resulting portal hypertension.
- Comparison of types of viral hepatitis
  Type A Hepatitis (HAV)
  - Transmission mode: fecal-oral route, usually through food or fluid ingestion
  - Incubation period: 3 to 5 weeks
  - Onset: May be asymptomatic; highly contagious during the 2 weeks before the onset of jaundice
  - Prognosis: low mortality, recovery within a few weeks

Type B Hepatitis (HBV)
- Transmission mode: blood, percutaneous, and permucosal route; oral route via saliva or through breastfeeding; sexual activity via blood, semen, saliva, or vaginal secretions; gay men are at high risk
- Incubation period: 2 to 5 months
- Onset: insidious and prolonged
- Prognosis: mortality as high as 10%, with another 10% of patients progressing to carrier status or developing chronic hepatitis. Hepatitis B infection is responsible for about 20% of all liver cancers.

Type C Hepatitis (HCV)
- Transmission mode: blood or blood product transfusion; found among IV drug users and renal dialysis patients and personnel; sexual intercourse; contaminated piercing and tattooing tools
- Incubation period: 1 week to several months
- Onset: Symptoms usually occur 6 to 7 weeks after transfusion; occurs in all age groups; is the most common form of posttransfusion hepatitis
- Prognosis: Hepatitis C infection is responsible for about 50%–60% of all liver cancers

Type D Hepatitis (HDV, Delta Hepatitis)
- Transmission mode: occurs along with HBV or may superinfect a chronic HBV carrier; cannot outlast a hepatitis B infection; may be acute or chronic
- Mode of transmission and incubation are the same as for HBV
- Occurrence in the United States is primarily among IV drug abusers and multiply transfused patients; the highest incidence exists in the Mediterranean, Middle East, and South America.
- Prognosis: Mortality rate is extremely high, with rates as high as 50% of fulminant hepatitis

Type E Hepatitis (HEV)
- Transmission mode: Fecal-oral, but fecal detection is difficult
- Incubation is the same as for HAV
- Occurrence is primarily in India, Africa, Asia, and Central America and may be found in recent travelers to these areas; it is more common in young adults and more severe in pregnant women

Incidence and Demographics
- In the United States, the estimated number of viral hepatitis cases is much higher than the number of reported cases. Hepatitis A is somewhat more common than hepatitis B or hepatitis C. Reported cases of hepatitis A and B have declined since 2003.

Risk Factors
- See comparison of types above for at-risk behaviors that increase exposure to viral contact.

Prevention and Screening
- Emphasize to patients and families the relationship between liver disorders and alcohol and drug abuse. Teach patients to abstain from excessive alcohol ingestion and injection drug use, which increase the risk for contracting hepatitis B, C, and D.
- Vaccines: Hepatitis A and hepatitis B are preventable diseases. Vaccines and medications are available to prevent the disease following known or suspected exposure.
- Hepatitis A vaccine provides long-term immunity after the recommended two doses.

- Hepatitis B vaccine (also protects against hepatitis D) requires three doses and is recommended in high-risk groups such as persons on renal dialysis or otherwise immunocompromised. Nurses are considered a high-risk category due to blood and body fluid exposure and needle-stick risk.
- Combination hepatitis A and hepatitis B vaccine is available in three doses and recommended for high-risk groups. The three-dose schedule requires an initial dose followed by the second dose at least 4 weeks later and third dose 6 months later.
- Postexposure prophylaxis may be recommended for nonimmunized household or sexual contacts of people with hepatitis A or hepatitis B. Hepatitis A prophylaxis is available in a single-dose injection given within 2 weeks following exposure. Hepatitis B vaccine may be given at the same time.

Assessment

HISTORY
- Assess for risk factors as mentioned above.
- Current health status, including anorexia, nausea, vomiting, abdominal discomfort, changes in bowel elimination or color of stools, muscle or joint pain, and fatigue. No manifestations are present during the incubation period, so early manifestations may be few. When present, the liver appears enlarged and tender. A dull, aching pain in the RUQ may be present as well as weight loss, weakness, anorexia, and constipation or diarrhea.
- Although the extent of damage and immune response vary among the different hepatitis viruses, the disease itself follows a predictable pattern as described below.
- *Preicteric (prodromal) phase:* "flulike" symptoms (e.g., anorexia, malaise, fatigue, chills, fever, GI disturbances, muscle aches, polyarthritis, and mild right upper quadrant [RUQ] pain).
- *Icteric phase* (occurs 5 to 10 days later): jaundice (elevated serum bilirubin levels), pruritus (bile salts accumulate in skin), clay-colored stools, brown urine, and decrease in prodromal manifestations wherein the appetite may improve. Note: Patients with hepatitis C may not demonstrate jaundice, therefore remaining undiagnosed for a longer period of time.
- *Posticteric/convalescent phase:* lasts several weeks. Serum bilirubin and enzymes return to normal; energy level increases; pain and GI disturbances subside.

PHYSICAL EXAM
- See icteric phases noted above.
- General head-to-toe assessment, noting temperature, mucous membrane and sclera coloring for jaundice, abdominal enlargement and tenderness, color of stool and urine.

DIAGNOSTIC STUDIES
- Liver function studies: ALT, AST, ALP, and GGT all may be elevated in cirrhosis.
- LDH/LDH5 increases.
- CBC with platelets: Expected are decreased counts of WBC, RBC, hemoglobin, hematocrit, and platelets, and deficiencies of folic acid and vitamin B12.
- Coagulation studies: prolonged prothrombin time (PT).
- Serum electrolytes: Malnutrition-related findings are seen with hyponatremia, hypophosphatemia, and hypomagnesemia.

- Serum bilirubin levels: Increases seen in both direct (conjugated) and indirect (unconjugated) bilirubin.
- Serum viral antigen-antibody to identify the infecting virus.
- Liver biopsy may be done to rule out other forms of liver disease. Using ultrasound, a biopsy needle is inserted into the liver and guided to the pathologic site. Nursing management highlights for liver biopsy include:
  - Prep the patient; assure a signed consent form is in the chart. Keep NPO 4 to 6 hours prior to procedure. Assess baseline vital signs, PT, and platelet count; administer vitamin K as ordered. Assist patient to empty bladder just prior to procedure. Place patient in supine position on right side of bed; turn head to left and extend right arm above head.
  - During procedure: Coach the patient to take several deep breaths and on cue to exhale and hold his or her breath for 10 to 15 seconds while the physician inserts a needle and obtains the tissue sample. There may be some pain or discomfort during this time.
  - Postprocedure: Apply direct pressure to the site immediately after needle removal and place patient on his or her right side to maintain pressure.
  - Provide comfort measures. Teach patient that right shoulder pain may occur as the local anesthetic effect diminishes. Monitor for bleeding. Patient should avoid food or fluids for 2 hours, then resume usual diet. The patient should avoid coughing, lifting, or straining for 1 to 2 weeks.

Nursing Management

- Nursing care focuses on preventing spread of infection and supporting efforts for patient comfort and self-care. Selected nursing priorities are described below.
- Prevent spread of infection: Use standard precautions including careful handwashing, contact isolation if fecal incontinence is present (with hepatitis A and hepatitis E); avoid skin contact with blood and other body fluids.
- Promote adequate nutrition by encouraging a diet of high calories and adequate carbohydrates to spare protein metabolism. Supplements such as Ensure or instant breakfast drinks may be helpful to meet caloric needs. Limit fat intake and provide small, frequent meals at times when patient is least nauseated and anorexic, such as in the afternoon and evening. At all times alcoholic drinks must be avoided.
- Provide good skin care and emotional support needed when jaundice is present. Avoid overheating, do not rub skin, keep skin lubricated with alcohol-free lotions, and instruct patient to wear loose cotton garments that allow moisture to evaporate from the skin; keep nails short to prevent scratching.
- Plan care activities according to patient level of fatigue to allow for adequate patient rest and sense of well-being. After jaundice has cleared, gradual increase in physical activities. This may require many months.
- Inject vitamin K subcutaneously if prothrombin time is prolonged. Avoid trauma that may cause bruising; limit invasive procedures, if possible; and maintain adequate pressure on needle-stick sites.
- Administer antiemetics for nausea. Avoid phenothiazines, such as chlorpromazine (Thorazine), which have a cholestatic effect and my cause or worsen jaundice.

NONPHARMACOLOGIC TREATMENT
- See Nursing Management above.

PHARMACOLOGIC TREATMENT
• See vaccinations and prophylaxis above.

Special Considerations
• Food handlers or childcare workers who are diagnosed with hepatitis A must contact the local health department to report possible community exposure. Patient identification is kept confidential. Persons exposed to the virus must receive prophylactic treatment to prevent a local epidemic of hepatitis.

Follow-up

EXPECTED OUTCOMES
• When the hepatitis course is uncomplicated, spontaneous recovery may begin within 2 weeks of the onset of jaundice. In most cases, clinical recovery occurs within 3 to 16 weeks.

COMPLICATIONS
• Death and liver cancer can result from certain types of hepatitis. Stress the importance of keeping follow-up appointments for vaccinations and lab/diagnostic testing.

CIRRHOSIS

Description
• Cirrhosis is progressive and irreversible, and is the end stage of chronic liver disease. Alcoholic (Laënnec's) cirrhosis is the most common type. Other types include biliary cirrhosis and posthepatic cirrhosis. Malnutrition commonly occurs with alcoholic cirrhosis.

Etiology
• An unknown cause or viral exposure initially triggers the gradual destruction of liver tissue, development of fibrous scar tissue, and discontinuation of liver metabolic functions. Resulting restricted blood flow through the liver to the inferior vena cava leads to portal hypertension (increased pressure in the portal venous system).
• Alcoholic cirrhosis (Laënnec's): Metabolic changes occur in the liver and result in fatty infiltration of hepatocytes (fatty liver).
• Biliary cirrhosis: Refers to liver or biliary pathway obstruction resulting in bile damage and liver destruction.
• Posthepatic cirrhosis results from advanced liver disease caused by chronic hepatitis B or C or unknown cause. Many liver cells die, liver size decreases, and the organ becomes nodular and fibrotic.

Incidence and Demographics
• Overall, cirrhosis is the 12th leading cause of death in the United States, 6th leading cause of death in adults ages 25 through 64 years; death rates in men are double the rate in women.
• Native Americans (men and women) have the highest incidence and mortality rate from cirrhosis and chronic liver disease, followed by Hispanic men and women. Contributory factors may include socioeconomic factors associated with higher alcohol consumption, patterns of drinking (in place of meals), and variations in alcohol metabolism among compared populations.

Risk Factors

- Alcohol ingestion, injection drug use, and/or viral hepatitis. Increased occurrence in certain ethnic groups.

Prevention and Screening

- Emphasize to patients and families the relationship between liver disorders and alcohol and drug abuse. Teach patients to abstain from excessive alcohol ingestion and injection drug use, which increase the risk for contracting hepatitis B, C, and D, disorders that can lead to cirrhosis.
- Early manifestations may be few; when present, the liver appears enlarged and tender. A dull, aching pain in the RUQ may be present as well as weight loss, weakness, anorexia, and constipation or diarrhea. As the disease progresses, the following manifestations occur:
  - *Portal hypertension:* Blood is shunted to adjoining lower-pressure vessels and veins become engorged in the esophagus, rectum, and abdomen. Increased capillary hydrostatic pressure results in ascites.
  - *Splenomegaly* (enlarged spleen): This results from portal hypertension, the shunting of blood to the splenic vein, and leads to increased blood cell destruction. The patient becomes anemic, leukopenic, and thrombocytopenic.
  - *Ascites:* The accumulation of plasma-rich fluid in the abdominal cavity results from portal hypertension, decreased serum proteins (hypoalbuminemia), and increased aldosterone. Edema results.
  - *Esophageal varices:* Enlarged thin-walled esophageal veins are another result of portal hypertension and carry a very high risk of rupture and massive hemorrhage. Esophageal bleeding is a medical emergency and management of airway and prevention of aspiration of blood are critical factors.
  - *Portal systemic (hepatic) encephalopathy:* As liver tissue dies, ammonia is no longer converted to urea and it accumulates in the blood (along with other possible neurotoxins) and causes cerebral edema. Other contributing factors are constipation, blood transfusion, GI bleeding, hypoxia, high-protein diet, severe infection, and surgery. Medications that increase this risk are sedatives, tranquilizers, narcotic analgesics, and anesthetics.
  - An early sign of hepatic encephalopathy is asterixis (liver flap), a fine muscle tremor, inability to maintain a fixed position of the extremities, and resulting jerking movements. Body jerking is most commonly seen in the upper extremities, and may affect the tongue and feet. Asterixis is triggered when the patient is instructed to extend the arms and dorsiflex the wrists. If present, asterixis causes a downward flapping of the hands. Additionally, neurological changes are evident and progress to confusion, disorientation, and incoherence. Cerebral edema leads to increased intracranial pressure and hypoxia and results in death.
  - *Hepatorenal syndrome* may develop in patients with advanced cirrhosis and ascites. This syndrome, renal failure with azotemia, may be triggered by GI bleeding, aggressive diuretic therapy, or an unknown cause.
  - *Spontaneous bacterial peritonitis:* This life-threatening condition may develop without known peritoneal contaminants and worsens ascites by increasing ascitic fluid, abdominal pain, fever, and encephalopathy.

Assessment

HISTORY
- Current health status, history of gallbladder or liver disease, GI complaints and anorexia, recent weight loss, excessive bleeding or bruising, jaundice or pruritus, edema, altered libido or impotence. Note duration of all abnormal findings.

PHYSICAL EXAM
- General head-to-toe assessment, noting bowel sounds, abdominal girth, percussion for liver borders, palpation for tenderness and size, and altered mentation.

DIAGNOSTIC STUDIES
- Liver function studies: ALT, AST, ALP, and GGT may be elevated.
- CBC with platelets: Expected are decreased WBC, RBC, hemoglobin, hematocrit, platelets, and deficiencies of folic acid and vitamin B12.
- Coagulation studies: prolonged PT.
- Serum electrolytes: Malnutrition-related findings are seen with hyponatremia, hypophosphatemia, and hypomagnesemia.
- Bilirubin levels: Increases are seen in both direct (conjugated) and indirect (unconjugated) bilirubin.
- Serum albumin at lowered levels.
- Serum ammonia at elevated levels.
- Serum glucose and cholesterol levels are abnormal.
- Abdominal ultrasound to assess liver size, ascites, and nodules.
- Doppler studies to evaluate blood flow through the liver and spleen.
- Esophagoscopy to determine presence of esophageal varices.
- Liver biopsy may be done to rule out other forms of liver disease. Using ultrasound, a biopsy needle is inserted into the liver and guided to the pathologic site. Nursing management highlights for liver biopsy include:
  - Prep the patient; assure a signed consent form is in the chart. Keep NPO 4 to 6 hours prior to procedure. Assess baseline vital signs, PT, and platelet count; administer vitamin K as ordered. Assist patient to empty bladder just prior to procedure. Place patient in supine position on right side of bed; turn head to left and extend right arm above head.
  - During procedure: Coach the patient to take several deep breaths and on cue to exhale and hold his or her breath for 10 to 15 seconds while the physician inserts a needle and obtains the tissue sample. There may be some pain or discomfort during this time.
  - Postprocedure: Apply direct pressure to the site immediately after needle removal and place patient on his or her right side to maintain pressure. Provide comfort measures. Teach patient that right shoulder pain may occur as the local anesthetic effect diminishes. Monitor for bleeding. Patient should avoid food or fluids for 2 hours, then resume usual diet. The patient should avoid coughing, lifting, or straining for 1 to 2 weeks.

Nursing Management
- There are many challenges to caring for the patient with cirrhosis and coordinating care among the healthcare team. Selected priority nursing challenges and key interventions are listed below.

- **Excess fluid volume:** Daily care—Provide a low-sodium diet (500 mg to 2,000 mg/day). Restrict fluids as ordered. Monitor weight, jugular vein distention (if present), abdominal girth, peripheral edema, intake and output, and urine color/specific gravity as an indicator of hydration. Report immediately: oliguria, face and eye edema, rising serum creatinine and BUN levels. These are indicators of hepatorenal syndrome or acute renal failure.
- **Disturbed thought processes:** Assess neurologic status and report even slight changes in handwriting, speech, and asterixis. Provide low-protein diet. Promote regular bowel elimination to promote protein and ammonia elimination. Provide a calm environment to reduce agitation and anxiety.
- **Imbalanced nutrition** (less than body requirements): Weigh daily, provide small meals with between-meal snacks. Work with dietitian planning a diet that is adequate in calories and nutrients and appealing for an anorexic patient.
- *Risk for bleeding:* (Note: Clotting is affected by vitamin K deficiency, impaired synthesis of coagulation factors, and increased platelet destruction due to splenomegaly.) Assess for hypovolemia due to hemorrhage, monitor vital signs, report tachycardia or hypotension; institute bleeding precautions (avoid rectal temperatures or enemas, injections, blowing nose, hard-bristle toothbrush; prevent constipation. Monitor platelet count, PT, and aPPT and report out-of-range values.) Note: Be aware of risk for bleeding esophageal varices and immediately report hematemesis, hematochezia (bright blood in the stool) or tarry stools, and signs of hypovolemia or shock. During an episode of bleeding, management of the airway and prevention of aspiration of blood are critical factors.
- *Impaired skin integrity:* Bile salts may deposit on the skin and cause pruritus. Avoid hot water when bathing patient, apply emollient or lubricants to keep skin moist; do not rub the skin, teach patient not to scratch and to keep nails trimmed and rub with knuckles instead; reposition every 2 hours, use alternating pressure mattress. Apply antihistamines, if ordered, with great caution due to risk for altered drug responses.

NONPHARMACOLOGIC TREATMENT

- Nutritional care is directed at slowing cirrhosis progression to liver failure and reducing complications. The approach changes as hepatic function fluctuates. For example, restrictions are placed on sodium to under 2 g/day and fluids to 1,500 mL/day based on urine output, diuretic therapy, and serum electrolyte levels. Protein may be restricted or eliminated with acute hepatic encephalopathy, and limited to 60 g/day for chronic encephalopathy. When encephalopathy abates and serum ammonia levels stabilize, protein intake is allowed as tolerated.
- To promote healing, a diet high in calories and moderate fat is allowed. Parenteral nutrition is administered when food intake is limited.
- As needed, B-complex vitamins such as thiamin, folate, and B12, and the fat-soluble vitamins A, D, and E are administered, as well as magnesium supplements.
- Paracentesis is aspiration of fluid from the peritoneal cavity. It is done to diagnose or to relieve respiratory distress and abdominal discomfort from ascites when diuretic therapy is not effective. Ascites fluid ranging in amount from 500 mL to 6L of fluid daily may be removed. Salt-poor albumin IV may be administered to maintain intravascular volume during large-volume paracentesis. Nursing care priorities for paracentesis include:
  - Describe the procedure to the patient and family. The procedure involves abdominal site cleansing and local anesthesia, and a small incision to allow a trocar or needle insertion to withdraw fluid into a connecting tube and collection bottle. Specimens are sent to the lab.

- Assess baseline weight and vital signs; have patient void; assist patient to a seated position on bedside or chair with feet supported. Assess blood pressure during the procedure, which may take several minutes to over an hour to complete.
- After the needle is removed, there may be fluid leakage at the site, so apply a small dressing.
- Carefully monitor vital signs, noting blood pressure changes and respiratory response to the procedure.

PHARMACOLOGIC TREATMENT
- Several groups of drugs are commonly prescribed, with an avoidance of known hepatotoxic medications (e.g., acetaminophen). Medications provide supportive care only.
- Diuretics (e.g., spironolactone [Aldactone], furosemide [Lasix])
- Laxatives (e.g., lactulose [Cephulac, Chronulac]) reduce ammonia-producing bacteria and lower colon pH, thus promoting ammonia excretion in feces and increased number of bowel movements.
- Neomycin, a locally acting antibiotic that reduces the number of ammonia-forming bacteria in the bowel.
- Beta-blocker nadolol (Corgard) may be given with isosorbide mononitrate (Ismo, Imdur, Monoket) to decrease hepatic venous pressure and therefore esophageal bleeding risk.
- Ferrous sulfate and folic acid to treat anemia.
- Vitamin K to decrease bleeding risk; when bleeding is acute, packed RBCs, fresh frozen plasma, or platelets may be administered.
- Antacids.
- Systemic antibiotics to treat *H. pylori*.
- Oxazepam (Serax), a benzodiazepine and antianxiety/sedative drug not metabolized by the liver, may be used to treat agitation and restlessness.

Special Considerations
- Care for the patient with cirrhosis is challenging. It is best managed with holistic care to address psychosocial and spiritual needs as well as the physiologic changes. The family should be involved in the care, particularly if risk behaviors are involved.

Follow-up

EXPECTED OUTCOMES
- Cirrhosis is progressive and irreversible; it signifies the end stage of chronic liver disease, and eventually leads to death. Provide referrals for home health services, dietary consultation, social services, and counseling as needed for patient and family. Suggest local or online support groups when available. When appropriate, discuss hospice services.

COMPLICATIONS
- See Expected Outcomes above.
- If esophageal varices bleed, this presents a life-threatening situation and requires intensive care management.
- Liver transplantation is indicated for some patients with irreversible, progressive cirrhosis and requires intensive care management.

CHOLECYSTITIS

Description
- Cholecystitis (inflammation of the gallbladder) is usually associated with cholelithiasis (stones in the gallbladder). Cholecystitis may be acute or chronic. Cholecystectomy (removal of the gallbladder) is among the most common surgical procedures performed in the United States.

Etiology
- Cholecystitis is most commonly associated with obstruction caused by gallstones or biliary sludge. Acalculous cholecystitis also can occur with prolonged immobility and fasting, parenteral nutrition, and diabetes mellitus. It also can result from bacteria reaching the gallbladder via the vascular or lymphatic route or chemical irritants in the bile.
- Cholelithiasis: The actual cause is unknown but develops when the balance of cholesterol, bile salts, and calcium in solution is altered and precipitates occur. Conditions that upset this balance include infection and altered cholesterol metabolism.

Incidence and Demographics
- It is estimated that 8% to 10% of adults in the United States have cholelithiasis. The incidence is higher in women, multiparous women, and persons over 40 years of age. Postmenopausal women on estrogen therapy are at slightly greater risk than women who are taking birth control pills. Other correlated risk factors include a sedentary lifestyle, family history, and obesity. Gallbladder disease is more common in Native Americans and Whites than in Asian Americans and Blacks.

Risk Factors
- See Incidence and Demographics above and Assessment section below.

Prevention and Screening
- The nurse should be responsible to recognize predisposing factors of gallbladder disease in general health screening. High-risk individuals should be taught early indicators and instructed to see their healthcare providers when early indicators occur. Earlier detection is advantageous so at-risk individuals can be managed with a low-fat diet and monitored more closely.

Assessment

HISTORY
- Risk factors: obesity, multiparity, infection, cancer, extensive fasting, pregnancy
- Medication risk factors: use of estrogen or oral contraceptives
- Other risks: surgery or other treatment; previous abdominal surgery

PHYSICAL EXAM
- Current lifestyle: sedentary, weight loss, anorexia, indigestion, fat intolerance, nausea and vomiting, dyspepsia, chills
- Elimination: clay-colored stools, steatorrhea, flatulence, dark amber foamy urine
- Subjective data: moderate to severe pain in right upper quadrant that may radiate to the back or scapula; pruritus

- Objective data: fever, restlessness (with acute attack), jaundice, icteric sclera, diaphoresis, tachypnea, splinting during respirations, tachycardia, palpable gallbladder, abdominal guarding and distention

DIAGNOSTIC STUDIES
- Serum liver enzymes and bilirubin (may increase); absence of urobilinogen in urine, increased urinary bilirubin; bleeding tendencies, leukocytosis; abnormal gallbladder ultrasound
- Endoscopic retrograde cholangiopancreatography (ERCP)

Nursing Management
- *Pain relief:* Pain is often very severe; give pain medications as required by the patient and before the pain becomes more severe. Observe for pain medication side effects.
- *Nausea and vomiting relief:* NPO status and gastric decompression. NG tube with suction may be necessary for severe symptoms to prevent further stimulation of the gallbladder; oral hygiene and nares care. Assess intake and output status. Administer antiemetics as needed, frequent mouth rinses, and remove any vomitus immediately from the patient's view. Maintain nutrition and fluid and electrolyte balance. Carefully assess for treatment effectiveness.
- *Comfort and emotional support:* Keeping the bed clean, assisting patient to comfortable positioning, and oral care are important. If pruritus occurs with jaundice, anti-itching measures are necessary. These may include baths with baking soda or Alpha Keri; soothing lotions, such as those containing calamine; antihistamines; soft, old linen; and moderate room temperatures that are not too hot or cold. Patient's nails should be kept short and clean and they should be taught to rub with their knuckles and not scratch with their nails if they cannot resist scratching.
- Assess for complications.
  - *Duct obstruction:* Report jaundice; clay-colored stools; dark, foamy urine; steatorrhea; fever; and increased WBC count.
  - *Bleeding tendencies:* Monitor prothrombin time. Closely assess injection sites and mucous membranes of the mouth, nose, and gingivae for prolonged bleeding.
  - *Infection:* Monitor vital signs and report temperature elevation with chills and jaundice.
- After ERCP: Assess for pancreatitis (abdominal pain and fever), perforation, infection, and bleeding. Keep on bedrest and NPO until gag reflex returns.
  - Post-op care priorities after laparoscopic surgery: Monitor for bleeding complications, make the patient comfortable, and prepare the patient for discharge. Note: Absorbed CO_2 used during surgery can irritate the phrenic nerve and diaphragm, causing some difficulty breathing. Place the patient in Sims' position (left side with right knee flexed) to help move the gas pocket away from the diaphragm. Encourage deep breathing, movement, and ambulation. Pain is usually minimal and can be relieved by NSAIDs or codeine. Many patients go home the same day, but some will stay overnight.
  - Patient and family teaching includes instructions to remove the bandages on the puncture site the day after surgery and that the patient may shower; to report signs and symptoms of redness, swelling, bile-colored drainage or pus from any incision; severe abdominal pain; nausea; vomiting; fever; or chills. Normal activities can be resumed gradually, and return to work usually occurs within 1 week of surgery. Instruct patient to resume usual diet; may need to be a low-fat diet for several weeks following surgery.

- Post-op care priorities after incisional cholecystectomy: Assessment priorities are adequate ventilation and prevention of respiratory complications due to the high (right subcostal) incision. Other nursing care is the same as general post-op care. If the patient has a T-tube inserted into the common bile duct during surgery, the nurse is responsible to maintain bile drainage and observe T-tube functioning and drainage. The T-tube purpose is to drain excess bile while the small intestine is adjusting to receiving a continuous flow of bile. The T-tube is connected to a closed gravity drainage system. Provide a sterile pouching system to protect the skin if the Penrose or Jackson-Pratt drain or the T tube is draining large amounts.
- The patient may be discharged in as soon as 2 to 3 days and should be instructed to avoid heavy lifting for 4 to 6 weeks. Usual sexual activities can be resumed when the patient feels ready, unless otherwise instructed.
- Ambulatory and home care for conservative (nonsurgical) therapy: symptom-based. Dietary teaching usually includes low-fat foods and weight reduction as needed. The patient may need to take fat-soluble vitamin supplements. Instruct the patient about self-assessments of duct obstruction (stool and urine changes, jaundice, and pruritus) and the importance of early reporting to the healthcare provider.

NONPHARMACOLOGIC TREATMENT
- Low-fat diet, weight reduction; less commonly, ERCP with sphincterotomy (papillotomy) or ECSW (extracorporeal shock-wave lithotripsy) may be used for biliary stone removal.

PHARMACOLOGIC TREATMENT
- See above for pain medications (morphine and NSAIDs). Conservative care also includes antiemetics, analgesics, anticholinergics (antispasmodics), and antibiotics for secondary infection. Sometimes fat-soluble vitamins (A, D, E, and K) are prescribed. Cholestyramine (Questran) may provide relief from pruritus related to bile salt.

Special Considerations
- Drugs used to dissolve gallstones are not used routinely due to the common use of laparoscopic cholecystectomy. Dissolution therapy includes ursodeoxycholic acid (UDCA), ursodiol (Actigall) and chenodeoxycholic acid (CDCA). Side effects are generally mild and include abdominal cramping, pain, and diarrhea, and rarely hepatoxicity. Dissolution of stones may take anywhere from 6 months to 2 years.

Follow-up

EXPECTED OUTCOMES
- The patient will appear comfortable and have pain relief and knowledge of activity level and dietary restrictions.

COMPLICATIONS
- Cholecystitis: gangrenous cholecystitis, subphrenic abscess, pancreatitis, cholangitis (inflammation of biliary ducts), biliary cirrhosis, fistulas, and rupture of the gallbladder, which can produce bile peritonitis.

PANCREATITIS

Description
- *Acute pancreatitis* is an inflammatory disorder that involves pancreatic self-destruction from its own enzymes through autodigestion. It can occur in a milder form (interstitial edematous pancreatitis) and be self-limiting. A more severe form, necrotizing pancreatitis, leads to death of pancreatic tissue. Acute pancreatitis is a serious disease.
- *Chronic pancreatitis* is characterized by gradual destruction of functioning pancreatic tissue.

Etiology
- Exact cause unknown; however, activated proteolytic enzymes, particularly trypsin, digest pancreatic tissue and activate other enzymes that digest the elastic tissue of blood vessel walls. Cellular damage and necrosis release activated enzymes and vasoactive substances that produce vasodilation, increase vascular permeability, and cause edema. Large volumes of fluid may shift from circulating blood into the retroperitoneal space, peripancreatic spaces, and the abdominal cavity.

Incidence and Demographics
- About 5,000 new cases of acute pancreatitis are reported each year in the United States. It is more common in middle age, and affects men and women equally. With mild cases, the mortality rate is 6%; with severe cases, it is 23%.

Risk Factors
- Certain factors are believed to lead to pancreatic autodigestion. These factors include gallstones, excessive alcohol intake, tissue ischemia or anoxia, trauma or surgery, ERCP, pancreatic tumors, late-stage pregnancy, elevated calcium levels, hypertriglyceridemia, and infectious agents. Also, thiazide diuretics, estrogen, sulfonamides, steroids, salicylates, and NSAIDs have been linked with pancreatitis. In some cases, the cause is unknown.

Prevention and Screening
- Teach patients who abuse alcohol about their increased risk for pancreatitis. Advise abstinence to reduce this risk, and refer to an alcohol treatment program or Alcoholics Anonymous.

Assessment

HISTORY
- Asses for biliary tract illness history and other clinical manifestations described below in Physical Exam.

PHYSICAL EXAM
- Acute pancreatitis presents with abrupt onset of severe epigastric and left upper quadrant (LUQ) pain, which may radiate to the back; nausea and vomiting; fever; decreased bowel sounds; abdominal distention and rigidity; tachycardia; hypotension; cold, clammy skin; possible jaundice; positive Turner's sign (flank ecchymosis) or Cullen's sign (periumbilical ecchymosis).
- Chronic pancreatitis presents with recurrent epigastric and LUQ pain that radiates to the back, anorexia, nausea and vomiting, weight loss, flatulence, constipation, and steatorrhea (excess fat in the feces caused by reduced pancreatic enzymes).

DIAGNOSTIC STUDIES
- Ultrasonography
- CT scan
- Endoscopic retrograde cholangiopancreatography (ERCP)
- Endoscopic ultrasonography
- Percutaneous fine-needle aspiration biopsy to differentiate from pancreatic cancer
- Lab tests for pancreatic enzymes (serum amylase, lipase, trypsinogen), which rise within hours to days of onset of acute pancreatitis
- Serum glucose (may increase)
- Serum bilirubin and serum alkaline phosphatase (may increase if bile duct blocked)
- Serum calcium (may decrease)
- WBC (rises with acute pancreatitis)

Nursing Management
- Nursing care priorities include managing pain, nutrition, and maintaining fluid balance.
- Selected implementations include:
  - *Pain:* Assess pain thoroughly and frequently, noting nonverbal cues of pain. Administer analgesics on a regular schedule to prevent pain, which may increase pancreatic enzyme secretion. Assist to a comfortable position, such as a side-lying position with knees flexed and head up 45 degrees, or other patient-preferred position of comfort. Maintain a calm, quiet, restful environment.
  - *Nutrition:* Keep patient NPO (as ordered) during acute pancreatitis to reduce pancreatic secretions and promote rest of the pancreas. Total parenteral nutrition (TPN) is initiated.
  - NG tube insertion may be ordered and attached to suction.
  - *Fluid balance:* Maintain IV fluid care to promote vascular volume.
- After serum amylase levels return to normal, bowel sounds are normal, and pain disappears, a low-fat diet and fluids are resumed, with alcohol being strictly disallowed. Maintain stool chart to note return of steatorrhea.

NONPHARMACOLOGIC TREATMENT
- None

PHARMACOLOGIC TREATMENT
- Medication therapy focuses on supportive care.
  - *Pain medications:* Generally opioids are required to manage the severe pain with acute episodes.
  - *Antibiotics* to treat or prevent infection.
  - *Pancreatic enzyme supplements* may be necessary for life with chronic pancreatitis (e.g., pancrelipase [Lipancreatin], which promotes nutrition and decreases the number of bowel movements). Administer and teach the patient and family to give with meals, be sure to follow prescribed diet, maintain a stool chart to include frequency and consistency, and record patient weight every other day.
  - *GI antisecretory medications* (e.g., H2 blockers and proton-pump inhibitors) may be given to neutralize or decrease gastric secretions.
  - *Octreotide (Sandostatin)* is a synthetic hormone given to suppress pancreatic enzyme secretion and relieve pain.

INTERVENTIONAL TREATMENT
- Surgery
  - If pancreatitis is caused by a lodged gallstone in the sphincter of Oddi, surgery may be required to remove it. Surgical procedures may include an endoscopic transduodenal sphincterotomy or cholecystectomy.
  - Drainage of pancreatic enzymes into the duodenum, pseudocyst removal or drainage, or pancreatic resection for pain relief may be required.

Special Considerations
- Alcohol withdrawal is a risk in the patient with acute pancreatitis. Monitor neurological status. Report increasing restlessness and change in mental status.

Follow-up

EXPECTED OUTCOMES
- In acute pancreatitis, some patients recover completely, others experience recurring attacks, and still others develop chronic pancreatitis. The patient, along with family members, needs teaching about hospital procedures and self-care at home following discharge. Information emphasis will include avoidance of alcohol, smoking, and stress. Use of pancreatic enzymes may be required and the regimen may require close instruction, as well.

COMPLICATIONS
- Possible complications include malabsorption, malnutrition, peptic ulcer disease, pancreatic pseudocyst or abscess, common bile duct stricture, diabetes mellitus, and pancreatic cancer. Narcotic (opioid) addiction related to frequent, severe pain episodes is not uncommon.
- Severe abdominal pain can precipitate shallow respirations, hypoventilation, and weak coughing attempts, which can lead to pooling of respiratory secretions, atelectasis, and pneumonia. Assess respiratory status every 4 to 8 hours; report tachypnea, adventitious, or absent breath sounds; oxygen saturation levels below 92%, $PaO_2 < 70$ mm Hg or $PaCO_2 > 45$ mm Hg.

PERITONITIS

Description
- Peritonitis results from a localized or generalized inflammatory process of the peritoneum and is a complication of many acute abdominal disorders. The patient with peritonitis is extremely ill and needs skilled supportive care.

Etiology
- Primary causes of peritonitis are organisms in the bloodstream or genital tract or bacteria in ascites (fluid) resulting from cirrhosis of the liver. Other causes are ruptured appendix or diverticula, trauma to abdominal organs, ischemic bowel disorders, GI obstruction, pancreatitis, peptic ulcer perforation, peritoneal dialysis, and postoperative complications. The resulting inflammatory response leads to massive fluid shifts (peritoneal edema) and adhesions as the body attempts to wall off the infection.

Incidence and Demographics

- None available. The overall mortality rate associated with peritonitis is about 40%. Those individuals who are younger and with less extensive bacterial contamination, and who receive early surgical intervention, have mortality rates of less than 10%.

Risk Factors

- Patients who use ambulatory peritoneal dialysis are at high risk for peritonitis.

Prevention and Screening

- Assess patients at risk for clinical manifestations.

Assessment

HISTORY
- Assess for occurrence of risk factors noted above in etiology.

PHYSICAL EXAM
- Careful abdominal assessment for pain location and quality, bowel sounds, increasing abdominal distention, abdominal guarding, nausea, fever, and hypovolemic shock.

DIAGNOSTIC STUDIES
- CBC, serum electrolytes, abdominal x-ray, abdominal paracentesis and fluid culture, CT scan or ultrasound, peritoneoscopy.

Nursing Management

- See Assessment above.
- Nursing diagnoses relevant to peritonitis include:
  - Acute pain
  - Risk for deficient fluid volume
  - Imbalanced nutrition: less than body requirements
  - Anxiety

NONPHARMACOLOGIC TREATMENT
- Monitor vital signs carefully, I&O, and electrolyte status to determine fluid replacement needs.
- IV fluids: Maintain patent IV line for vascular fluid replacement and antibiotic therapy.
- Semi-Fowler's position with knees flexed to increase comfort. Provide rest and a quiet environment.
- NPO status: NG tube insertion with suction connection may be planned to decrease gastric distention and further leakage of bowel contents into the peritoneum. Low-flow oxygen may be needed.
- Prep for surgery, to include parenteral nutrition, is likely.

PHARMACOLOGIC TREATMENT
- Antibiotics for fighting infection
- Sedatives for anxiety
- Antiemetics to provide relief from nausea and vomiting and prevent further fluid and electrolyte loss
- Analgesics (e.g., morphine) for pain

POSTOPERATIVE CARE
- NPO status
- NG tube to low-intermittent suction
- Semi-Fowler's position
- IV fluids with electrolyte replacement
- Parenteral nutrition as needed
- Antibiotic therapy
- Blood transfusions as needed
- Sedatives and opioids

Special Considerations
- Post-op care after open surgery includes assessment of drainage via drains inserted to remove purulent and excessive fluid.

Follow-up
EXPECTED OUTCOMES
- Goals:
  - Resolution of inflammation
  - Relief of abdominal pain
  - Freedom from complications (adhesions, shock, infection)
  - Normal nutritional status

COMPLICATIONS
- Life-threatening abscess and fibrous adhesions may lead to follow-up obstruction. Septicemia and septic shock can develop without prompt and effective treatment.

REFERENCES

American Nurses Credentialing Center. (2007). *Medical-surgical nursing review and resource manual* (2nd ed.). Silver Spring, MD: Author.

Lehne, R. A. (2010). *Pharmacology for nursing care* (7th ed.). St. Louis, MO: Saunders Elsevier.

LeMone, P., & Burke, K. (2008). *Medical-surgical nursing: Critical thinking in client care* (4th ed.). Upper Saddle River, NJ: Pearson Education.

Lewis, S., Dirksen, S., Heitkemper, M., Bucher, L., & Camera, I. (2011). *Medical-surgical nursing: Assessment and management of clinical problems* (8th ed.). St. Louis, MO: Elsevier Mosby,

Lewis, S., Heitkemper, M., Dirksen, S., O'Brien, P., & Bucher, L. (2007). *Medical-surgical nursing: Assessment and management of clinical problems* (7th ed.). St. Louis, MO: Mosby Elsevier.

3

Renal and Genitourinary (GU) System

Paula Harrison Gillman, MSN, RN-C, ANP-BC, GNP-BC

GENERAL APPROACH

- The kidneys are important organs that maintain water, salt, and electrolyte balance; remove wastes from the blood; play an important role in acid–base regulation; and secrete several endocrine hormones that help regulate blood pressure and stimulate red blood cell production.
- Each kidney is made up of about 1 million functional units called nephrons, many more than are needed to do the work of kidneys.
- The kidneys receive about one-fifth of the cardiac output each minute (1 L of blood).
- Glomerular filtration rate (GFR) is the volume of filtrate that enters Bowman's capsule per unit of time.
- Average GFR in an adult is 180 L/day, resulting in about 1.5 L/day of urine output.
- GFR declines with age due to loss of functional nephrons and decreased renal blood flow. Older adults also have less muscle mass, thus reducing the amount of creatinine to be cleared, making the serum creatinine a poor estimate of the adequacy of renal function.
- Renal blood flow is regulated by both intrarenal and extrarenal mechanisms.
- Autoregulation refers to the inherent ability of the afferent and efferent arterioles to dilate or constrict.
- External regulation occurs via changes in mean arterial pressure and effects of the sympathetic nervous system.
- Release of renin by the kidney also affects systemic circulation by stimulating the conversion of angiotensinogen to angiotensin I (a potent vasoconstrictor).

RED FLAGS

- Hematuria is never normal and can indicate infection or cancer of the GU system.
- Postmenopausal vaginal bleeding or discharge may be evidence of endometrial cancer.
- Persistent vague abdominal symptoms (discomfort, bloating) in a woman with ovaries should prompt an investigation into the possibility of ovarian cancer.
- Men develop increased difficulty with voiding as they age due to prostatic hyperplasia. These same symptoms, however, may be indicators of prostate cancer.

Common Disorders of the Renal/GU System

ACUTE RENAL FAILURE (ARF)

Description
- Renal failure that occurs in days to weeks.
- Marked by an abrupt rise in blood urea nitrogen (BUN) and creatinine.
- Elevated BUN and creatinine is called azotemia.

Etiology
- Divided into three types depending on where the cause is located.
- Prerenal failure: problem occurs before the kidney, resulting in reduced blood flow to the kidney, thus reducing renal clearance.
  - Hypovolemia from dehydration, vomiting, diarrhea, hemorrhage
  - Vascular redistribution such as in shock or CHF
  - Renal artery stenosis or embolism
- Intrinsic renal failure: occurs within the kidney.
  - Acute tubular necrosis (ATN): ischemic injury (most common)
  - Acute glomerulonephritis (see Box 13–1 below)
  - Interstitial nephritis
  - Contrast dye
  - Nephrotoxic drugs (aminoglycosides, nonsteroidal anti-inflammatory drugs [NSAIDs], angiotensin-converting enzyme [ACE] inhibitors, ampicillin, and others)
  - Disease processes that affect the kidneys: rheumatoid arthritis, systemic lupus erythematosus (SLE), leukemia, myeloma
- Postrenal failure: problem occurs past the level of the kidney, resulting in obstruction to urine drainage
  - Benign prostatic hyperplasia (BPH): most common
  - Renal stones
  - Retroperitoneal tumors/cancer
  - Urethral stricture
  - Neurogenic bladder

Box 13-1. Acute Glomerulonephritis

Glomerulonephritis can follow an acute streptococcal infection (APSGN) and causes hematuria, proteinuria, and red cell casts in the urine, accompanied by edema and hypertension. The condition was first recognized in the 18th century as a complication of scarlet fever. Incidence has decreased in the United States, but remains high in areas where skin infections are common, such as tropical climates. APSGN occasionally requires renal biopsy for diagnosis. Goal of treatment is to control edema and blood pressure until kidney function recovers.

Incidence and Demographics
- Occurs in 100 persons per million in the general population.
- Diagnosed in 1% of hospital admissions.
- Occurs in one-third of critical care admissions.
- Men and women are affected equally.

Risk Factors
- In addition to etiological causes above, certain conditions make persons more vulnerable to renal insult.
  - Age: older kidneys have less reserve
  - Diabetes mellitus
  - Hypertension

Prevention and Screening
- Prevention of ARF centers on avoidance of precipitating causes: contrast dye in high-risk persons, dehydration, etc.
- ACEIs should be avoided in persons who have known volume depletion or in those with renal artery stenosis.
- Control of diseases that commonly lead to chronic kidney disease (CKD), such as diabetes and hypertension
- Calcium channel blockers have been shown to prevent renal failure in persons receiving cyclosporine.
- No routine screening is performed for this condition in the general population.
- Evaluation of persons at risk includes BUN and creatinine and urinalysis

Assessment
HISTORY
- Persons with acute renal failure may appear critically ill or have mild to minimal symptoms.
- Prerenal failure
  - Thirst, decreased urine output, dizziness or orthostatic hypotension
  - Altered mental status in elders
  - Sources of volume loss: excessive sweating, diarrhea, vomiting, hemorrhage, polyuria
  - Symptoms of congestive heart failure (CHF): orthopnea, paroxysmal nocturnal dyspnea (PND), shortness of breath
- Intrinsic failure
  - Hematuria, edema, new-onset hypertension
  - History of throat or skin infections
  - Recent hypotension such as with sepsis, hemorrhage, surgery
  - Exposure to nephrotoxins or new medications
  - Allergic interstitial nephritis usually occurs with fever, arthralgias, rash, and history of exposure to NSAIDs or antibiotics

- Postrenal failure
  - Older men with history of obstructive urinary symptoms: urgency, frequency, nocturia, hesitancy, straining, retention
  - Flank pain or hematuria
  - History of any GU surgery or abdominal or pelvic malignancy

PHYSICAL EXAM
- Postural hypotension and tachycardia with volume depletion
- Mucous membrane moisture
- Elevated jugular venous pressure
- Heart: murmurs or gallop
- Pulmonary: rales with volume overload
- Abdomen: costovertebral angle (CVA) tenderness, distended bladder, pelvic mass, digital rectal exam for evidence of prostatic enlargement

DIAGNOSTIC STUDIES
- Laboratory
  - Urinalysis with microscopic
  - Urine microalbumin
  - BUN
  - Serum creatinine; large reductions in glomerular filtration rate may occur while the serum creatinine remains within normal range (see Chronic Kidney Disease below)
  - Cystatin C (new biomarker of early kidney injury; can identify a problem while creatinine is still normal)
  - Complete blood count (CBC)
  - Blood chemistries
  - Urine chemistries (sodium, creatinine, osmolality)
- Imaging
  - Renal ultrasound with Doppler
- Procedures
  - Renal biopsy when glomerular causes are suspected

Differential Diagnosis
- CHF
- Systemic vasculitis
- Chronic kidney disease
- Urinary tract infection
- Nursing management
- Nonpharmacologic treatment
- Fluid replacement for hypovolemia
- Discontinue potentially offending medications: NSAIDs, antibiotics, ACE inhibitors

Nursing Management

NONPHARMACOLOGIC TREATMENT
- None

PHARMACOLOGIC TREATMENT
- Diuretics for volume overload

- Dopamine: renal vascular vasodilator at low doses
- Fenoldopam (Corlopam): selective dopamine agonist that increases renal blood flow and provides renal protection to critically ill persons at risk for renal failure

INTERVENTIONAL TREATMENT
- Urinary catheter placement to relieve obstruction
- Renal replacement therapy (hemodialysis, peritoneal dialysis), continuous venovenous hemodiafiltration (CVVHD)

Special Considerations
- Most causes of ARF in hospitalized patients are iatrogenic.
- It is important to follow trends in creatinine because absolute numbers may be in the normal range even with significant decline in renal function.

Follow-up

EXPECTED OUTCOMES
- Patient will have normal BUN and creatinine and acid–base balance.
- Patient will have signs of normal fluid balance.
- Patient will maintain normal urine output.

COMPLICATIONS
- Fluid and electrolyte abnormalities including hyperkalemia, hypercalcemia, metabolic acidosis
- Volume overload leading to CHF, myocardial infarction (MI), arrhythmias
- Hypoxia occurring during hemodialysis is very detrimental to persons with underlying pulmonary disease.
- Nausea, vomiting, and anorexia occur with uremia.
- Infections occur in 33% of persons with ARF.
- Neurologic signs of lethargy, confusion, cognitive deficits, disturbances in sleep-wake cycle
- Death

CHRONIC KIDNEY DISEASE (CKD)

Description
- Progressive decline in renal function that occurs over months to years
- Classified in five stages (see Table 13–1)

Etiology
- 65% of end-stage renal disease (ESRD) is due to diabetes mellitus (DM) and hypertension (HTN).
- Untreated causes of acute renal failure (see section above)
- Polycystic kidney disease
- Atherosclerotic renovascular disease

Table 13-1. Classification of Chronic Kidney Disease

Stage	Description	GFR mL/min/1.73m^2
1	Persistent albuminuria with normal or ↑ GFR	≥ 90
2	Persistent albuminuria with mildly ↓ GFR	60–89
3	Moderately ↓ GFR	30–59
4	Severely ↓ GFR	15–29
5	Renal failure/dialysis	< 15

Adapted from National Kidney Foundation Kidney Disease Outcomes Quality Initiative (KDOQI). (2002). KDOQI clinical practice guidelines for chronic kidney disease: evaluation, classification and stratification. *American Journal of Kidney Disease*, 39(2 suppl 1):S1–S266.

Incidence and Demographics
- Affects 11% of the population
- More than 50 million people worldwide have early to moderate (Stages 1–3) renal impairment.

Risk Factors
- Age: over 60
- Race: Black
- Diabetes mellitus
- Hypertension
- Autoimmune disease
- Exposure to nephrotoxic drugs
- Family history
- See risk factors for ARF (above)

Prevention and Screening
- Control of underlying disease processes: DM and HTN
- Proper use of renal-protective drugs: ACE inhibitors, angiotensin receptor blockers (ARBs), and calcium channel blockers
- Avoidance of nephrotoxic drugs and contrast dye in at-risk patients

Assessment

HISTORY
- Decline in renal function is asymptomatic until approximately 50% of nephrons are lost (Stage 3).
- Possible signs and symptoms are listed in Table 13–2

Table 13-2. Signs and Symptoms of Renal Failure

GFR mL/min	> 50	20–50	< 20	< 10
Signs/ Symptoms	None except underlying disease	Elevated BUN & creatinine Metabolic acidosis ↑ Potassium Polyuria Anemia Fatigue	↓ Calcium ↑ Phosphate Metabolic acidosis Fluid overload	Uremia Nausea, vomiting Heart failure Pruritus Fatigue Insomnia

PHYSICAL EXAM
- Vital signs: hypertension
- Funduscopic eye exam
- Neck: carotid bruits
- Heart and lung exam for signs of volume overload
- Abdominal pelvic exam: masses, enlarged prostate, renal artery bruits
- Extremities: edema, peripheral nerve involvement

DIAGNOSTIC STUDIES
- Urinalysis with microscopic exam.
- Urine microalbumin: early and sensitive marker of kidney damage.
- BUN: Disproportionate elevation is seen with volume depletion.
- Serum creatinine: Large reductions in glomerular filtration rate (GFR) may occur while the serum creatinine remains within normal range (see Box 13–2).
- Creatinine clearance either calculated or measured by 24-hour urine (see Box 13–3).
- CBC: Anemia will occur due to reductions in erythropoietin production.
- Blood chemistries: hyperkalemia, hypocalcemia, hyperphosphatemia, acidosis
- Parathyroid hormone (PTH): Hypercalcemia from hyperparathyroidism occurs later.
- Imaging
  - Renal ultrasound: kidneys usually smaller than normal (< 9 cm).

Box 13–2. Comparison of Creatinine Clearance

The following patients have a "normal" creatinine by laboratory assessment; however, the elderly woman has clearance that is half that of the man. This example illustrates the importance of calculating creatinine clearance to assess renal function, especially in older adults.

Patient	80-year-old female	60-year-old male
Body weight	50 kg body weight	70 kg body weight
Serum Cr	1.1	1.1
Cr Clearance	32	70

Box 13–3. Calculating Creatinine Clearance

Simplified 4-Variable MDRD formula (Levey, 1999)
$$GFR = 186.3 \times (SCR)^{-1.154} \times (\text{age in years})^{-0.203} \times 1.212 \ (\text{if patient is Black}) \times 0.742 \ (\text{if female})$$

Cockcroft-Gault Equation (Cockcroft, 1976)
$$CrCl = [(140 - \text{age}) \times IBW] / (SCR \times 72) \ (\times 0.85 \text{ for females})$$

Nursing Management

NONPHARMACOLOGIC TREATMENT
- Nutritional restrictions on sodium, potassium, protein may be necessary.
- Fluid restrictions may be necessary with advanced failure and volume overload.
- Avoid potentially harmful medications and substances: NSAIDs, contrast dyes, illegal drugs.
- Stop smoking.

PHARMACOLOGIC TREATMENT
- Much pharmacologic management is aimed at control of the underlying disease processes, usually DM and HTN.
- Lipid management is usually a target of therapy to reduce morbidity from atherosclerotic disease, but has inconclusive benefits on the kidneys themselves.
- ACE inhibitors and ARBs slow progression in both diabetic and nondiabetic CKD.
- Phosphate binders are given to reduce elevated phosphate levels.
- Erythropoietin and calcitriol, two hormones produced by the kidney, often are replaced.

INTERVENTIONAL TREATMENT
- Hemodialysis (HD) or peritoneal dialysis for Stage 5 disease with intractable volume overload or electrolyte imbalances.
- Renal transplantation has a survival benefit, but not all patients qualify as transplant candidates.

Special Considerations
- Home hemodialysis appears to be associated with better survival and greater quality of life than in-center HD or peritoneal dialysis.

Follow-up

EXPECTED OUTCOMES
- Patient will voice understanding and comply with dietary and fluid restrictions.
- Patient will maintain a normal sleep-wake cycle.
- Patient will demonstrate adequate control of underlying disease processes as indicated:
  - BP < 125/75 mm Hg
  - HbA1C < 7.0%

COMPLICATIONS
- The leading cause of death in persons with CKD is cardiovascular disease, regardless of the stage of CKD
- Cardiac arrhythmias
- Volume overload
- Anemia
- Malnutrition
- Metabolic acidosis
- Sleep disturbances
- Itching, hiccups, nausea, anorexia

URINARY TRACT INFECTION (UTI)

Description
- Infection of the urethra, bladder, or ureters.
- Infection may extend to the kidneys, resulting in pyelonephritis (see Box 13–4).

Box 13–4. Pyelonephritis

Infection of the ascending urinary tract that has reached the renal pelvis. Severe cases often lead to sepsis, which may result in multiorgan dysfunction syndrome (MODS) and death. Symptoms may be similar to those seen in lower tract infection, only usually the patient is much more ill with higher fever. Treatment is with IV antibiotics based on results of urine or blood cultures and sensitivities.

Etiology
- Most commonly caused by *E. coli* or other gram-negative bacteria from the gastro-intestinal tract.
- Women have a short urethra in close proximity to the perirectal area, making colonization possible.
- Relatively uncommon in men, but may occur due to prostatitis or in older men with prostatic hyperplasia.

Incidence and Demographics
- 8 to 10 million in the United States each year.
- More common in women.
- 20% of women in the United States develop a UTI at some time; 20% of those will have recurrent infections.

Risk Factors
- Female gender
- Diabetes mellitus
- Urinary instrumentation and catheterization
- Any cause of neurogenic bladder
- Women
  - Increased sexual activity, diaphragm and spermicide use
  - Pregnancy
  - Postmenopausal status
  - History of UTI
  - Delayed voiding
- Men
  - Homosexuality
  - Lack of circumcision
  - HIV infection
  - BPH or urethral stricture

Prevention and Screening

- No routine screening is performed in asymptomatic persons.
- Voiding after intercourse (for women).
- Meticulous perineal care.
- Consumption of cranberries or their juice.
- Prompt voiding when urge occurs and attention to completely emptying the bladder.
- For women, wiping front to back after using the toilet.

Assessment

HISTORY

- Most common symptoms: dysuria, urgency, frequency, nocturia, suprapubic pressure/cramping
- Older adults may have atypical symptoms such as confusion, anorexia, or no symptoms at all.
- Occasionally fever in younger persons
- Past history of UTIs
- For pyelonephritis
  - Acute onset of high fever, chills, flank pain, headache, malaise, and often hematuria

PHYSICAL EXAM

- Vital signs: fever
- Abdomen: tenderness, bladder distention, mass
- Back: costovertebral angle (CVA) tenderness
- Pelvic exam in women
- Genital exam in men

DIAGNOSTIC STUDIES

- Urinalysis with microscopic exam
- Urine culture and sensitivity (C&S): not indicated in young, healthy persons with first UTI
- If pyelonephritis is suspected: CBC and blood cultures may be indicated
- Selected tests with suspicion of sexually transmitted illnesses (STIs): cultures for gonorrhea and Chlamydia, wet mount of vaginal secretions in women

Differential Diagnosis

- Diabetes
- STIs
- Bladder or urinary tract cancer
- Renal calculi
- Vaginitis
- Prostatitis
- Pyelonephritis

Nursing Management

NONPHARMACOLOGIC TREATMENT

- Increased water/fluid consumption

PHARMACOLOGIC TREATMENT
- Antibiotic therapy as indicated by C&S or based on patient status.
- Uncomplicated UTI in a young, healthy, nonpregnant woman is treated with trimethoprim-sulfamethoxazole (Bactrim DS) b.i.d. for 3 days.
- Phenazopyridine HCL (Pyridium) 100 mg t.i.d. may be prescribed for a short time to relieve pain or bladder spasms.
  - Note: Warn patient that urine will turn orange and stain clothing.

Special Considerations
- Asymptomatic bacteruria is a colony count > 100,000 bacteria/mL urine without symptoms of UTI or white blood cells (WBCs) on microscopic exam.
- Occurs in 15% to 50% of institutionalized older adults.
- Treatment with antibiotics is indicated only in persons who are immunosuppressed, such as with HIV or malignancy.
- UTI should be suspected in any older patients (especially women) who present with any vague symptoms.
- Postmenopausal women may have their risk reduced by using vaginal estrogen.

Follow-up

EXPECTED OUTCOMES
- Patient will complete full course of antibiotic therapy and maintain adequate hydration.
- Patient will verbalize precautions to prevent further UTIs.

COMPLICATIONS
- Ascending urinary tract infection and sepsis may result.
- Recurrent infection if treatment is incorrect or too short in duration.
- Repeated infections increases likelihood of infection with resistant organisms.

URINARY INCONTINENCE (UI)

Description
- Involuntary loss of urine
- One of the most common health problems affecting older patients

Etiology
- Age-related changes in urinary function
- Decreased bladder capacity
- Increased involuntary bladder contractions
- Increased nocturnal urine production
- Acute UI
- UTI
- Immobility
- Fecal impaction
- Delirium
- High blood glucose
- Alcohol use in excess
- Medications (anticholinergics, diuretics, psychotropics, benzodiazipines, narcotics)

- Five types of chronic UI:
  - Stress incontinence: loss of urine during episodes of increased intra-abdominal pressure, such as coughing, sneezing, or laughing.
  - Urge incontinence: associated with abnormal bladder contractions and often called overactive bladder. Common causes are cystitis, urethritis, tumors, central nervous system disorders like stroke and Parkinson's disease.
  - Overflow incontinence: chronically full bladder (inadequate emptying) leads to excessive pressure and involuntary emptying. Most common in patients with diabetes, spinal cord injuries, those taking anticholinergic medications or persons with an obstruction to emptying (BPH or uterine prolapse).
  - Functional incontinence: loss of urine that occurs due to inability or unwillingness to get to a toilet. Can be seen in persons after cerebrovascular accident, with severe arthritis or pain, or persons with dementia.
  - Mixed-type incontinence: combination of two or more types of incontinence.

Incidence and Demographics
- Occurs in more that 30% of community-dwelling older adults (mostly women).

Risk Factors
- Gender: women more likely to have stress incontinence; men more likely to have overflow or urge incontinence due to BPH
- Age
- Excess weight
- Smoking

Prevention and Screening
- Maintain a healthy weight
- Don't smoke
- Practice Kegel exercises
- Avoid bladder irritants like caffeine
- Eat more fiber
- Exercise
- Screening for UI is accomplished by asking about symptoms of the condition. Because of the potential impact on socialization, screening questions should always be asked in post-menopausal women and older males.

Assessment

HISTORY
- Questions to determine type of incontinence
- Bladder habits
- Past medical and surgical history (especially diabetes, CHF, urinary tract infections, CVA, Parkinson's disease, mobility and neurological problems or cognitive impairment)
- Obstetrical history
- Functional assessment
- Impact of the incontinence on caregivers, socialization
- Related problems, such as skin breakdown
- Bladder diary to include frequency and volume of incontinence, timing, and associated symptoms or circumstances

PHYSICAL EXAM
- Abdominal, rectal, and pelvic exam
- Neurological exam
- Gait and balance

DIAGNOSTIC STUDIES
- Urinalysis
- Urine culture and sensitivity
- Urodynamic testing as indicated

Nursing Management

NONPHARMACOLOGIC TREATMENT
- Determine willingness and capability of the patient and caregiver to cooperate with prescribed therapy
- Bladder retraining
- Pelvic floor exercises
- Biofeedback
- Scheduled toileting for patients with cognitive impairment
- Avoiding bladder irritants such as caffeine
- Limit fluid intake after dinner
- Pessary for women with pelvic prolapse
- In and out catheterization for atonic bladders and overflow incontinence
- Condom caths for men
- Pads and protective garments

PHARMACOLOGIC TREATMENT
- Antichoinergics: diminish bladder contractions in urge incontinence
- Oxybutinin (Ditropan)
- Solifenacin (Vesicare)
- Tolterodine (Detrol)
- Topical estrogen: rejuvenates vaginal and urethral tissue and may improve bladder control
- Imiptramine (Tofranil): tricyclic antidepressant that is sometimes used to treat mixed incontinence

INTERVENTIONAL TREATMENT
- Radiofrequency therapy: heats the tissue to increase firmness and integrity
- Bulking material injections: collagen or similar is injected into tissues surrounding the urethra
- Sacral nerve stimulator
- Surgical procedures include sling procedure, bladder neck suspension, artificial urinary sphincter

Special Considerations
- Many older women and men consider urinary leakage to be a normal part of aging and will not mention their symptoms unless asked.
- Urinary incontinence is a major reason for admission to long-term-care facilities.
- Older persons may experience confusion or increased risk of falls as a side effect of bladder medications. Monitoring is crucial to prevent complications.

Follow-up

EXPECTED OUTCOMES
- Patient will have improved control of urine with therapy.
- Patient will verbalize behavioral therapies to minimize urine loss.

COMPLICATIONS
- Patients with uncontrollable incontinence usually incur tremendous expense, as well as social isolation.
- Urinary incontinence places an added burden on caregivers who may be over-stressed already.

ATROPHIC VAGINITIS

Description
- Inflammation of vaginal tissue due to thinning and lack of lubrication

Etiology
- Related to reduced estrogen levels

Incidence and Demographics
- Symptoms occur in up to 40% of postmenopausal women.
- Only 20%–25% seek medical attention.

Risk Factors
- Post-menopausal status
- Oophorectomy
- Medications or hormones that reduce estrogen levels
- Pelvic radiation or chemotherapy

Prevention and Screening
- Screening is by symptom assessment in at-risk women.
- Topical or systemic estrogen replacement can prevent or relieve symptoms, but decisions to treat must be individualized due to possible risks of therapy.

Assessment

HISTORY
- Vaginal dryness, itching or burning
- Dyspareunia
- Leukorrhea or yellow, malodorous discharge
- Dysuria
- Hematuria
- Urinary frequency
- Urinary tract infection
- Stress incontinence
- Use of perfumes, powders, soaps, panty liners, spermicides and lubricants
- Tight-fitting clothing

PHYSICAL EXAM
- External genitalia: decreased elasticity and turgor, sparse pubic hair, dryness and possible fusion of labia minora
- Vaginal epithelium: pale, smooth and shiny; possibly friable with patchy erythema
- Cystocele, urethral polyps, eversion of urethral mucosa, rectocele or pelvic prolapse

DIAGNOSTIC STUDIES
- Serum hormone levels
- Pap smear
- Wet mount
- Ultrasonography of uterine lining
- Urinalysis

Nursing Management

NONPHARMACOLOGIC TREATMENT
- Vaginal lubricants and moisturizers

PHARMACOLOGIC TREATMENT
- Systemic or local estrogen replacement
- Thickens and revascularizes the epithelium
- Alleviates symptoms
- Contraindications: estrogen-sensitive tumors, end-stage liver disease, past history of estrogen-related thromboembolism

Special Considerations
- Many older women may attribute symptoms to aging and not realize that treatment is available.
- Though vaginal estrogen relieves local symptoms, systemic estrogen also decreases postmenopausal bone loss and reduces hot flashes.

Follow-up

EXPECTED OUTCOMES
- Patient will have improved comfort with intercourse.
- Patient will get relief from urinary symptoms with treatment.

COMPLICATIONS
- Unopposed estrogen therapy in women with a uterus increases the risk of endometrial carcinoma.
- Estrogen therapy may increase risk of breast cancer and thromboembolism, thus therapy must be individualized.

URINARY TRACT CANCER (BLADDER OR KIDNEY)

Description
- Bladder cancer is the most common GU malignancy.
- Renal cell carcinoma (RCC) often lacks early warning signs, but may have diverse clinical manifestations due to the tumor's effects on other organ systems (paraneoplastic syndromes).

Etiology
- 90% originate in the epithelial lining of the bladder (transitional cell).

Incidence and Demographics
- Bladder cancer is most common in persons 50 to 70 years old.
- Bladder and renal cell cancers occur more commonly in men.
- Whites develop bladder cancer twice as often as other ethnic groups.
- American Cancer Society estimated that in 2009 there were nearly 58,000 cases of kidney malignancies diagnosed in the United States, accounting for nearly 13,000 deaths.
- Renal cell carcinoma is the 10th leading cause of cancer deaths in men in the United States
- Incidence of RCC in the United States is slightly higher among Blacks.

Risk Factors
- Cigarette smoking
- Exposure to industrial dyes, rubber, chemicals, benzene, or paint
- Dietary consumption of fried meats and animal fats
- Obesity increases risk of renal cell cancer, especially in women
- Phenacetin-containing analgesics
- von Hippel-Lindau (VHL) disease: inherited disease associated with RCC

Prevention and Screening
- No routine screening tests are recommended in the general population.
- Avoidance of risk factors is important for prevention.
- Fruit and yellow-orange vegetables appear to moderately reduce the risk of bladder cancer.
- Citrus fruits and cruciferous vegetables may have a protective effect.

Assessment

HISTORY
- Dysuria, frequency, urgency, or painless hematuria with bladder cancer
- Hematuria, flank pain, and palpable mass in flank or abdomen: most common presentation of renal cell cancer
- Other presentations: weight loss, fever, hypertension, hypercalcemia, night sweats, malaise
- Renal cell carcinoma is commonly associated with paraneoplastic syndromes, which are numerous

PHYSICAL EXAM
- Hypertension
- Supraclavicular adenopathy
- Flank or abdominal mass with bruit
- 30% of renal cell carcinomas present with metastatic disease (lung, soft tissues, bone, liver, cutaneous sites, central nervous system [CNS])

DIAGNOSTIC STUDIES
- Urinalysis
- Urine C&S
- CBC
- Electrolytes

- Renal profile
- Liver profile
- Erythrocyte sedimentation rate (ESR)
- Cystoscopy
- Imaging studies
  - CT scan
  - Ultrasound
  - MRI

Differential Diagnosis

- Benign renal tumor
- Renal cyst
- Metastasis from another primary tumor
- Urinary tract infection (as cause of hematuria)

Nursing Management

PHARMACOLOGIC TREATMENT
- Treatment of bladder cancer is based on staging of the cancer.
  - BCG instillation immunotherapy is often used for superficial bladder tumors.
  - Combination of chemotherapy and radiation therapy may be used for invasive disease.
  - Cystectomy.
- Treatment of renal cell cancer also is based on staging and may involve a combination of treatment options.
  - Surgery: nephrectomy or nephron-sparing and thermal ablation for smaller tumors
  - Radiation
  - Chemotherapy
  - Hormonal therapy
  - Immunotherapy

Special Considerations

- More than 50% of early stage RCCs are cured.
- In 25% to 30% of patients, RCC is asymptomatic and found incidentally on a radiologic study.
- BCG immunotherapy is effective in up to two-thirds of superficial bladder tumors.

Follow-up

EXPECTED OUTCOMES
- Patient will maintain weight within normal range.
- Patient will get adequate rest and pace activities to avoid fatigue.
- Patient will maintain normal urinary output.
- Immunocompromised patients will verbalize precautions to minimize the risk of infection.

COMPLICATIONS
- Severe, sharp, band-like back pain may be an early warning sign of metastasis to the spinal cord.

- As many as one-third of patients with localized disease may have metastasis after nephrectomy, thus necessitating close follow-up.
- Virtually any organ system may be affected by a paraneoplastic syndrome associated with RCC.

BENIGN PROSTATIC HYPERPLASIA (BPH)

Description
- Benign, age-related enlargement of the prostate gland that constricts the urethra and prevents outflow of urine
- Can lead to bladder outlet obstruction, urinary retention, and a distended bladder

Etiology
- Hyperplasia of stromal and epithelial cells resulting in expansion in the periurethral region of the prostate, compressing the urethral canal
- Adenomatous prostatic growth begins at about age 30, but most men are over 50 before they experience clinical symptoms.

Incidence and Demographics
- Estimates of symptomatic benign hyperplasia are 10% to 30% for men in their early 70s and increase with age.

Risk Factors
- Increasing age
- Increased levels of active testosterone (DHT)

Prevention and Screening
- No screening indicated for BPH
- Usually diagnosed incidentally either due to an elevated prostate-specific antigen (PSA) level or by digital rectal exam (DRE; done for prostate cancer screening)
- Smoking may have a protective effect, but risks of cigarette smoking far outweigh any benefits for this condition.

Assessment

HISTORY
- Obstructive voiding symptoms
  - Hesitancy
  - Decreased force of stream
  - Dribbling
  - Retention
- Irritative voiding symptoms
  - Dysuria
  - Frequency
  - Urgency
  - Nocturia

PHYSICAL EXAM
- Abdominal exam for distended bladder, renal tenderness or mass
- Digital rectal examination (DRE) to assess size, consistency, symmetry, and tenderness of prostate

DIAGNOSTIC STUDIES
- Urinalysis
- Prostate-specific antigen (PSA)
- Ultrasound assessment of postvoid residual urine
- Transrectal ultrasound

Differential Diagnosis
- Prostate cancer
- Other cause of urethral obstruction
- Impaired bladder contractility
- Diabetes mellitus, CHF, or other condition causing increased nocturnal voiding

Nursing Management

NONPHARMACOLOGIC TREATMENT
- Avoid drugs that may aggravate symptoms: anticholinergics, decongestants, diuretics.
- Limit fluid intake after dinner.
- Limit or avoid caffeine and alcohol.
- Frequent voiding or double voiding.

PHARMACOLOGIC TREATMENT
- Alpha-adrenergic blockers such as terazosin, doxazosin, and tamsulosin (Flomax): decrease bladder outlet resistance
- 5α-reductase inhibitors such as finasteride (Proscar) and dutasteride (Avodart): reduce serum dihydrotestosterone, thus reducing the volume of the prostate by 20% to 25%
  - Full response may take 6 to 12 months
  - Usually well-tolerated, but 5% have sexual dysfunction

INTERVENTIONAL TREATMENT
- Transurethral resection of prostate (TURP)
- Open prostatectomy
- Transurethral needle ablation (TUNA)
- Transurethral microwave therapy (TUMT)
- Laser therapy
- High-intensity focused ultrasonography (HIFU)

Special Considerations
- Alpha-adrenergic blockers can cause hypotension, especially with position changes, making older men more prone to falls and fractures.

Follow-up

EXPECTED OUTCOMES
- Patient will be able to empty bladder effectively.

- Patient will identify signs of worsening urinary retention and seek immediate medical assistance.
- Patient will experience minimal sleep disruption from urinary pattern.

COMPLICATIONS
- Urinary retention can lead to UTIs, and in severe cases hydronephrosis.

PROSTATITIS

Description
- Inflammation of the prostate gland in men

Etiology
- Divided into 4 types:
  - Acute bacterial prostatitis: *E.coli, Klebsiella, Proteus*
  - Chronic bacterial prostatits: usually asymptomatic, but may present as a UTI
  - Chronic prostatits without infection: recurrent pelvic or rectal pain with no infection
  - Asymptomatic inflammatory prostatitis

Incidence and Demographics
- 8% of urology visits
- 1% of primary care visits

Risk Factors
- Increasing age
- Increased levels of active testosterone (DHT)

Prevention and Screening
- Good hygiene
- Adequate fluid consumption
- Safe sex practices

Assessment of Acute Bacterial Prostatitis

HISTORY
- Fever, chills, sweats
- Urgency, frequency and dysuria

PHYSICAL EXAM
- Genital exam
- Digital rectal examination (DRE) to assess size, consistency, symmetry, and tenderness of prostate; prostatitis causes a tender, boggy prostate

DIAGNOSTIC STUDIES
- Urinalysis
- Urine culture and sensitivity
- Possible ultrasound, x-ray or CT

Nursing Management

NONPHARMACOLOGIC TREATMENT
- Drink plenty of fluids
- Adequate rest

PHARMACOLOGIC TREATMENT
- Antibiotics based on urine culture and sensitivity or empiric ciprofloxacin
- Analgesics for pain

Special Considerations
- Prostatits can cause an elevated prostate specific antigen (PSA)

Follow-up

EXPECTED OUTCOMES
- Patient will experience relief of urinary symptoms upon completion of antibiotics.

COMPLICATIONS
- Chronic prostatitis may lead to problems with painful ejaculation or erectile dysfunction.

ERECTILE DYSFUNCTION (ED)

Description
- Problems getting or sustaining an erection that is adequate for sexual intercourse

Etiology
- ED may be due to problems in any of these areas:
  - Psychological
  - Neurologic: cerebrovascular accident, spinal cord injury, multiple sclerosis
  - Endocrine: diabetes (produces neurovascular abnormalities); hypogonadism (testosterone deficiency)
  - Vascular: atherosclerosis
  - Local anatomy: Peyronie's disease
  - Prescription medications (SSRIs, beta blockers)
  - Recreational drugs

Incidence and Demographics
- Prevalence ranges from 40% to 70% and increases with age

Risk Factors
- Advanced age
- Comorbid disease as listed above
- Relationship problems

Prevention and Screening
- Men routinely should be asked about problems with erectile function.
- Good health practices to avoid development of chronic diseases that may impair erectile dysfunction (DM, atherosclerosis, etc.).

Assessment

HISTORY
- Other medical conditions; vascular disease, diabetes mellitus (DM), neurologic disease, liver or kidney disease
- List of medications
- Habits: recreational drugs, alcohol, smoking
- History of pelvic/GU surgery or radiation
- History of pelvic, genital, or spinal cord trauma
- Quality of relationship/patient and partner expectations

PHYSICAL EXAM
- General appearance and affect
- Secondary sexual characteristics (gynecomastia, hair loss)
- Peripheral vascular assessment
- Cardiopulmonary exam
- Neurologic exam
- Abdominal and rectal exam

DIAGNOSTIC STUDIES
- Testosterone and prolactin levels
- Hemoglobin A1C to screen for DM
- Liver/kidney function tests
- Lipid panel for risk factor assessment

Nursing Management

NONPHARMACOLOGIC TREATMENT
- Withdrawal of offending medications
- Vacuum constriction devices
- Sex therapy

PHARMACOLOGIC TREATMENT
- PDE5 inhibitors prevent the breakdown of cyclic GMP
- Silidenafil (Viagra)
- Vardenafil (Levitra)
- Tadalafil (Cialis)
- Hormonal therapy and dopamine agonists
- Intracavernous injection therapy
- Intrauretheral therapy
- Topical agents

Special Considerations
- Many men are reluctant to discuss problems with ED.
- Men who demonstrate poor compliance with anti-hypertensive medications may have problems with ED.
- All PDE5 inhibitors are contraindicated with use of nitroglycerine.
- Vardenafil is contraindicated in patients taking doxazosin (Cardura), terazosin (Hytrin), or tamsulosin (Flomax).

- Tadalafil is contraindicated in patients using doxazosin or terazosin, but may be taken with tamsulosin at the 0.4-mg dose.

Follow-up

EXPECTED OUTCOMES
- Patient will discuss difficulty with ED if desired.
- Patient will experience satisfactory erection with prescribed treatment.

COMPLICATIONS
- Concurrent use of nitrates and PDE5 inhibitors can result in severe hypotension.

PROSTATE CANCER

Description
- Very common cancer occurring in older men
- Usually slow-growing with a favorable prognosis

Etiology
- Most tumors are adenocarcinomas.

Incidence and Demographics
- Approximately 218,000 new cases of prostate cancer diagnosed in 2010, with about 32,000 deaths.
- 1 in 6 men will be diagnosed with prostate cancer in their lifetimes..
- Incidence is highest in Blacks.

Risk Factors
- Age
- Family history
- HTN
- Low vitamin D levels
- Folic acid supplements (> 1 mg/day)
- High alcohol intake
- Diet high in trans fats
- History of STIs
- Obesity
- Elevated levels of testosterone
- Exposure to Agent Orange

Prevention and Screening
- Possible protective role for vitamin B6, selenium, vitamin E, lycopene, and soy foods.
- Cruciferous vegetables may be protective.
- Regular exercise.
- 5α-reductase inhibitors.
- Vegetarian diets have been associated with a lower incidence of prostate cancer.
- Preliminary study found correlation between coffee consumption and a lower risk of aggressive prostate cancer.

- Screening is by annual DRE and PSA blood test in appropriate individuals, but screening PSA has recently come under scrutiny due to studies showing no mortality benefit.

Assessment

HISTORY
- Usually asymptomatic in early stages.
- May present with symptoms of BPH.
- Pain in the hips, back, or pelvis may indicate metastasis.

PHYSICAL EXAM
- DRE may be normal or reveal an asymmetric, hard, or nodular gland.

DIAGNOSTIC STUDIES
- PSA: more important to look at PSA velocity than absolute value (see Box 13–5)
- Urinalysis or urine C&S with urinary symptoms
- Transrectal ultrasound and biopsy

Box 13–5. PSA Velocity

PSA velocity looks at the rate of change in the PSA rather than the absolute value. Laboratory norms consider a "normal" PSA to be < 4.0. However, if the PSA doubles in a year (for example: 0.5 to 1.0 to 2.0 in a 2-year period), this would indicate a rapidly increasing PSA, which might signify a growing cancer.

Differential Diagnosis
- BPH
- Prostatitis
- Urethral stricture
- UTI
- Bladder of renal cancer

Nursing Management

NONPHARMACOLOGIC TREATMENT
- "Watchful waiting" or "active surveillance" indicated for some persons.
- Treatment decisions depend on the following:
  - Stage of disease
  - Gleason score
  - PSA level
  - Age of patient
  - General health and life expectancy
  - Feelings about treatments and possible side effects

PHARMACOLOGIC TREATMENT
- Chemotherapy
- Hormonal therapy

INTERVENTIONAL TREATMENT
- Radiation therapy
- Brachytherapy (internal radiotherapy)
- High-intensity focused ultrasound (HIFU)
- Cryosurgery
- Radical prostatectomy

Special Considerations
- Most important clinical prognostic indicators are stage of disease, pretreatment PSA, and Gleason score.
- Prostate cancer is more prevalent in developed countries, possibly owing to longer life expectancy and more consumption of red meat.

Follow-up

EXPECTED OUTCOMES
- Patient will regain normal urinary elimination and sexual function after treatment of cancer.
- Patient will express satisfaction with control of pain throughout period of illness.

COMPLICATIONS
- Most common sites of metastasis are bone and lymph nodes.
- Can cause problems with urination or erectile dysfunction

OVARIAN AND ENDOMETRIAL CANCER

Description
- Cancer of the female reproductive tract can arise in the vulva, vagina, cervix, uterus (endometrium), fallopian tubes, or ovaries.
- This section will cover ovarian and endometrial cancer.

Etiology
- Most ovarian cancers (90%) arise from the epithelium of the ovary and are thus classified as "epithelial."
- Most endometrial cancers are adenocarcinomas.

Incidence and Demographics
- Approximately 26,000 cases of ovarian cancer are diagnosed each year and roughly 16,000 women die, making it the leading cause of death from gynecologic cancers.
- Lifetime risk for ovarian cancer is 1.6% in the general population, 5% if a first-degree relative is affected, and 25% to 60% in women with certain BRCA1 or BRCA2 gene mutations.
- Endometrial is the most common gynecologic cancer in the United States, with 35,000 women diagnosed each year, but death rates are lower than for ovarian and cervical cancer.

Risk Factors
- Ovarian
  - Age
  - Obesity

- Family history of ovarian, breast, or colorectal cancer
- Nulliparity
- Infertility
- Postmenopausal estrogen replacement
- Possibly use of talcum powder in genital area
- Endometrial
  - Age
  - Nulliparity
  - Infertility
  - Unopposed postmenopausal estrogen replacement
  - Early menarche
  - Late menopause
  - Polycystic ovary syndrome
  - Endometrial hyperplasia
  - Obesity
  - HTN
  - Diabetes
  - High-fat diet
  - Tamoxifen
  - 40% more common in Whites, but Black women have twice the death rate

Prevention and Screening

- Ovarian
  - Multiparous
  - Early age at first pregnancy (before 25) and older age at final pregnancy
  - Breastfeeding
  - Combined oral contraceptives
  - Tubal ligation
  - Low-fat diet
  - Routine screening of general population is not recommended because there is no cost-effective test with adequate sensitivity and specificity
- Endometrial
  - Regular exercise
  - Pregnancy and breastfeeding
  - Diet low in saturated fats and high in fruits and vegetables
  - Soy foods
  - Routine screening of general population is not recommended

Assessment

- Ovarian cancer symptoms are very vague. Abdominal distention is the most common complaint. Other complaints may include:
  - Abdominal pain or mass
  - Bloating
  - Back pain
  - Urinary urgency
  - Constipation, diarrhea, gas, nausea
  - Dyspareunia
  - Abnormal vaginal bleeding

- Fatigue
- Weight loss
- Endometrial cancer symptoms
  - Postmenopausal vaginal bleeding
  - Postmenopausal vaginal discharge
  - Abnormal menstrual periods
  - Fatigue, shortness of breath, or other symptoms of anemia
  - Pelvic pain or cramping

  PHYSICAL EXAM
  - Pelvic with bimanual examination
  - Complete abdominal exam with rectal for stool occult blood

  DIAGNOSTIC STUDIES
  - Transvaginal ultrasound
  - Abdominal/pelvic CT scan
  - Ovarian
    - CA-125 tumor marker (not effective in all cases)
  - Endometrial
    - CBC with blood loss
    - Pap smear may be normal or abnormal
    - Endometrial curettage (may require dilation)
    - Hysteroscopy

Nursing Management

NONPHARMACOLOGIC TREATMENT
- None

PHARMACOLOGIC TREATMENT
- Chemotherapy (see Interventional Treatment below)

INTERVENTIONAL TREATMENT
- Treatment is based on staging and type of cancer
  - Ovarian
    - Oophorectomy for women at Stage I who have not completed childbearing.
    - For Stages II–IV, TAH and BSO is standard surgical intervention.
    - Debulking surgery if tumor has spread outside the ovary.
    - Chemotherapy.
  - Endometrial
    - Abdominal hysterectomy with bilateral salpingo-oophorectomy

Special Considerations

- Ovarian cancer has a poor prognosis because of the vague presentation and usually late diagnosis. More than 60% of women are diagnosed at stage III or IV, when it has spread beyond the ovaries and pelvic region.
- Having one type of reproductive cancer increases the risk of other types, making regular follow-up critical.

Follow-up

EXPECTED OUTCOMES

- Patient will maintain weight within normal range.
- Patient will get adequate rest and pace activities to avoid fatigue.
- Patient will express feelings about loss of fertility as applicable.
- Immunocompromised patients will verbalize precautions to minimize the risk of infection.

COMPLICATIONS

- Metastasis
- Ascites
- Intestinal obstruction
- Uterine perforation during endometrial biopsy
- Death

REFERENCES

Bachmann, G. A., & Nevadunsky, N. S. (2000). Diagnosis and treatment of atrophic vaginits. *American Family Physician, 6*(1), 3090–3096.

Brinkman, M., & Zeegers, M. P. (2006). Use of selenium in chemoprevention of bladder cancer. *Lancet Oncology, 7*(9), 766–774.

Cockcroft, D. W., & Gault, M. H. (1976). Prediction of creatinine clearance from serum creatinine. *Nephron, 16*(1), 31–41

Dirks, J. H., de Zeeuw, D., Agarwal, S. K., Atkins, R. C., Correa-Rotter, R., D'Amico, G., ..., Weening, J. J. (2004). Prevention of chronic kidney and vascular disease: Toward global health equity—the Bellagio 2004 Declaration. *Kidney International, 98,* S1–S6.

Djulbegovic, M., Beyth, R. J., Neuberger, M. M., Stoffs, T. L., Vieweg, J., Djulbegovic, B., & Dahm, P. (2010). Screening for prostate cancer: Systematic review and meta-analysis of randomised controlled trials. *British Medical Journal, 341,* c4543.

Freidman, S. (2006). Urinary function. In S. E. Meiner & A. G. Lueckenotte (Eds.), *Gerontological nursing* (pp. 630–652). St. Louis, MO: Mosby-Elsevier.

Geetha, D. (2010). *Poststreptococcal glomerulonephritis.* Retrieved from http://emedicine.medscape .com/article/240337-overview

Giri, M. (2004). Choice of renal replacement therapy in patients with diabetic end stage renal disease. *EDTNA/ERCA Journal, 30*(3), 138–142.

Lakin, M. (2009). *Erectile dysfunction.* Retrieved from http://www.clevelandclinicmeded.com/ medicalpubs/diseasemanagement/endocrinology/erectile-dysfunction/

Levey, A. S., Bosch, J. P., Lewis, J. B., Greene, T., Rogers, N., & Roth, D. (1999). A more accurate method to estimate glomerular filtration rate from serum creatinine: A new prediction equation. Modification of Diet in Renal Disease Study Group. *Annals of Internal Medicine, 130*(6), 461–470.

Mills, E. J. (Ed.) (2005). *Handbook of medical-surgical nursing* (4th ed.). Philadelphia: Lippincott Williams & Wilkins.

National Cancer Institute. (n.d.). *Bladder cancer.* Retrieved from http://www.cancer.gov/cancertopics/ types/bladder

National Cancer Institute. (n.d.). *Endometrial cancer.* Retrieved from http://www.cancer.gov/ cancertopics/types/endometrial

National Cancer Institute. (n.d.). *Ovarian cancer.* Retrieved from http://www.cancer.gov/cancertopics/ types/ovarian

National Cancer Institute. (n.d.). *Prostate cancer.* Retrieved from http://www.cancer.gov/cancertopics/ types/prostate

National Cancer Institute. (n.d.). *SEER Stat Fact Sheets: Prostate.* Retrieved from http://seer.cancer.gov/ statfacts/html/prost.html#incidence-mortality

National Kidney Foundation Kidney Disease Outcomes Quality Initiative (KDOQI). (2002). KDOQI clinical practice guidelines for chronic kidney disease: Evaluation, classification and stratification. *American Journal of Kidney Disease, 39*(2suppl 1), S1–S266.

Ouslander, J. G. (2003). Urinary incontinence. In W. R. Hazzard (Ed.), *Principles of geriatric medicine and gerontology.* New York: McGraw-Hill.

Peacock, P. R. (2010). *Acute renal failure.* Retrieved from http://emedicine.medscape.com/article/ 777845-overview

Remedy Health Media, LLC. (2011). *Urinary tract infection overview.* Retrieved from http://www .urologychannel.com/uti/index.shtml

Sachdeva, K. (2010). *Renal cell carcinoma.* Retrieved from http://emedicine.medscape.com/article/ 281340-overview

U.S. Renal Data System. (2001). *USRDS annual data report: Atlas of end-stage renal disease in the US.* Bethesda, MD: National Institutes of Health, National Institute of Diabetes and Digestive and Kidney Disease.

4

Musculoskeletal Disorders

Nancy Henne Batchelor, MSN, RN-BC, CNS

GENERAL APPROACH

- Includes bones, muscles, tendons, ligaments, and cartilage
- Has key role in maintenance of healthy function
- Allows movement
- Produces blood cells

BONE NEOPLASMS

Description

- Primary: rare
  - Emerge from connective and supportive tissue cells
  - Rare after age 30
- Metastatic: due to relapsed cancer
  - Common sites to metastasize from:
    - Thyroid
    - Colon
    - Breast
    - Lung
    - Prostate
    - Melanoma
    - Kidney

- Bone exposed to radiation treatment is more likely to develop bone cancer later.
- Symptoms
  - General symptoms
    - Decreased range of motion (ROM) due to swelling
    - Joint effusion
    - Tenderness and warmth on palpation
    - Superficial blood vessels
  - Osteosarcoma
    - Pain
    - Swelling
    - Sunburst appearance on x-ray
  - Chondrosarcoma
    - Intermittent or dull pain
    - Lobular appearance on x-ray
  - Ewing's sarcoma
    - Pain
    - Swelling
    - Fatigue
    - Anemia
    - Leukocytosis
    - "Onion skin" appearance on x-ray

Etiology

- Osteosarcoma
  - 35% of reported cases of bone cancer
  - Usually ages 10 to 30
  - 10% after age 60
  - More common in males than in females
  - Sites: distal femur, proximal tibia, humerus, pelvis
- Chondrosarcoma: cancer of cartilage cells
  - Most common type of bone neoplasm
  - Usually over 20 years old (30 to 60)
  - Males and females equally affected
  - Sites: pelvis, legs, arms, trachea, larynx, chest wall
  - Slow-growing, locally invasive
- Ewing's sarcoma: forms in bone cavity
  - Ages 4 to 25
  - 80% younger than 20 years old
  - Higher incidence in Whites
  - Sites: long bones of leg, arm, pelvis; extends into soft tissue

Incidence and Demographics

- Estimated new cases per year: 2,380
- Expected deaths per year: 1,470

Risk Factors

- Osteosarcoma
  - Paget's disease
  - Parathyroid hormone injection

- Osteoporosis
  - Radiation therapy
- Chondrosarcoma
- Ewing's sarcoma

Assessment

HISTORY
- Pain with lifting
- Limping
- Bone pain

PHYSICAL EXAM
- Tenderness, swelling, redness at tumor site
- Limited motion

DIAGNOSTIC STUDIES
- X-ray: increase or decrease in bone density
- Bone scan: identifies extent of tumor, helps with planned therapy
- CT/MRI: soft-tissue injury and exact location
- Complete blood count (CBC)
- Chemistry profile: increased alkaline phosphatase
- Bone biopsy; arteriogram; chest, lung scan: identify metastases

Nursing Management
- Provide support
- Pain relief
- Prevention of pathologic fractures

NONPHARMACOLOGIC TREATMENT
- Radiation

PHARMACOLOGIC TREATMENT
- Chemotherapy
- Immunotherapy
- Hormone therapy

INTERVENTIONAL TREATMENT
- Surgery to remove malignant tissue

Follow-up

EXPECTED OUTCOMES
- Pain relief
- Prevention of pathologic fractures

FRACTURES

Description
- Break in continuity of the bone
- Classified by location, type, or direction or patterns of fracture line
- Vary in intensity according to location and type
- More common in people who have sustained trauma and in older adults
- Can occur in any of the 206 bones
- Occurs when bone is subjected to more kinetic energy than can be absorbed

Etiology
- Direct blow
- Crushing force: compression
- Sudden twisting motion: torsion
- Severe muscle contraction
- Disease causing weak bones: pathologic

Incidence and Demographics
- In 2006, there were 316,000 hospital admissions for hip fractures in older adults, an increase of 7% from 2005.
- High-risk recreation or employment-related activities result in fractures for individuals with healthy bones
- Most common fracture sites for older adults
  - Hip
  - Femur
  - Wrist

Risk Factors
- Trauma
- Osteopenia, osteoporosis
- Malnutrition
- Neoplasm
- Medications
- Abuse
- Osteogenesis imperfecta
- Age
- Deconditioning

Prevention and Screening
- Trauma prevention
- Safety equipment
- Screening for risks in the older adult
  - Osteoporosis
  - Activity levels
  - Cognitive and affective disorders
  - Sensory impairments
  - Risk for falls

- Educational programs
  - Workplace and farm safety
  - Ergonomic principles
- Promotion of bone health
  - Exercise program
  - Avoid obesity
  - Calcium intake

Assessment

PHYSICAL EXAM
- Pain
- Skin temperature
- Pulses
- Deformity
- Edema
- ROM
- Skin color
- Touch
  - **5 Ps** of neurovascular assessment
    - **Pain:** scale
    - **Pulses:** compare bilaterally
    - **Pallor:** warm and blue: venous policy; pale and cool: arterial compromise
    - **Paralysis or paresis:** distal to fracture site; limited ROM: nerve damage
    - **Paresthesia**

DIAGNOSTIC STUDIES
- X-ray
- CBC, chemistry panel, coagulation studies: assess blood loss, renal function, muscle breakdown, risk of bleeding or clotting
- Bone scan: determine fracture site by increased uptake

Nursing Management

NONPHARMACOLOGIC TREATMENT
- Emergency care
  - Stabilize
    - Maintain immobilization: traction, casting, or splint
    - Prevent complications: circulation checks, position change
    - Restore function
  - Splint
    - Maintain alignment
    - Prevent dislocation
    - Relieve pain: ice, elevation, alternative pain management modalities
    - Prevent complications

PHARMACOLOGIC TREATMENT
- Nonsteroidal anti-inflammatory drugs (NSAIDs)
- Narcotics
- Patient-controlled analgesia (PCA)
- Epidural
- Request p.r.n. medications prior to severe pain
- Offer routinely for 24 to 48 hours post injury and surgery
- Reassure patient re: addiction
- Unrelieved and escalating pain may indicate complications

INTERVENTIONAL TREATMENT
- Internal fixation
- External fixation
- Electronic bone stimulation

Special Considerations
- Older adults
- Wrist and hip fractures most common
- Usually result from fall
- Pathological fractures caused by osteoporosis usually occur prior to fall
- Delay in surgical repair leads to complications
  - Atelectasis
  - Deep vein thrombosis
  - Urinary tract infection
  - Pressure ulcers

Follow-up

EXPECTED OUTCOMES
- Bone healing: hematoma formation in 48 to 72 hours
- Cellular proliferation: osteoblast multiplication and differentiation into fibrocartilaginous callus
  - Callus formation: at level of fracture
  - Ossification: mature bone replaces callus
  - Remodeling: excess callus resorbed, bone thickens and strengthens

COMPLICATIONS
- Respiratory insufficiency, acute respiratory distress syndrome (ARDS)
  - Fat embolus: bone marrow releases fat, which enters venous system and pulmonary vessels; pulmonary vessels are blocked; surfactant inactivated
  - Symptoms: respiratory distress, tachypnea, air hunger, hypoxia, fever, decreased level of consciousness, tachycardia, restlessness
- Venous thromboembolism
  - Due to immobility, prolonged surgery, hypercoagulability, vessel injury
- Compartment syndrome
  - Restricted blood flow within an anatomical compartment
  - Symptoms: edema, pain, engorgement, no pulses, paresthesia, pallor, paralysis
- Pressure ulcers
  - Can be due to friction secondary to prosthetic devices

- Infection
  - Risk increases with:
    - Diabetes mellitus
    - Chronic obstructive pulmonary disease (COPD)
    - Preexisting infection
    - Open fracture
- Joint dislocation
  - Due to joint overextension
  - Symptoms: pain, decreased ROM, nausea, vomiting
- Heterotrophic ossification
  - Growth of bone tissue where it is not normally present
  - Symptoms: pain, rubor, swelling, fever
- Osteogenesis or avascular necrosis
  - Bone tissue death due to impaired circulation

OSTEOARTHRITIS (OA)

Description
- Loss of articular cartilage in articulating joints and hypertrophy of bones at the articular margins
- Two types:
  - Idiopathic
    - Associated with increasing age
    - May be inherited as autosomal recessive trait with genetic defects that cause destruction of joint cartilage
    - Due to articular injury
    - Wear and tear on joints
    - Improper joint alignment
  - Trauma
    - Mechanical stress
    - Occupational/hobbies
    - Professional athletics
    - Running
    - Gymnastics
    - Joint instability
    - Congenital defects
    - Inflammatory disease
    - Metabolic disorders
    - Selected medications
- Symptoms:
  - Pain
    - Deep ache
    - Aggravated by joint motion or use
    - Relieved by rest
    - May be persistent with disease progression
    - May be accompanied by paresthesias
    - May be referred to other body parts

- Joint stiffness
  - Occurs after inactivity/rest
- Decreased ROM
- Crepitus/grating with movement
- Joint enlargement due to bony overgrowth

Etiology
- Noninflammatory process
  - Enzymatic degradation causes loss of proteoglycans and collagen from cartilage.
  - Bone becomes exposed due to cartilage loss.
  - Weight-bearing joints are affected.
- Factors associated with OA
  - Joint integrity
  - Genetic predisposition
  - Local inflammation
  - Mechanical forces
  - Cellular/biochemical processes

Incidence and Demographics
- Leading cause of disability and pain in the elderly
- May affect individuals at about age 40
- Manifestations present between 50 and 60
- Men and women affected equally until age 55
  - More common in women after age 55
  - Slowly progressive

Risk Factors
- Tends to run in families
- Obesity
- Lack of exercise
- Medical conditions:
  - Hemophilia
  - Avascular necrosis
  - Chronic gout
  - Pseudogout
  - Rheumatoid arthritis

Prevention and Screening
- Maintain normal weight.
- Maintain regular, moderate exercise program.
- Use of glucosamine and chondroitin supplements for symptom reduction.

Assessment
HISTORY
- Family history of OA
- Occupation
- Recreational activities
- Ability to carry out activities of daily living (ADLs)

- Self-care activities
- Joint pain
- AM stiffness
- Joint deformity
- Fatigue
- General weakness
- Anorexia
- Cold intolerance
- Paresthesias

PHYSICAL EXAM
- Height/weight
- Gait
- Joints: symmetry, size, color, shape, appearance
- Deformities
- Cold, clammy extremities
- Shiny skin
- Limited movement
- Temperature
- Stiffness
- Heberden's nodes
- Bouchard's nodes

DIAGNOSTIC STUDIES
- CT scan
- MRI
- Bone density
- X-ray
- Erythrocyte sedimentation rate
- Rheumatoid factor

Nursing Management

NONPHARMACOLOGIC TREATMENT
- Physical therapy for ROM
- Joint rest
- Assistive devices
- Weight loss

COMPLEMENTARY THERAPY
- Bioelectromagnetic therapy
- Yoga
- Nutritional supplements
  - Boron
  - Zinc
  - Copper
  - Selenium
  - Manganese
  - Flavonoids

- Glucosamine
- Chondroitin
- Herbal therapy
  - Evening primrose oil

PHARMACOLOGIC TREATMENT
- NSAIDs—instruct about GI side effects
- Cox-2 inhibitors
- Antimalarials
- Acetaminophen: preferred for the older adult because of less chance for toxicity and GI side effects of NSAIDs
- Narcotics if pain is unrelieved by over-the-counter medications
- Topical antiseptics
- Capsaicin
- Heating rubs
- Intra-articular injections
  - Sodium hyaluronate (Hyalgan, Synvisc)
  - Steroid injections: can hasten rate of cartilage breakdown if given more often than every 4 to 6 months

INTERVENTIONAL TREATMENT
- Synovectomy: removal of swollen synovial
- Arthrodesis: joint fusion for severe destruction of joint surfaces
- Reconstructive surgery: joint replacement
  - Reserved for patients with severely restricted ROM and pain at rest
- Arthroscopy: debridement and lavage of involved joint
- Osteotomy: incision into/transaction of bone for joint realignment when significant bony overgrowth or osteophyte formation has occurred

Special Considerations
- Can be debilitating; decreases quality of life.
- Encourage weight loss for obese patients.
- Promote exercise, independence, empowerment, and safe environment.
- Implement fall protocol if individual is a fall risk.

Follow-up

EXPECTED OUTCOMES
- Decreased pain
- Increased or maintained mobility
- Improved quality of life
- Fall prevention
- Self-care with ADLs or adaptation

COMPLICATIONS
- Joint pain and stiffness may affect ability to maintain activities
- Increased disability
- Decreased quality of life

OSTEOMYELITIS

Description
- Acute or chronic infection of the bone
- Infections in adjacent bone or soft tissue
- Can lead to tissue death or necrosis
- Offending organisms
  - *Staphylococcus epidermis*
  - *Staphylococcus aureus* (90%)
  - *Pseudomonas aeruginosa*
  - *Escherichia coli*
  - *Mycobacterium tuberculosis*
  - *Neisseria gonorrhoeae*
- Symptoms:
  - Fever
  - Malaise
  - Edema at site
  - Abscess
  - Warmth
  - Fracture
  - Tenderness
  - Chills
  - Movement or joint limitations at site
  - Low back pain
  - Fatigue
  - Nausea
- Problem: symptoms develop over time and may go unnoticed for up to 1 week

Etiology
- Direct extension: from trauma or surgery
- Seeding through bloodstream: hematogenetic
- Skin infections secondary to peripheral vascular disease (PVD)

Incidence and Demographics
- 2 in 10,000

Risk Factors
- Immune compromise
- Diabetes mellitus
- Peripheral vascular disease
- Malignancies
- Prosthetic hardware within bone
- Sickle cell disease
- Renal failure with dialysis
  - IV drug abuse
  - Age: elderly at higher risk

Assessment

HISTORY
- Onset may be acute, subacute or chronic
- General complaints
- Fever
- Fatigue
- Malaise
- Joint limitations

PHYSICAL EXAM
- Edema at site
- Limited joint movement
- Warmth
- Tenderness

DIAGNOSTIC STUDIES
- CBC: decreased hemoglobin, increased white blood count (WBC) and erythrocyte sedimentation rate (ESR)
- C-reactive protein increases dramatically with inflammation and bacterial infection
- Reportable levels: 0.3–20 mg/dL
- Blood culture to identify offending organism
- X-ray
  - Early: nondefinitive
  - Later: shows tissue swelling and bone loss
- MRI: useful for surgical localization
  - Identifies soft tissue vs bone marrow involvement
- Bone scan: increased concentration of radioactivity at infection site
- Ultrasonography identifies soft-tissue abscess, fluid collection, and periosteal elevation
- Needle aspiration: sample of fluids and cells
- Bone biopsy

Nursing Management

NONPHARMACOLOGIC TREATMENT
- Treat underlying cause to prevent loss of function.
- Gear treatment to prevent nonhealing of wound, sepsis, immobility, amputation.
- Immobilization of affected bone; no weight-bearing.
- Surgery to incise and drain (I&D).
- If chronic: remove diseased bone.
- May require multiple I&Ds, sterile dressing changes.
- Physical therapy:
  - Maintain function.
  - Teach use of assistive devices.
- Nutrition:
  - High protein, high calorie, high vitamins A, B, C to promote healing.
- Teaching:
  - Support for affected area: increase circulation and proper alignment
  - Disease process
  - Medications

- Signs of inflammation and changes indicating worsening of disease
- Care of IV lines: for prolonged antibiotic therapy

PHARMACOLOGIC TREATMENT
- Pain control: NSAIDs, narcotics
- Antibiotics: broad spectrum until organism is identified
  - Usually 4 to 6 weeks IV, followed by p.o.

Special Considerations
- Physical therapy to maintain activity level and proper use of assistive devices
- Nutrition consult to determine caloric need for healing
- Social service referral for outpatient treatment options—antibiotic therapy and physical therapy

Follow-up

EXPECTED OUTCOMES
- Healed bone
- Safety in ambulation when using assistive device
- Weight maintenance without loss of muscle

COMPLICATIONS
- May become chronic
- Requires incision and drainage and repeated debridements if abscess
- Delayed identification/treatment may result in:
  - Chronic infection
  - Chronic pain
  - Chronic draining sinuses
  - Loss of function
  - Amputation
  - Death

OSTEOPOROSIS

Description
- Metabolic bone disease resulting in loss of bone mass
- Increased bone fragility
- Increases fracture risk
- Aging is primary cause
- Types
  - Primary
  - Secondary
    - Cushing's disease
    - Bariatric surgery
    - Medications
      - Anticonvulsants
      - Thyroid hormone
      - Glucocorticoids

- Furosemide
- Antipsychotics

Etiology

- Disturbance in normal balance between osteoblastic (bone-building) and osteoclastic (bone resorbing) activity.

Type I (Postmenopausal)

- Estrogen promotes osteoblast activity and increases new bone formation.
- Estrogen enhances calcium absorption and stimulates the thyroid to secrete calcitonin.
- Loss of estrogen post-menopause results in decreased bone mineral density and fragile bone.

Type II

- Results from the normal aging process.
- Declines in number and activity of osteoblasts.
- Affects trabecular and cortical bone.

Incidence and Demographics

- Most common metabolic bone disorder
- Approximately 44 million people in United States are affected
- Women are affected more commonly and at younger ages than men
- Most frequent fracture sites are hip, wrist, and vertebrae
- Bone loss in men results from decreasing testosterone levels and estrogen levels

Risk Factors

- Risk depends on how much bone mass is achieved between ages 25 and 35 and how much is lost later.
  - **Nonmodifiable**
    - Age
      - Women see effects postmenopause.
      - Men see effects 15 to 20 years later.
      - Men: Decrease in testosterone and estrogen contribute to bone loss.
    - Race
      - White or Asian
      - Bone mass positively correlates with amount of skin pigmentation
      - Dark-skinned people have greater bone density
    - Metabolic disorders
    - Cushing's syndrome
      - Thyrotoxicosis
      - Hyperparathyroidism
      - Homocytinuria
      - Affect nutritional states and bone mineralization
    - Family history
  - **Modifiable**
    - Nutritional deficiencies
      - Calcium
      - Vitamin D
      - With decreased intake, calcium is removed from skeleton, weakening bone tissue
    - Acidosis due to high-protein diet or diet soda with high phosphate
      - Kidney tries to buffer excess acid, relying on calcium withdrawn from bone
      - Osteoclast function is stimulated

- Cigarette smoking
  - Decreases blood supply to bone.
  - Osteoblast production slowed by nicotine.
  - Calcium absorption impaired by nicotine.
  - Bone density is decreased.
- Alcohol
  - Excessive drinking is toxic to osteoblast activity.
  - Alcohol intoxication suppresses bone formation.
  - Excess alcohol increases parathyroid hormone levels and reduces calcium reserves.
  - Excess alcohol increases cortisol levels, which decrease bone formation and increase bone breakdown.
  - Increased alcohol intake may cause nutritional deficiencies.
- Female athletes
  - Decreased estrogen production
  - Poor nutrition
  - Intense training
  - Eating disorders
  - Amenorrhea
- Sedentary lifestyle
  - Bone metabolism decreases without weight-bearing exercise
  - Blood flow to bone decreases without weight-bearing, including standing, walking and running
  - Growth-producing nutrients to cells decrease
  - Osteoblast growth and activity decreases
- Medications
  - Increase calcium excretion
    - Antacids with aluminum
    - Corticosteroids
    - Anticonvulsants
    - Heparin: increases bone resorption causing osteoporosis
    - Antiretroviral therapy: decreases bone density

Prevention and Screening

Screening
- Bone mineral density every 2 years for screening
- Women 50 and over
- Men 70 and over
- Individuals with conditions that predispose to decreased bone density

Prevention
- Identification of risk factors
- Modification of detrimental lifestyle factors
- Reinforcement of positive lifestyle choices
- Calcium- and vitamin D–rich diet
- Exercise—strength and weight-bearing
- Education
- Safety measures to prevent fractures
- Fall prevention programs
- Home assessment

Assessment

HISTORY
- Age
- Menstrual history
- Exercise
- Risk factors
- Medications
- Activity level
- Family history
- Diet

PHYSICAL EXAM
- Height
- Spinal curves
- Low back pain

DIAGNOSTIC STUDIES
- DEXA scan: T score below –2.5 standard deviations (SD) of the young adult mean
- Bone density of lumbar spine and hip
- Serum or urine markers of bone remodeling
- X-ray: identifies osteoporotic changes after 30% bone mass loss

Nursing Management

NONPHARMACOLOGIC TREATMENT
- Health promotion
  - Calcium intake
  - Exercise: regular and weight-bearing, 20 minutes 4 times per week
    - Increases blood flow to bone
    - Allows growth-producing nutrients to enter the cells
- Health-related behaviors
  - Diet: optimal calcium intake before age 30 to 35 increases peak bone mass
  - Foods
    - Milk, milk products
    - Sardines, clams, oysters, salmon
    - Dark green leafy vegetables: broccoli, spinach, bok choy, greens
  - Supplements
    - Calcium and vitamin D
    - Complementary therapies
    - Aid in pain relief; physical, emotional, and mental stress
    - Increase body's energy system to maintain state of well-being
    - Yoga, biofeedback, massage and reflexology

PHARMACOLOGIC TREATMENT
- Estrogen replacement for postmenopausal women
- Androgen replacement for men with low testosterone
- Bisphosphonates: alendronate (Fosamax), ibandronate (Boniva), risedronate (Actonel), zoledronate (Zometa)
- Calcium: 1,500 mg/day

- Vitamin D: 800 IU/day
- Calcitonin
- Selective estrogen receptor modulators: raloxifene (Evista)
- Teriparatide (Forteo)

Follow-up

EXPECTED OUTCOMES
- Pain relief
- Prevention of further bone loss
- Increased mobility, strength, and stability
- Fracture prevention
- Improved quality of life

COMPLICATIONS
- Pathologic fractures
- Decreased function and mobility

SOFT-TISSUE AND JOINT INJURIES

Description
- Contusions
  - Least serious
  - Rupture of small blood vessels with bleeding into soft tissue
  - Result in bruise
- Lacerations
  - Torn skin
- Strains
  - Stretching injury due to mechanical overload
  - Occurs at muscle belly or its tendon attachment
  - Results in swelling, tenderness
- Sprains
  - Injury to ligament surrounding a joint
  - Results from overstretching or tear
  - Symptoms: joint instability, discoloration, heat, pain, edema, rapid swelling

Table 14–1. Grading of Sprains

Severity	Degree of Damage	Symptoms	Recovery
Grade 1	Ligament stretch	Mild pain, swelling, tenderness	1–3 weeks
Grade 2	Tear 20%–75%	Mod. pain, swelling, tenderness, decreased ROJM/function, joint instability	3–6 weeks
Grade 3	Complete tear, rupture	Severe swelling, tenderness, joint instability, loss of ROJM, unable to bear weight	Several months

- Dislocations
  - Displacement or separation of bone ends of a joint
  - Injury occurs to ligament and joint capsule

Etiology
- Accidental
  - Overuse
  - Sports injuries
  - Impact
  - Motor vehicle accidents (MVA)
  - Falls
- Nonaccidental, inflicted
  - Abuse: blunt trauma
- Most common: MVA, falls, bicycle and pedestrian injuries

Incidence and Demographics
- Most commonly reported injuries
- 50% work-related injuries
- Most common work-related: back injury
- Most common sprain: ankle
- Most common muscle strain: cervical and lumbar

Risk Factors
- Age
- Inactive lifestyle
- Overuse
- Sports injury
- Overweight

Prevention and Screening
- Healthy behaviors
  - Proper warm-ups for sports
  - Proper training
  - Supervision
  - Proper equipment and surfaces
  - Refrain from competition in presence of pain or injury
  - Trauma prevention: safety education

Assessment

HISTORY
- Circumstances leading to injury
- Mechanism of injury
- Previous injury

PHYSICAL EXAM
- Check for redness, warmth
- Inspect and palpate for swelling, tenderness around a joint
- Compare extremities for deformity or asymmetry

- Assess ROM: determine baseline
  - Assess active, passive, and resisted movement
- Assess for neurological impairment or progression

DIAGNOSTIC STUDIES
- X-rays: fracture vs. soft-tissue injury
- MRI for further assessment

Nursing Management

Contusions

NONPHARMACOLOGIC TREATMENT
- Ice × 48 hours; capillary constriction impedes blood and edema.
- Warm moist heat increases circulation and resorbs edema.

PHARMACOLOGIC TREATMENT
- NSAIDs

Lacerations

NONPHARMACOLOGIC TREATMENT
- Stop the bleeding.
- Wash wound with soap and water.
- Follow with saline flush.
- Suture, surgical glue or steristrip depending on severity.
- Pressure bandage or splint.

PHARMACOLOGIC TREATMENT
- Tetanus booster (TDAP preferred)

Sprains and Strains

NONPHARMACOLOGIC TREATMENT
- PRICE
  - Protect
    - Immobilize and prevent weight-bearing
    - Splint, wrap, brace, or cast for grade 2 or 3 sprain
  - Rest
    - 24 to 48 hours to prevent further damage
  - Ice
    - Decreases pain, nerve conductivity
    - Slows metabolism at injury site
    - Decreases cell death and inflammation
    - 10 to 15 minutes 3 to 4 times a day for 3 to 4 days
  - Compress
    - Control edema through direct pressure
    - Increases venous return
    - 4 to 5 days
  - Elevate
    - Above level of heart to promote blood flow and decrease swelling

PHARMACOLOGIC TREATMENT
- NSAIDs

Dislocations

NONPHARMACOLOGIC TREATMENT
- Protection
- Prevent vascular or nerve damage
- Reduction: within 15 to 30 minutes

PHARMACOLOGIC TREATMENT
- Dependent upon pain level
- NSAIDs to narcotics

Special Considerations
- Seek immediate care for function or sensation loss, pallor, or pain disproportionate to injury.

Follow-up

EXPECTED OUTCOMES
- Decreased pain
- Joint protection
- Return of ROM, strength, and mobility

COMPLICATIONS
- Recurring pain, swelling, bruising or inability to bear weight may indicate underlying fracture
- Dislocations

RHEUMATOID ARTHRITIS (RA)

Description
- Systemic inflammatory disease with autoimmune component.
- Inflammatory process begins in the synovial membrane and joint capsule.
- Inflammatory response perpetuated by infiltration of lymphocytes, macrophages, and neutrophils.
- Cartilage is destroyed by enzyme production.
- Inflammation of connective tissue, primarily in the joints.
- Symptoms:
  - Fatigue
  - Anorexia
  - Weight loss
  - Generalized aching
  - Stiffness
  - Swollen glands

Etiology
- Host tissues are attacked by autoantibodies (rheumatoid factors).
- Autoantibodies bind with target antigens in the blood and synovial membranes, forming immune complexes.
  - B cells make too much rheumatoid factor.
  - T cells: responsible for inflammation; too many in RA.
  - Cytokines: control state of inflammation; levels too high in RA.
  - Interleukin 1 and 6: too much in RA.
- Result in damage to cartilage.

Incidence and Demographics
- Occurs in 1% to 2% of the total population; 0.5% to 1% of U.S. population.
- 75% of cases are female.
- Onset usually between 20 and 40 years.
- Incidence increases with age up to 70 years.
- Onset insidious and subtle.
- Course: variable, with exacerbations and remissions.

Risk Factors
- Increased risk if family member has been diagnosed.

Assessment

HISTORY
- Complaints of joint stiffness, pain, swelling, fatigue, weight loss, anorexia

PHYSICAL EXAM
- Subcutaneous nodules: bony prominences
- Symmetrical bilateral joint involvement
- Crepitus
- Contractures
- Muscle atrophy

DIAGNOSTIC STUDIES
- Rheumatoid factor: present in 75% of individuals with RA
  - High levels: severe disease
- Antinuclear antibodies
- Anticitrulline antibody
- ESR elevated
  - Used as indicator of disease or inflammatory activity when evaluating effectiveness of treatment
- Synovial fluid exam: identify changes with inflammation
  - Cloudiness
  - Decreased viscosity
  - Increased protein level
- WBCs: 3,000 to 50,000
- CBC: anemia with decreased WBC due to spleen enlargement and elevated platelets
- X-ray
  - Early identification shows soft-tissue swelling
  - Later: joint space narrowing and erosions

Nursing Management

NONPHARMACOLOGIC TREATMENT
- Maintain joint function.
- Decrease joint damage.
- Decrease deformity.
- Rest for flares, except in older clients: need to maintain activity to minimize complication of immobility.
- Exercise.
- Protection:
  - Schedule activities and planned rest periods.
- Heat: decrease inflammatory process and increase motion.

PHARMACOLOGIC TREATMENT
- NSAIDs: decrease inflammatory process, manage symptoms
- Cox-2 inhibitors
- Disease-modifying antirheumatics:
  - Alter disease course
  - Reduce joint destruction
  - Clinical improvement evident after several weeks to months
  - Do not slow bone erosion or facilitate healing
  - Used in conjunction with NSAIDs
- Immunosuppressants
  - Methotrexate (Rheumatrex)
    - Given weekly: drug of choice for aggressive disease
    - In conjunction with NSAIDs
    - Benefits seen within 2 to 4 weeks
  - Cyclosporine (Sandimmune)
  - Mycophenolate
  - Azathioprine
  - Cyclophosphamide (Cytoxan)
  - Sulfasalazine
  - Tumor necrosis factor inhibitors
- Antimalarials
  - Hydroxychloroquine (Plaquenil)
  - Chloroquine
  - Quinacrine
  - Require 6 months of therapy before seeing desired response
- Chelating agents
  - D-penicillamine
- Gold compounds
- Corticosteroids
  - Prednisone
    - Low dose to reduce pain and inflammation
    - May slow development and progression of bone erosion
- RA biologics (disease-modifying antirheumatic drugs [DMARDs])
  - Produced from living cells
  - Slow disease progression
  - IV or self-injection

INTERVENTIONAL TREATMENT
- Synovectomy: temporary relief of inflammation and pain, slow destructive process, helps preserve function
- Arthrodesis: joint fusion: stabilize joints
- Arthroplasty: for those with gross deformity or joint destruction
- Experimental therapies

Special Considerations
- For older adults with RA, safety is critical while maintaining dignity.
- Holistic treatment in symptom control.
- Family may need to intervene in caregiving when individual is incapacitated.

Follow-up

EXPECTED OUTCOMES
- Maintain joint function.
- Slow or stop joint damage.
- Reduce inflammation.
- Improve well-being.
- Maintain independence.
- Control pain.

COMPLICATIONS
- Anti-inflammatory response secondary to steroid therapy
- Risks with long term use of NSAIDs and COX 2s
- Inflammatory process in:
  - Lungs: pleuritis
  - Heart: pericardial effusion
  - Blood vessels: vasculitis
  - Eyes: Sjogren's syndrome, scleritis

REFERENCES

Black, J. M., & Hawks, J. H. (2009). *Medical-surgical nursing: Clinical management for positive outcomes* (8th ed.). St. Louis, MO: Saunders Elsevier.

Cleveland Clinic Foundation. (2009). *Osteomyelitis.* Retrieved from http://my.clevelandclinic.org/ disorders/osteomyelitis//hic_osteomyelitis.aspx

Genentech USA. (2010). *Rheumatoid arthritis vs osteoarthritis.* Retrieved from http://www. rheumatoidarthritis.com/understanding-ra/ra-vs-osteoarthritis.aspx

Genentech USA. (2010). *Treating RA.* Retrieved from http://www.rheumatoidarthritis.com/treating-ra/ default.aspx

National Institutes of Health. (2009). *Handout on Health: Rheumatoid arthritis.* Retrieved from http:// www.niams.nih.gov/Health_Info/Rheumatic_Disease/default.asp#ra_10

National Institutes of Health. (2009). *Rheumatoid arthritis.* Retrieved from http://www.niams.nih.gov/ Health_Info/Rheumatic_Disease/default.asp

National Institutes of Health. (2010). *Handout on Health: Osteoarthritis.* Retrieved from http://www .niams.nih.gov/Health_Info/Osteoarthritis/default.asp#7

National Institutes of Health. (2011). *Osteoporosis in men.* Retrieved from http://www.niams.nh.gov/ Health_Info/Bone/Osteoporosis/Men.asp

National Institutes of Health. (2011). *What people recovering from alcoholism need to know about osteoporosis.* Retrieved from http://www.niams.nh.gov/Health_Info/Bone/Condiions_Behaviors/ default.asp

Osborn, K. S., Wraa, C. E., & Watson, A. B. (2010). *Medical surgical nursing: Preparation for practice.* Upper Saddle River, NJ: Pearson Health Science.

15

Metabolism and Endocrine System

Deborah Jane Schwytzer, MSN, RN-BC, CEN

GENERAL APPROACH

- The endocrine system is involved in maintaining the homeostasis of the organs and tissues of the human body through the release of hormones. Hormones are chemical substances that serve to stimulate or inhibit various body processes.
- Hormones interact at target or receptor cells to regulate the body's responses to the internal and external environment, control growth and development, adapt to changes in the body, and assist in reproductive functions.
- The major endocrine glands, the hormones they secrete, and their functions are listed in Table 15–1.
- General hormone regulation to maintain homeostasis is the result of negative and positive feedback systems that signal the release of hormones. For example, a high serum glucose level will stimulate the release of insulin from the islet cells of the pancreas to restore a normal glucose level. Conversely, a low glucose level will stimulate the release of glucagon to increase serum glucose levels and restore physiological homeostasis.
- Conditions and disease processes may cause hyposecretion or hypersecretion of a hormone. In either case, physiological changes will be noted.

Table 15–1. Major Endocrine Glands

Gland	Hormone Secreted	Function
Pituitary—anterior	Thyroid-stimulating hormone (TSH)	Stimulates the synthesis and release of thyroid hormones T3 and T4.
	Adrenocorticotropic hormone (ACTH)	Stimulates release of hormones such as glucocorticoids from the adrenal cortex. ACTH also stimulates production of cortisol by the adrenal glands. Cortisol, a so-called "stress hormone," is vital to survival. It helps maintain blood pressure and blood glucose levels.
	Follicle-stimulating hormone (FSH) Luteinizing hormone (LH)	FSH promotes sperm production in men and stimulates the ovaries to enable ovulation in women. LH regulates testosterone in men and estrogen in women. LH and FSH work together to facilitate normal function of the ovaries and testes.
	Prolactin (PRL)	Stimulates the production of breast milk.
Pituitary—posterior	Oxytocin	Stimulates uterine contractions, breast milk release, and smooth muscles of the prostate for ejection of secretions.
	Antidiuretic hormone (ADH)	Stimulates kidneys to reabsorb water for maintenance of BP and fluid volume; also stimulates peripheral vasoconstriction.
Thyroid	Thyroxine (T4)	Increases ATP production in the mitochondria and cell nuclei.
	Triiodothyronine (T3)	Works with T4 to increase ATP production in the mitochondria and cell nuclei.
	Calcitonin	Regulates the calcium ion in body fluids by targeting bone and kidney cells.
Parathyroid	Parathyroid hormone (PTH)	Maintains concentrations of calcium ions by decreasing excretion in the kidneys and promoting reabsorption in the intestines.
Adrenal—medulla	Epinephrine	Increases glucose levels and rate and force of cardiac contractions; causes vasoconstriction in skin, kidneys, and mucous membranes and vasodilatation in skeletal muscles and coronary and pulmonary arteries.
	Norepinephrine	Increases rate and force of cardiac contractions and causes vasoconstriction.
Adrenal—cortex	Mineralocorticoids	Help to maintain sodium and water in the body to control blood pressure and fluid volume.
	Glucocorticoids	Enhance carbohydrate metabolism, assist in immune response, and are released in response to stress.

Pancreas—islet cells	Insulin Glucagon	Responsible for carbohydrate metabolism and regulation of glucose levels.
Gonads—testes and ovaries	Testosterone Estrogen Progesterone	Regulate body growth, promote the onset of puberty and secondary sexual characteristics, and maintain reproductive functioning.

- In general, a thorough, systematic history and physical assessment of the patient should be completed to identify potential endocrine dysfunction. The physical assessment should specifically include assessment of the physical features such as height, weight, fat and hair distribution, skin color and pigmentation distribution, and muscle mass. Because the thyroid gland and testes are the only potentially palpable endocrine organs, these organs should be assessed for size, shape, symmetry, and presence of nodules. Auscultation of the blood pressure bilaterally should be assessed for fluid volume status. The chest should be assessed for the rate and rhythm of the heart. The psychosocial history should be completed with a focus on recent coping, behavioral or emotional changes, which may indicate a hormonal imbalance. Laboratory studies that focus on hormone and metabolite levels such as direct hormone level measurement, simulation/suppression tests, assays, and urine tests can be used along with imaging (MRI and CT scans) of some of the endocrine structures to assess functioning.

RED FLAGS

- Any dysfunction in any of the endocrine glands or hormone receptor sites can cause an alteration in one or more body systems. A thorough health history and physical assessment should be completed to assess the extent of the effects.
- Because of age-related variables such as acute and chronic illnesses, changes in activity and diet, multiple medications that may affect hormone function, and decreasing hormone clearance, it is difficult to identify abnormal functioning of the endocrine system in the aged population. Typically, decreasing functioning is observed in the thyroid and pancreas as well as the gonads as a result of aging.
- Patients must understand that the need for endocrine hormone replacement therapy is often a life-long process to avoid increased morbidity and mortality. They must also understand the importance of telling their healthcare providers if they use any over-the-counter or herbal products because these can alter the effectiveness of some of hormones.

Disorders of the Endocrine System

HYPERTHYROIDISM—GRAVES' DISEASE

Description
- A condition resulting from excessive overproduction of thyroid hormones by the thyroid gland. Thyroid hormones triiodothyronine (T3) and thyroxine (T4) are released in response to thyroid-stimulating hormone (TSH) to regulate the body's metabolism. Excessive secretion of thyroid hormone results in a hypermetabolic state that affects most of the body systems. The seriousness of the disease depends on the degree of hypersecretion.

Etiology

- The cause of hyperthyroidism is unknown. It is hypothesized that an autoimmune response or hereditary factors may contribute to the development of the condition.
- The effects of hyperthyroidism include increased metabolic rate and alteration in the sympathetic nervous system response to stimuli. Increases in cardiac output, peripheral blood flow, oxygen consumption, and appetite without weight gain, as well as body temperature changes, result from the increased metabolic rate.

Incidence and Demographics

- Graves' disease occurs at any age but is most common in persons between the ages of 20 and 40. It is rare in the elderly (over 65 years of age) and is more common in women.
- Increased incidence of hyperthyroidism also is seen in countries and populations with increased iodine intake, such as in the United States, where much of the food is fortified with iodine and countries who depend on much of their food sources from fish and kelp, such as Asian countries.

Risk Factors

- Increased iodine intake
- Family history of thyroid conditions

Prevention and Screening

- Populations with high iodine intake and individuals with a family history of thyroid disease should be screened.
- Education about the risks of elevated intake of iodine-rich foods and water fortified with iodine can assist in the prevention of hyperthyroidism.

Assessment

HISTORY
- Subjective complaints of heat intolerance, excessive perspiration, and increased appetite with concurrent weight loss.
- Complaints of generalized fatigue and muscle weakness may be present. Physical exertion may result in a complaint of chest pain, palpitations, or shortness of breath.
- Patient may complain of discomfort when wearing anything snug around the neck such as necklaces or collars.
- Abdominal cramping and frequent bowel movements.
- Decreased libido.
- If thyroid hormone levels will be tested, assess medication history. Iodine-containing medications such as oral contraceptives and recently administered diagnostic contrast dyes can cause falsely elevated serum thyroid hormone levels while aspirin, corticosteroids, and phenytoin (as well as recent severe illness or malnutrition) can cause falsely decreased thyroid levels.
- Family history of thyroid disease.

PHYSICAL EXAM
- Enlarged thyroid gland (thyroid goiter) on inspection and palpation. Presence of bruit over the thyroid gland may be noted.

- Visual changes such as blurred or double vision (diplopia) and exophthalmos (protruding eyes) may be noted. Eyelid retraction, infrequent blinking, and the presence of periorbital edema may be noted. Cornea injury may be present as a result of decreased lacrimal secretions.
- Cardiovascular status should be assessed for increased heart rate, elevated blood pressure, jugular vein distention, and peripheral edema. These may be indications of heart failure as a result of the increased demands on the heart.
- Cardiac dysrhythmias such as atrial fibrillation and tachycardias may be noted.
- Increased bowel sounds and peristalsis, splenomegaly, and hepatomegaly may be found on abdominal assessment.
- Skin assessment may reveal smooth, warm, moist skin. Hair will be silky and fine but with a patchy distribution.
- Generalized muscle weakness may be noted, along with peripheral dependent edema.
- Nervous system changes may reveal a generalized nervousness, restlessness, and lack of ability to concentrate. Fine tremors may be noted along with hyperreflexia.
- Emotional lability, depression, and apathy also may be present.

DIAGNOSTIC STUDIES
- Serum thyroid antibody studies can reveal an autoimmune process as the cause of symptoms.
- Elevated T4 and decreased thyroid-stimulating hormone (TSH) levels indicate hyperthyroidism.
- Radioactive iodine uptake (RAIU) thyroid scan can differentiate between Graves' disease and thyroiditis.

Nursing Management

NONPHARMACOLOGIC TREATMENT
- Surgical removal of all or part of the thyroid may be necessary. A subtotal thyroidectomy or total thyroidectomy may be necessary to prevent airway or esophageal obstruction if the gland is significantly enlarged. Efforts to reduce the function and size of this high vascular gland should be initiated prior to surgery to prevent hemorrhage.
- Nutritional therapy will be necessary to treat the deficits that result from the increased metabolic rate of hyperthyroidism. A high-calorie diet of 4,000 to 5,000 kcal/day may be ordered to meet the patient's increased nutritional needs.

PHARMACOLOGIC TREATMENT
- Propylthiouracil (PTU) and methimazole (Tapazole) block the synthesis of thyroid hormone and thus decrease symptoms over time. Emphasize the need to maintain therapeutic levels by administering the medication at the same time each day and to monitor for signs of hypothyroidism.
- Sodium iodine and potassium iodine (SSKI, Thyro-Block, Pima) inhibit the synthesis and release of thyroid hormone. These preparations are contraindicated in patients with known hypersensitivities to iodine, shellfish, or contrast dyes.
- Radioactive iodine therapy involves the ingestion of a radioactive iodine isotope (I-131) to destroy thyroid cells, resulting in a decrease in production of thyroid hormone. Because it is difficult to control the amount of thyroid cells destroyed, patients may become hypothyroid and require replacement thyroid hormone therapy for life.

Special Considerations
- Older adults must be monitored for the development of heart failure.
- Hyperthyroidism usually can be treated on an outpatient basis unless surgical intervention is required.
- Patients undergoing thyroidectomy should be monitored for signs and symptoms of potential parathyroid damage occurring during surgery. Damage to the parathyroid gland may lead to hypocalcemia and the development of tetany.

Follow-up

EXPECTED OUTCOMES
- Patient will report increased activity tolerance with a decrease in cardiac symptoms. Heart rate should return to normal range and no shortness of breath should be experienced. Sleeping pattern should allow for periods of adequate sleep.
- Patient should experience weight gain with normal bowel elimination pattern.
- Heat intolerance should decrease.
- Patient should acknowledge that medications and treatment are life-long requirements.
- If surgical intervention was needed, wound care and gradual return to normal activity level should be explained.
- Patients receiving I-131 treatment should be able to describe signs and symptoms of hypothyroidism.

COMPLICATIONS
- If Graves' disease remains uncontrolled or a physiologic stress such as trauma, surgery, infection, or diabetic ketoacidosis (DKA) occurs, a life-threatening condition known as thyrotoxic crisis (thyroid storm) can develop. This condition stresses organ systems to their capacity. The cardiac system will begin to fail due to the increased myocardial oxygen demand, resulting in systemic hypertension, myocardial infarction, and heart failure. The enlarged thyroid gland can press on the trachea, resulting in respiratory distress. The metabolic hyperactivity also can result in insomnia, anxiety, and psychosis. This syndrome requires the provision of supportive care, frequently in an ICU, as a result of the effects on all body systems. Cardiac monitoring and treatment of cardiac decompensation, maintenance of adequate oxygenation, and fluid/volume replacement may be required.

HYPOTHYROIDISM

Description
- A condition resulting from a decrease in thyroid hormone produced by the thyroid gland, which decreases the metabolic rate and heat production. This decrease will be seen in multiple body systems.

Etiology
- Symptoms of hypothyroidism usually have a slow onset with symptoms occurring over an extended period of time.

- Primary hypothyroidism, which accounts for approximately 99% of all cases, is due to antibody or cell-mediated destruction of the thyroid gland. Other causes include infection, iodine deficiencies, external radiation of the gland (whether through treatment of hypothyroidism or exposure), and congenital or idiopathic effects.
- Secondary hypothyroidism (central hypothyroidism) is caused by insufficient secretion of TSH from the pituitary gland, decrease in the secretion of thyroid-releasing hormone (TRH) as a result of disease of the hypothalamus, or peripheral resistance to thyroid hormone.

Incidence and Demographics
- Hypothyroidism can occur at any age but is more common between 30 and 60 years of age.
- The incidence is 5 to 7 times higher in women.

Risk Factors
- Insufficient intake of iodine or exposure to high doses of radiation.
- Some medications, such as amiodarone used for cardiac dysrhythmias, can contain high levels of iodine. A thorough medication history should be obtained on all patients.

Prevention and Screening
- Public education about the need for an adequate dietary intake of iodine will help to prevent hypothyroidism.
- Routine assessment of signs and symptoms of hypothyroidism should be completed in individuals with a genetic predisposition for hypothyroidism as well as those individuals in areas of low iodine intake.
- Individuals with high exposure to radiation should be screened regularly. Education about the dangers of excessive exposure, use of protective equipment, and awareness of the signs and symptoms of hypothyroidism should be provided.

Assessment
HISTORY
- History of pituitary or thyroid disease or surgeries
- Use of iodized salt
- History of neck or head radiation
- Respiratory difficulties
- Increasing lethargy and fatigue due to slowed metabolism
- Excessive weight gain
- Constipation
- Reproductive changes such as menorrhagia and infertility in females and decreased libido in males

PHYSICAL EXAM
- Lethargy and altered level of consciousness
- Course, dry, easily lost hair
- Course, dry, edematous skin
- Thyroid enlargement or goiter will be present as a result of compensatory attempt to increased hormone levels
- Bradycardia and hypotension
- Hypothermia
- Periorbital edema and facial puffiness with tongue swelling

DIAGNOSTIC STUDIES

• Thorough history and physical assessment
• Laboratory tests will reveal decreased T4 and free T4 levels with normal T3 levels. There will be an increased TSH level as the pituitary gland tries to stimulate thyroid gland function.

Nursing Management

NONPHARMACOLOGIC TREATMENT

• Dietary restriction of foods known to inhibit the utilization of thyroid hormones (such as spinach, peaches, carrots, and cabbage) should be emphasized.
• Surgical removal of the thyroid gland or subtotal thyroidectomy may be necessary in cases of large goiter size that may obstruct the airway or esophagus.

PHARMACOLOGIC TREATMENT

• Hormone replacement therapies will be initiated. Medications such as levothyroxine (T4; Synthroid, Levothroid) or triiodothyronine (T3; Cytomel) can be used to enhance thyroid hormone levels and thus increase metabolic rate. Dosage must be individualized according to the patient's sensitivity to thyroid hormone, degree of thyroid dysfunction, age, body size, and other comorbidities. Thyroid medications can potentiate the affects of anticoagulants and digitalis and alter response to insulin.

Special Considerations

• Many of the symptoms of hypothyroidism are frequently attributed to normal aging in the older population.
• Thyroid medications can enhance the risk of iodine toxicity. Dietary restriction of iodized salt and any preparation with iodine should be avoided.
• Patients with a history of cardiac disease must be monitored very closely because the increase in metabolic rate induced by thyroid replacement therapy can increase myocardial oxygen demand and cause angina, cardiac dysrhythmias, and respiratory complications.

Follow-up

EXPECTED OUTCOMES

• Patients will understand the signs and symptoms of hypothyroidism and hyperthyroidism and the need to report any changes in condition to their primary care providers as soon as they occur. Patients will wear medical alert jewelry (such as a bracelet).
• Patients will understand the importance of medication administration on a daily basis in the morning 1 hour before a meal or 2 hours after a meal, and that medication is needed for life. Patients will also understand the importance of using the same brand of medication to avoid potential variance in chemical properties between manufacturers.
• Patient weight will stabilize, vital signs will be within normal range, and patient will be able to perform activities of daily living without fatigue, shortness of breath, or dysrhythmias.
• Skin will be elastic and hair loss will subside. There will be no evidence of skin breakdown.
• Patient will verbalize the need to maintain a high-fiber diet with increased fluid intake to facilitate bowel elimination.

COMPLICATIONS
- Myxedema coma is a life-threatening complication of untreated or longstanding hypothyroidism. Symptoms include mental sluggishness, drowsiness, and lethargy that progress to a severely altered level of consciousness and coma. Patients also will exhibit a subnormal temperature, hypotension, and slowed respiratory rate. This condition can be precipitated by infection; trauma; drugs such as opioids, tranquilizers, and barbiturates; and exposure to extreme cold. Treatment includes the support of vital functions while IV thyroid hormone replacement is administered.

HYPERPARATHYROIDISM

Description
- A condition resulting from excessive secretion of parathyroid hormone (PTH) from the parathyroid gland. Because parathyroid hormone helps to regulate the calcium and phosphate levels in the body through resorption from bone and renal tubules, the elevated levels of PTH result in increased serum calcium levels.

Etiology
- There are three classifications for hyperparathyroidism.
  - Primary hyperparathyroidism is caused by increased secretion of PTH, which leads to disorders of calcium, phosphate, and bone metabolism. It is most commonly caused by a benign tumor in the parathyroid gland (adenoma).
  - Secondary hyperparathyroidism is believed to be a compensatory response to conditions that cause hypocalcemic conditions. Calcium is the primary stimulator of PTH secretion. Conditions commonly associated with low calcium levels include malabsorption syndromes, vitamin D deficiency, chronic renal failure, and hyperphosphatemia.
  - Tertiary hyperparathyroidism is the result of enlargement of the parathyroid gland and loss of the negative feedback mechanism in response to circulating serum calcium levels. Thus, the secretion of PTH occurs despite normal serum calcium levels.
  - The increase in PTH leads to increased resorption of calcium from the kidneys and release of calcium from the bones resulting in bone decalcification and renal calculi formation. The decreased bicarbonate can lead to metabolic acidosis.

Incidence and Demographics
- Hyperthyroidism is more common in women.
- Primary hyperparathyroidism has a greater incidence between the ages of 30 and 70 years of age and in individuals who have previously undergone head or neck radiation; 75% of cases are the result of primary hyperparathyroidism.
- Secondary hyperparathyroidism can occur in any age group but is more common in persons with poor dietary intake or digestive diseases.
- Tertiary hyperparathyroidism usually occurs in individuals who have received a kidney transplant after extended periods of dialysis.

Risk Factors
- Poor nutritional intake
- Renal transplantation
- Chronic renal failure
- Pituitary cancer
- Postmenopause

Prevention and Screening
- Regular screening of calcium levels as part of a routine annual exam is important for individuals over 50 years of age.
- Many individuals will be asymptomatic, so a thorough assessment of risk factors should be completed.

Assessment

HISTORY
- Polyuria
- Anorexia
- Constipation
- Weakness and fatigue
- Nausea, vomiting, and abdominal pain
- Bone pain and pathologic fractures

PHYSICAL EXAM
- Muscle weakness and atrophy
- Skeletal deformities
- Hyperactive deep tendon reflexes in advanced stages of hyperparathyroidism
- Bone fractures with no apparent cause
- Altered mental status, including confusion and disorientation
- Paresthesia
- Renal calculi

DIAGNOSTIC STUDIES
- PTH radioimmunoassay level
- Serum calcium elevated and phosphorus levels low
- Renal calcium level
- Bone density studies for bone loss
- MRI, CT scan, or ultrasound can detect a parathyroid adenoma

Nursing Management

NONPHARMACOLOGIC TREATMENT
- Complete or partial surgical parathyroidectomy
- Autotransplantation of normal parathyroid tissue near sternocleidomastoid muscle to allow PTH secretion to continue
- Diet high in calorie and fluid intake with low calcium and vitamin D intake

PHARMACOLOGIC TREATMENT
- Phosphorus supplementation to inhibit calcium absorption in the GI tract
- Bisphosphates such as alendronate (Fosamax) and calcitonin to inhibit bone resorption
- Estrogen or progestin therapy in postmenopausal women to retard demineralization of bone and reduce serum calcium levels
- Diuretics to increase urinary excretion of calcium
- Calcimimetic medications such as cinacalcet (Sensipar), which increases the sensitivity of the calcium receptor on the parathyroid gland, thus decreasing PTH secretion and serum calcium levels.

Special Considerations
- If surgical intervention is needed, airway must be closely monitored for potential compromise.
- Hypercalcemic states increase potential for digitalis toxicity. Patients with a cardiac history prescribed digitalis should be monitored closely until serum calcium levels are controlled.
- If all parathyroid glands are removed, the patient must be treated with calcium supplements if signs or symptoms of hypocalcemia, such as tingling in the hands or mouth, or tetany develops.

Follow-up

EXPECTED OUTCOMES
- Patients will be free of or have minimal bone pain.
- Patients will have increased mobility, understand the need for activity, and be free of physical injury.
- Patients will verbalize understanding of the disease process and report symptoms of elevated calcium levels if pharmacological treatment has been prescribed.

COMPLICATIONS
- Demineralization of bone with pathologic fractures and osteoporosis
- Renal calculi, renal insufficiency, urinary tract infections, and renal failure as a result of the extracellular calcium deposited in soft tissues and the kidneys
- GI complications can result in the development of cholelithiasis, pancreatitis, and peptic ulcer disease resulting from the hypercalcemic state

HYPOPARATHYROIDISM

Description
- A condition resulting from abnormally low levels of parathyroid hormone (PTH) from the parathyroid gland. Because parathyroid hormone helps to regulate calcium and phosphate levels in the body through resorption from bone and renal tubules, low levels of PTH result in decreased serum calcium levels and increased phosphate levels.

Etiology
- The most common cause of hypoparathyroidism is the surgical removal of part or all of the parathyroid gland. The reduced levels of PTH result in a hypocalcemic state due to decreased absorption of calcium from the GI tract and regulation in the kidneys.
- Destruction of the parathyroid gland and the decreased levels or absence of PTH can be the result of an idiopathic or autoimmune disease.

Incidence and Demographics
- Hypoparathyroidism is a rare condition that may occur at any age. Surgically induced hypoparathyroidism can occur very quickly, while autoimmune-induced hypothyroidism is slow in onset.

Risk Factors

- Neck surgery
- Hypomagnesemia, which impairs PTH synthesis
- Radioactive iodine (I-131) treatment for Graves' disease
- Presence of antiparathyroid antibodies, which will destroy parathyroid gland tissues

Prevention and Screening

- Screening of individuals with risk factors listed above helps prevent acute complications of hypocalcemia.

Assessment

HISTORY

- Past history of neck surgery or radiation
- Presence of GI symptoms such as abdominal pain, nausea, vomiting, diarrhea, or anorexia
- Signs of hypocalcemia such as numbness and tingling in extremities, increased muscle tension and stiffness
- Painful, tonic spasms of smooth and skeletal muscles
- Headache
- Irritability
- Difficulty with balance and frequent falls
- Throat tightness or difficulty swallowing

PHYSICAL EXAM

- Constriction of facial muscles in response to a light tap on the facial nerve in front of the ear (Chvostek's sign)
- Carpal spasm in response to inflated blood pressure cuff on arm (Trousseau's sign)
- Laryngospasm and vocal hoarseness
- Involuntary muscle spasms
- Dry, thin, patchy hair
- Ridged fingernails

DIAGNOSTIC STUDIES

- Decreased serum calcium level
- Decreased serum PTH levels
- Increased serum phosphate levels

Nursing Management

NONPHARMACOLOGIC TREATMENT

- EKG monitoring to assess for the development of heart blocks.
- Rebreather mask or paper bag for rebreathing of exhaled carbon dioxide can be used to increase carbonic acid levels in the blood and lower the body pH to temporarily reduce muscle cramps and tetany.
- Diet rich in calcium, low in phosphorus, high in fiber and fluids.

PHARMACOLOGIC TREATMENT
- Emergency treatment of tetany will require IV calcium (calcium chloride, calcium gluconate, or calcium gluceptate), which must be given slowly to prevent hypotension, cardiac dysrhythmias, and potential for cardiac arrest.
- Oral calcium and vitamin D supplements (Calcitrol) are given to increase calcium levels and enhance the absorption of calcium.
- Phosphate-binding agents are used to assist in the excretion of phosphates.

Special Considerations
- Calcium given IV can cause irritation and inflammation of the veins. Extravasation can cause cellulitis, necrosis, and tissue sloughing.

Follow-up

EXPECTED OUTCOMES
- Patient will be free from injury due to falls. Ambulatory assistive devices may be needed until calcium levels return to normal.
- Progressive ambulation with frequent rest periods may be needed. Patient should gradually build up tolerance to predisease state.
- Patient will verbalize understanding of disease process, medication regimen, and symptoms that should be reported to the healthcare provider.
- Patient will understand dietary requirements. Foods high in calcium and vitamin D such as milk, cheese, almonds, collard greens, beans, and peanuts should be encouraged.

COMPLICATIONS
- Severe tetany can be life-threatening, resulting in airway obstruction and cardiac dysrhythmias.

HYPERCORTISOLISM—CUSHING'S SYNDROME

Description
- A condition resulting from hyperfunction of the adrenal gland cortex causing elevated serum cortisol or adrenocorticotropic hormone (ACTH) levels. Cortisol is a hormone responsible for maintaining normal electrical excitability of the heart, blood glucose levels, nerve cell conduction, and adequate circulatory volume as well as anti-inflammatory response. It also assists in the metabolism of proteins, fats, and carbohydrates.

Etiology
- There are three categories of Cushing's syndrome.
  - Iatrogenic Cushing's syndrome is due to chronic therapy or use of glucocorticoids.
  - Primary Cushing's syndrome is caused by excessive cortisol production from adrenal neoplasms such as adenomas and carcinomas. The tumors are usually only present in one adrenal gland; 50% of the tumors are malignant and have a 50% mortality rate even with appropriate treatment.
  - Secondary Cushing's syndrome is more common than primary and is commonly caused by adrenal hyperplasia resulting in excessive production of adrenocorticotropic hormone (ACTH) from the anterior pituitary. Ectopic tissue from an ACTH-producing cancer of the lung, bronchus, or pancreas also can cause hyperplasia of the adrenal cortex.

Incidence and Demographics

- Iatrogenic is the most commonly occurring Cushing's syndrome.
- Secondary Cushing's syndrome resulting from pituitary disease is more common in women but Cushing's syndrome resulting from excessive ACTH secretion is more common in males.

Risk Factors

- Long-term exogenous cortisol usage
- Familial autoimmune disorder

Prevention and Screening

- Patients with a family history of pituitary, adrenal, pancreatic, or pulmonary tumors should be screened frequently for symptoms for Cushing's syndrome to prevent long-term complications.

Assessment

HISTORY

- Changes in memory, attention span, or mood
- Sleep disturbances
- Changes in appearance
- Anorexia
- Weight gain
- Menstrual irregularities

PHYSICAL EXAM

- Central obesity
- Thin extremities with noticeable muscle wasting
- Round face (moon face)
- Acne and red cheeks
- Fat pads on back of neck and shoulders (buffalo hump)
- Thin, fragile skin
- Purplish red striae
- Petechial hemorrhages and bruising
- Edema of lower extremities
- Awkward gait and weakness
- Gynecomastia and testicular atrophy in males
- Hypertension

DIAGNOSTIC STUDIES

- Physical assessment
- 24-hour urine collection for free cortisol; levels of 50 to 100 mcg/day is an indication of Cushing's syndrome
- Elevated serum cortisol level
- Decreased serum potassium and chloride levels and metabolic alkalosis
- CT scan and MRI of pituitary and adrenal glands for tumor presence

Nursing Management

NONPHARMACOLOGIC TREATMENT
- Daily weights to assess treatment effectiveness
- Fluid restriction to decrease potential of fluid overload, hypertension, and respiratory complications such as pulmonary edema
- Surgical removal of adrenal gland or pituitary gland based on the underlying cause.
- Radiation therapy if patient is not a good surgical candidate

PHARMACOLOGIC TREATMENT
- Discontinuation or alteration of exogenous corticosteroids as needed. Medications can be gradually decreased to discontinuation or dosage may be reduced.
- Medications that inhibit adrenal function can be used. Mitotane (Lysodren) can be used in patients who are not good surgical candidates because it chemically destroys the function of the adrenal gland. The medication suppresses cortisol production, alters peripheral metabolism of cortisol, and decreases plasma and urine corticosteroid levels. Other medications can be used to inhibit cortisol synthesis such as ketoconazole (Nizoral) and aminoglutethimide (Cytadren).

Special Considerations
- Elderly patients may require the assistance of community resources due to the complexity of treatment regimen and safety risks.
- Steroids must be tapered to prevent potentially life-threatening adrenal insufficiency.

Follow-up

EXPECTED OUTCOMES
- Patients will have no signs of infection due to either surgical intervention or medication regimen.
- Patients will be able to perform activities of daily living at previous level.
- Weight will be stable with fluid and electrolyte balance restored.
- Patients will verbalize a positive body image and self-concept.
- Patients will be able to verbalize understanding of the disease process and identify what will exacerbate the disease. Patients will identify symptoms that should be reported to their healthcare providers immediately.
- Patients will understand their treatment regimens and verbalize expected outcomes as well as complications that should be reported as soon as possible.

COMPLICATIONS
- Adrenal crisis, a life-threatening condition, can develop as a result of rapid withdrawal of cortisol with surgical intervention or withdrawal of medications without tapering. Symptoms of hypotension, tachycardia, and decreased level of consciousness can indicate adrenal crisis.
- Care must be given to prevent potential infection due to the decreased immune response and inhibition of inflammation in patients with Cushing's syndrome.

ADRENAL INSUFFICIENCY—ADDISON'S DISEASE

Description
- A condition resulting from decreased production of cortisol, aldosterone, and androgen as a result of adrenal cortex dysfunction.

Etiology
- Causes of adrenal insufficiency can include an autoimmune process resulting in slow destruction of the adrenal tissue; infective processes such as seen with tuberculosis, histoplasmosis, acquired immunodeficiency syndrome (AIDS); and destructive hemorrhage into the adrenal gland. Sudden discontinuation of high-dose steroid therapy also can cause Addison's disease.

Incidence and Demographics
- Relatively uncommon
- Can occur at any age, but most commonly before 50 years of age
- Addison's disease as a result of an autoimmune response is found in White women

Risk Factors
- Steroid therapy
- History of tuberculosis (TB), AIDS, or antineoplastic chemotherapy
- Patients with history of bilateral adrenalectomy must be carefully treated with replacement therapy to prevent adrenal crisis.
- Polyendocrine deficiency syndrome, a disease process that involves alterations in multiple endocrine glands

Prevention and Screening
- Monitoring of patients with known risk factors
- Populations in countries of high TB incidence should be educated about the signs and symptoms of adrenal dysfunction to avoid development of Addison's disease.

Assessment

HISTORY
- Recent infection
- History of steroid use
- History of adrenal or pituitary surgery
- Poor activity and stress tolerance
- Weakness and fatigue
- Anorexia, nausea, vomiting and diarrhea due to altered metabolism
- Craving for salt
- Cold intolerance
- Altered menses in females and impotence in males

PHYSICAL EXAM
- Signs of dehydration such as tachycardia, altered level of consciousness, dry skin with poor skin turgor
- Dry mucous membranes
- Weight loss

- Weak peripheral pulses
- Postural hypotension
- Hyperpigmentation
- Loss of axillary and pubic hair due to decrease in androgen levels
- Signs of depression and irritability

DIAGNOSTIC STUDIES
- History and physical
- Decreased serum cortisol levels
- Altered serum electrolytes: hyperkalemia and hyponatremia
- Hypoglycemia
- Elevated ACTH levels
- ECG indicating tachycardia

Nursing Management

NONPHARMACOLOGIC TREATMENT
- Monitoring and support of vital functions during time of crisis

PHARMACOLOGIC TREATMENT
- IV infusion of 5% dextrose in 0.9% sodium chloride to replace fluid volume
- Replacement of corticosteroids and mineralocorticoids
- Fludrocortisone (Florinef), a mineralocorticoid that promotes kidney reabsorption of sodium and excretion of potassium, can be used to correct electrolyte balance; electrolyte levels should be monitored frequently

Special Considerations
- Patients with diabetes Type 1 will need to monitor their glucose levels more frequently and increase their insulin dosage to maintain their target glucose level.
- Patients with Type 2 diabetes will also need to monitor their glucose levels and increase their dosage of oral medication or possibly be placed on insulin temporarily to maintain their target glucose level.

Follow-up

EXPECTED OUTCOMES
- Patients will understand disease process and signs and symptoms of changes in condition.
- Patients know to report the following immediately to their healthcare provider: weight gain, bleeding and bruising, weakness, dizziness, lethargy, or changes in blood pressure or pulse.
- Patients know to consult their healthcare provider before taking any over-the-counter, herbal, or alternative medications.
- Patients will understand medication regimen and that treatment is a lifelong process. Patients should wear medical alert jewelry (such as a MedicAlert® bracelet) indicating disease and treatment plan.
- Patients will understand dietary needs to promote immune system function and foods that increase sodium and decrease potassium levels.
- Patient activity tolerance returns to stable level.

COMPLICATIONS
- Acute adrenal crisis is a life-threatening condition that requires aggressive management of shock and administration of high-dose hydrocortisone to reverse hypotension and severe electrolyte imbalances.
- Hyperglycemia

DIABETES INSIPIDUS

Description
- Diabetes insipidus (DI) is characterized by excretion of large quantities of dilute urine. DI can be of multiple origins. Central or neurogenic DI is the result of a decrease in the amount of antidiuretic hormone (ADH) being excreted by the posterior pituitary gland. Nephrogenic or renal origin is the result of a decrease in responsiveness of the kidneys to ADH. Diabetes insipidus can be a chronic or transient condition depending on the cause.

Etiology
- The classification of diabetes insipidus is based on the underlying pathology. Central DI occurs as the result of interference with the synthesis, transport, or release of ADH from the pituitary gland. This can be due to a tumor, head trauma, brain surgery, or an infection of the central nervous system. Nephrogenic DI occurs as a result of a condition or medication that interferes with renal response to ADH. Medications such as lithium and demeclocycline; renal damage; and hereditary renal diseases can decrease the renal tubule response to ADH. Electrolyte imbalances such as hypokalemia and hypercalcemia also can cause nephrogenic DI. Psychogenic conditions such as structural lesions in the thirst center or psychiatric problems can lead to excessive water intake and psychogenic DI.

Incidence and Demographics
- DI can occur at any age.
- There is a familial or idiopathic malfunction in 50% of individuals who develop DI.

Risk Factors
- Overdose in psychiatric patients using medications such lithium can lead to DI.
- Tumors of the pituitary may lead to excessive production and release of ADH.
- Recent head trauma, cerebral infection, metastatic tumors from the lung or breast.
- Cerebrovascular hemorrhage or cerebral aneurysm.

Prevention and Screening
- Screening of individuals with a history of any risk factors.
- Prevention can include teaching patients to drink in response to thirst. Restriction of salt and caffeine-containing products can prevent polyuria.

Assessment

HISTORY
- Abrupt onset of excessive urination (polyuria), excessive thirst (polydipsia), and nocturia (excessive urination at night)
- Recent head trauma, brain surgery, infection, or history of renal disease
- Constipation
- Use of prescription medications such as lithium or demeclocycline

PHYSICAL EXAM
- Urinary output of 4 to 15 liters per day.
- Urine is clear to pale yellow.
- Signs of dehydration may be present such as dry lips and mouth, decreased tear formation, skin tenting, and dizziness. Decreased bowel sounds may be present.
- Tachycardia, orthostatic changes in pulse rate and blood pressure, and muscle weakness may be noted if significant dehydration is present.

DIAGNOSTIC STUDIES
- Urinalysis reveals a low specific gravity of < 10.5, urine osmolality < 300 mOsm/kg, and serum sodium > 145 mEq/L.
- Positive water deprivation test: prescribed decrease in fluid intake does not result in increased concentration of urine.
- Decreased urine output with the administration of exogenous vasopressin.
- Decreased level of ADH.

Nursing Management

NONPHARMACOLOGIC TREATMENT
- Monitoring of fluid volume intake and output to assess effectiveness of therapy.
- Replace water intake with either oral or intravenous solutions of D5W or hypotonic solutions to replace output.
- Low-sodium and low-protein diet to decrease excretion of solute.

PHARMACOLOGIC TREATMENT
- Hormone replacement with desmopressin acetate (DDVAP) or other vasopressin preparations such as aqueous vasopressin (Pitressin), vasopressin tannate, or lysine vasopressin (Diapid).
- Carbamazepine (Tegretol) and chlorpropamide (Diabinese) can be used to enhance the effect of ADH in the renal tubules.
- Thiazide diuretics such as hydrochlorothiazide (HydroDIURIL) and chlorothiazide (Diuril) can be used to slow the glomerular filtration rate and allow for increased kidney reabsorption of water.

Special Considerations
- Client should wear medical alert jewelry indicating diagnosis and treatment plan.

Follow-up

EXPECTED OUTCOMES
- Patient will verbalize understanding of the signs and symptoms of DI and the expected results of treatment. An understanding of prescribed medications and ability to self-administer them is necessary.
- Urine output will decrease with treatment to equal oral intake.
- Patient will acknowledge need to drink fluids equal to urine output.
- Weight will return to precondition baseline. Patient will acknowledge need to weigh self daily, on the same scale and at the same time of day, and report any weight loss.
- Patient will be free of signs and symptoms of dehydration.
- Patient and family will demonstrate coping mechanisms appropriate for chronic illness.
- Patient will verbalize the need to restrict the use of caffeinated products, which increase diuresis.

COMPLICATIONS
- Hypovolemia as a result of the inability to replace fluid volumes lost.
- Decreased mentation can lead to the inability to respond to the sensation of thirst in dehydration.

SYNDROME OF INAPPROPRIATE ANTIDIURETIC HORMONE (SIADH)

Description
- SIADH is a condition of posterior pituitary gland dysfunction and excessive secretion of antidiuretic hormone (ADH) into the central circulation, resulting in excessive water retention and hyponatremia.

Etiology
- SIADH occurs when ADH secretion is activated by factors other than hypovolemia or hyperosmolarity. The feedback mechanism that inhibits the posterior pituitary from excessive secretion of ADH in response to decreased serum osmolality fails, resulting in renal reabsorption of water. Suppression of the renin-angiotensin mechanism causes excessive renal sodium excretion. These conditions result in fluid overload, water intoxication, cellular edema, and dilutional hyponatremia.
- SIADH can lead to life-threatening complications due to severe electrolyte imbalances and water intoxication. Water intoxication can lead to cerebral edema, coma, and death.

Incidence and Demographics
- SIADH can occur as a result of many conditions that may affect the hypothalamus such as head trauma, hydrocephalus, encephalitis, meningitis, pituitary surgery, cerebrovascular accident, intracranial bleeding, or increased intracranial pressure.
- Malignant tumors that secrete endogenous ADH such as oat cell lung cancer, pancreatic cancer, leukemia, and Hodgkin's lymphoma can cause symptoms of SIADH.
- Trauma, stress, pain, acute psychosis, or anything that activates the limbic system can stimulate the hypothalamus to secrete ADH.
- Positive pressure ventilation or any condition that increases intrathoracic pressure and stimulates the baroreceptors to trigger the hypothalamus to secrete ADH can precipitate the development of SIADH.

Risk Factors
- Recent head trauma, cranial surgery, any disease or mechanical process that can increase intracranial pressure and affect the posterior pituitary gland.
- Many cancers such as bladder, prostate, gastrointestinal tract, sarcomas, Hodgkin's disease, and small cell lung cancer, as well as some chemotherapies, can secrete an ectopic supply of ADH.

Prevention and Screening
- Knowledge of the precipitating disease process can potentially lead to the early correction of factors and prevent the development of SIADH.

Assessment

HISTORY
- Recent head trauma or surgery
- History of malignant tumors of the lungs, pancreas, or brain
- Complaint of headache, fatigue, nausea, weight gain without edema, seizures, abdominal cramping, muscle aching
- Recent alterations in urinary pattern; any noticeable increase or decrease in urinary output
- Recent chemotherapy
- History of fatigue, weakness, headaches, nausea, vomiting, or seizure

PHYSICAL EXAM
- Altered level of consciousness, confusion, or seizure
- Muscle weakness or twitching
- Decreased urinary output with concentrated, dark amber urine
- History of excessive weight gain with no overt edema noted

DIAGNOSTIC STUDIES
- Urinalysis will demonstrate a high urine osmolality and specific gravity.
- Blood serum study results will reveal a low serum osmolality and decreased hematocrit, BUN, and sodium level.
- ADH levels will be elevated.

Nursing Management

NONPHARMACOLOGIC TREATMENT
- Limit fluid intake to approximately 600 to 800 mL/day to prevent further hemodilution.
- Daily weights and accurate assessment of intake and output to monitor effectiveness of therapies.
- Monitor serum sodium levels and urine osmolality and specific gravity to assure normalization.
- Monitor level of consciousness, cognition, muscle strength, nutritional intake, and comfort level. Patient may need assistance in the management of dietary and fluid restrictions.

PHARMACOLOGIC TREATMENT
- Hypertonic saline IV solution (3% to 4.5%) or oral intake to replace electrolytes and fluids.
- Replacement of electrolytes, particularly sodium and potassium, is necessary to prevent cardiac dysrhythmias.
- Diuretics may be used to enhance elimination of excessive fluid from body, particularly in patients with cardiac symptoms.
- Phenytoin (Dilantin) may be used to limit or prevent seizures and decrease further release of ADH in patients with low sodium levels.
- Demeclocycline (Declomycin) may be prescribed for chronic SIADH; it may cause nephrogenic diabetes insipidus by blocking the action of ADH at the distal and proximal tubules, thus utilizing a side effect of Demeclocycline for diuresis.

Special Considerations

- Due to fluid overload status, the safety needs of the patient should be prioritized. The patency of the patient's airway must be maintained if seizures occur. Ambulation may require assistance due to muscle strength and mentation changes. Range-of-motion exercises should be instituted for the patient who is bedridden to limit the complications of immobility.
- Seizure precautions, such as padded side rails and suction equipment availability, may be needed.
- Because fluid overload is a significant concern in the client with SIADH, intravenous infusions and piggybacks should be administered in the smallest volume possible. Collaboration with the pharmacist may be needed to determine these parameters.

Follow-up

EXPECTED OUTCOMES
- Level of consciousness and cognition will remain in intact.
- Patient will remain free of seizures.
- Excessive fluid will be eliminated and lab values will return to normal.
- Patient will be able to verbalize the symptoms of SIADH and symptoms to report to the healthcare provider.
- Patient will verbalize an understanding of the medications, need for fluid restriction, and meal planning to maintain fluid restriction and appropriate sodium intake.
- Patient will demonstrate ability to weigh self and report any weight gain.

COMPLICATIONS
- Seizures may occur because of fluid overload and alterations in sodium and potassium serum levels. Precautions should be initiated as soon as the need is identified.
- Water excess may lead to pulmonary edema and congestive heart failure, particularly in the patient with underlying cardiac and pulmonary disease. Patient's cardiovascular and respiratory status should be monitored frequently and changes reported to the healthcare provider.

DIABETES MELLITUS—TYPE 1

Description

- Diabetes is a chronic disorder of the pancreas resulting in inappropriate carbohydrate, protein, and fat metabolism due to an imbalance of insulin supply and demand. Type 1 diabetes is a condition in which the pancreatic islet cells are destroyed, resulting in a very low or total lack of circulating insulin. Patients with type 1 diabetes are dependent on insulin injections for prevention of hyperglycemia and ketosis. Type 1 diabetes was previously referred to as insulin-dependent diabetes or juvenile diabetes because of the early onset of symptoms and the need for insulin replacement therapy.

Etiology

- In the genetically predispositioned person, some triggering event such as an infection causes autoantibodies to be produced that destroy the beta cells of the pancreas. This destruction of cells leads to the reduction and eventual absence of insulin production after 90% of the cells have been destroyed.

- Beta-cell destruction can take years but once a sufficient proportion is lost, onset of type 1 diabetes mellitus is usually rapid.

Incidence and Demographics
- It is estimated that approximately 1 million people in the United States have type 1 diabetes mellitus.
- Onset can occur at any age but typically occurs before 20 years of age.
- Diabetes is the seventh leading cause of death in the United States and is the leading cause of new cases of blindness in adults, kidney failure, and nontraumatic lower limb amputations due to peripheral neuropathies, circulatory changes, and wound-healing difficulties.

Risk Factors
- Evidence suggests a genetic predisposition to the development of diabetes.
- In the individual with such a predisposition, environmental factors such as viral infection, exposure to toxins, and dietary factors such as cow's milk have been investigated as potential triggers for the development of type 1 diabetes, but the triggering event remains unclear.

Assessment

HISTORY
- Glucosuria (glucose in urine), which causes an osmotic diuresis
- Polyuria (frequent urination), the result of the osmotic diuresis
- Nocturia (frequent nighttime voiding) associated with the polyuria
- Dehydration as a result of the diuresis and volume depletion
- Polydipsia (frequent thirst) resulting from the dehydration
- Polyphagia (increased hunger) as a result of the loss of calories because glucose is excreted in the urine
- Losing weight without trying due to loss of calories and dehydration
- Feeling tired and fatigued due to altered metabolism of carbohydrates, proteins, and lipids

PHYSICAL EXAM
- Dry skin and mucous membranes
- Fruity breath odor due to presence of ketones
- Rapid, deep respirations (Kussmaul respirations)
- Nausea, vomiting, and abdominal pain
- Signs of dehydration such as poor skin turgor, sunken eyes, low blood pressure, and tachycardia as a result of dehydration and diuresis

DIAGNOSTIC STUDIES
- Urinalysis to assess presence of glucose and ketones in urine.
- *Fasting plasma glucose test* (FPG) involves fasting overnight before an early morning blood draw. A result of 126 mg/dL or higher suggests the presence of diabetes.
- *Oral glucose tolerance test* (OGTT) involves fasting overnight, having a fasting blood sugar drawn in the early morning, then ingestion of a sugary solution and a second blood specimen drawn 2 hours later. A serum blood glucose level of 200 mg/dL or greater may indicate the presence of diabetes. Blood glucose levels of 139 mg/dL or lower indicate a normal OGTT.

- *Hemoglobin A1c test* (HbA1c) reflects the average blood glucose levels over the prior 6 to 8 weeks. Hemoglobin A1c, sometimes referred to as glycosylated hemoglobin or glycohemoglobin, is a component of hemoglobin to which glucose is bound. Levels of HbA1c are not influenced by daily fluctuations or the current blood glucose concentration, so HbA1c is a useful indicator of how well the blood glucose level has been controlled in the recent past and may be used to monitor the effects of diet, exercise, and drug therapy on blood glucose in people with diabetes. Testing for the HbA1c level involves no special preparations for the patient. No diet or medication changes are needed and the sample of blood can be drawn at any time. The normal HbA1c level is less than 5.7% of total hemoglobin. HbA1c levels of 6.5% or higher indicate the presence of diabetes or poor glucose control in the patient known to have diabetes.
- Diagnosis should be based on the results of any of the above tests or repeat test taken 24 hours apart in the absence of unequivocal hyperglycemia.
- Other blood studies such as lipid profile, renal studies to assess kidney function, and thyroid studies may be needed to establish a baseline for follow-up as well as to assess for the presence of complications.

Nursing Management

NONPHARMACOLOGIC TREATMENT
- Goals should focus on the prevention of long-term complications such as renal failure, cardiovascular disease, and blindness as well as short-term episodes of hypoglycemia, hyperglycemia, and diabetic ketoacidosis (DKA).
- Frequent monitoring of blood glucose levels, both self-monitoring and laboratory assessments, are used to adjust insulin as needed and to monitor effectiveness of the treatment plan.
- Establish target glycemic and metabolic goals such as HbA1c < 6.0%, blood pressure < 130/80 mm Hg, low-density lipoprotein (LDL) < 100 mg/dL, high-density lipoprotein (HDL) > 40 mg/dL for men and > 50 mg/dL for women, and triglycerides < 150 mm/dL.
- Meal plans should be developed to meet individual nutritional needs, control blood glucose and lipids, and maintain appropriate weight. Caloric intake may need to be adjusted with changes in activity level. Control of timing and amount of food is essential for maintaining blood glucose control and insulin regimens.
- An exercise regimen is very important in the treatment plan of patients with diabetes. The program should be designed to fit the individual patient's fitness level and interests to enhance compliance, and adapted for any risk factors and complications currently present.
- Pancreatic transplantation may be considered, although donor pancreases are in short supply and patients will require immunosuppressive therapy to prevent rejection or destruction of transplanted beta cells.

PHARMACOLOGIC TREATMENT
- Effective management of type 1 diabetes requires insulin replacement. The specific type and dosage must be individualized to maintain an appropriate blood glucose level throughout a 24-hour period. Patients (or their parents or caregivers in the case of young children) must be instructed and able to demonstrate the ability to self-monitor blood glucose, administer appropriate insulin dosage in the correct manner, and monitor for side effects. Patients or caregivers must also understand how to adjust dosage during periods of stress, illness, or physiologic changes. An insulin pump may be considered as an alternative to an injection schedule.
- Insulin preparations (see Table 15–2)
- When amylin analogs (pramlintide [Symlin]) are used, a significant reduction in insulin dosage is often required.
- Angiotensin-converting enzyme (ACE) inhibitors, antihyperlipidemic, and other medications may be needed to treat or prevent potential cardiac, renal, and peripheral complications

Table 15–2. Insulin Preparations

Preparation	Name	Onset (hours)	Peak (hours)	Duration (hours)
Rapid-acting	Lispro (Humalog)	0.25	1–1.5	3–4
	Insulin Aspart (NovoLog)			
	Insulin Glulisine (Apidra)	0.25–0.5	1	
Short-acting	Regular	0.5–1	2–4	5–7
	Regular Humulin (R)			
	Novolin R			
Intermediate-acting	Insulin NPH	2	6–8	12–16
	Humulin N			
Long-acting	Insulin Detemir (Levemir)	2	16–20	24+
	Insulin Glargine (Lantus)	3–4		10.4–24
Premixed Combinations	Humulin 50NPH/50Regular	0.5	3	18–24
	Humulin 70NPH/30Regular	0.5	4–8	
	NovoLog Mix			
	75 Aspart Protamine/25aspart	0.25	4–8	

Special Considerations

- Due to the need for the strict management of diabetes and the potential for development of comorbidities, it is essential to stress compliance with the prescribed regimen of medication, diet, and activity. A consideration of the patient's specific needs, developmental stage, and abilities must be included in the patient teaching plan. Not only should the specifics of the medication administration and potential side effects be included, but emphasis on foot care and the treatment of hypoglycemia and hyperglycemia should also be included.
- Visual and manual dexterity difficulties should be taken into consideration when planning discharge teaching and follow-up care.
- Comorbidities and potential for complications generally increase as patients age.

Follow-up

EXPECTED OUTCOMES
- Patient's blood glucose levels will be maintained within normal limits with prescribed treatment regimen.
- Patient will be able to monitor blood glucose and urine ketone levels and treat appropriately.
- Patient will recognize signs and symptoms of high or low blood sugar levels and verbalize appropriate treatment measures. Candy, fruit juices, glucose tablets, and other sugar sources should be kept available for treatment of hypoglycemia. Patient should also verbalize the effects of alcohol on blood sugar control.
- Patient will understand and be able to plan meals with appropriate nutritional intake for an individual with diabetes. When food intake is impaired, such as with symptoms of nausea and vomiting, insulin should be administered as directed and glucose self-monitoring should be completed more frequently. Treatment adjustments should be completed in collaboration with the healthcare provider.
- Patient will know how to administer and store insulin and supplies appropriately. A plan to rotate injection or pump cannula insertion sites should be established to prevent tissue damage and altered absorption. When mixing two prescribed insulins, regular insulin should be drawn first to avoid contamination of the longer-acting insulin.
- Patient will understand the importance of exercise and its effects on food and insulin requirements, and adjustment of insulin dosage as needed.
- Patient will understand the need for consistent follow-up with healthcare providers and to report any changes in their status.
- Patient will verbalize understanding of potential complications to be monitored for and measures to prevent the development of complications.

COMPLICATIONS
- Hyperosmolar hyperglycemic state (HHS) is a life-threatening complication of diabetes, the result of a seriously elevated blood glucose level > 600 mg/dL. HHS can occur as a result of inadequate treatment; increased insulin need due to acute disease processes such as infection, burns, gangrene, myocardial infarction, or stroke. Chronic illnesses such as renal and cardiac diseases, hypertension, and alcoholism as well as exercise, stress, and therapeutic procedures such as surgery, dialysis, and hyperalimentation solutions can precipitate HHS. Because of the development of a hyperosmolar and dehydration state, potassium, sodium, and chloride ions will be decreased in the

circulating volume. Urinalysis will reveal the presence of glucose but no ketones. Treatment of HHS involves the aggressive administration of IV regular insulin to decrease serum glucose by 50 to 70 mg/dL/hour, as well as 0.9% NaCl intravenous fluids to treat hypovolemic and hemoconcentration state. Electrolyte replacement to reestablish an appropriate hemodynamic state and to prevent cardiac dysrhythmias, improve skeletal and smooth muscle function, and maintain endocrine function is also essential. Because of the severe hyperglycemic state in HHS, severe neurological effects potentially can occur such as seizures, shock, coma, and death.

- Diabetic ketoacidosis (DKA), a life-threatening complication of type 1 diabetes, is the result of inadequate treatment. Insulin needs can increase due to illness, infection, exercise or stress, alcohol, use of cocaine as well as medications such as glucocorticoids, sympathomimetic medications, and total parenteral nutrition (TPN). DKA also can be the first indication of the presence of type 1 diabetes. Because of the development of a hyperosmolar state, metabolic acidosis, and depletion of potassium and sodium ions in the decreased circulating volume, serum glucose levels elevate to > 300 mg/dL; plasma pH decreases to < 7.3; plasma bicarbonate decreases to < 15 mEq/L; serum potassium, sodium, and chloride levels decrease; and serum ketones are present. Urinalysis will reveal the presence of ketones and glucose (see Figure 15–1). Treatment of DKA involves the administration of an IV drip of regular insulin to reduce blood glucose levels, 0.9% NaCl intravenous fluids to treat hypotension and increase urine output to a minimum of 30 mL/hr, and electrolyte replacement to return the body to homeostasis.

Figure 15–1. Diabetic Ketoacidosis Etiology

DKA Etiology

Destruction of beta cells
↓
Inability to appropriately metabolize
carbohydrates, proteins, and fats
↓
Catabolism
↓
Increase in fatty acids
↓
Ketosis

- Blindness due to diabetic retinopathy as a result of the alterations in blood flow and ischemia in the blood-retina barrier is the leading cause of blindness in persons with diabetes between the ages 24 and 74 years.
- Kidney failure as a result of diabetic nephropathy occurs in 20% to 40% of all persons with diabetes. Diabetic nephropathy is thought to be due to the extended state of hyperglycemia and the fibrotic changes that occur in the glomerulus and tubules that allow for the excretion of albumin. Hypertension as a comorbidity also contributes to the decline in renal function.

- Hypertension, coronary artery disease, myocardial infarction (MI), and stroke are major complications of the diabetic disease process as a result of atherosclerotic changes in the blood vessels and alterations in the microcirculation. It is estimated that 20% to 60% of all persons with diabetes will develop hypertension, which is a major contributor to the increased mortality rate of persons with diabetes due to MI.
- Peripheral vascular insufficiency, intermittent claudication, and ulcerations are common diabetic complications. Because of decreased blood flow to the lower legs and resulting inadequate oxygenation, poor wound healing can lead to gangrene, the most common reason for nontraumatic amputation of toes and lower extremities in patients with diabetes.
- Diabetic neuropathies develop in the periphery and viscera. Neuropathies occur primarily in the extremities (peripheral neuropathies) but can occur anywhere. Peripheral neuropathies typically cause complaints of decreased sensation with aching, burning, or feeling of being cold, particularly in the feet and lower legs. Visceral neuropathy occurs in the autonomic nervous system. The pain and altered function of the areas depend on the location involved. Changes in sweating, constriction of the pupils, and autonomic response in the myocardium to control heart rate occur as a result of neuropathologies. Changes in gastrointestinal functioning typically include gastroparesis, constipation, and diarrhea as well as genitourinary dysfunctions such as urinary retention and decreased sexual functioning.
- Infection also is a major potential complication. Hyperglycemia, altered circulatory status, alterations in the function of neutrophils, and reduced sensation due to neuropathies significantly increase risk for development of infections.

DIABETES MELLITUS—TYPE 2

Description
- A chronic disorder of the pancreas resulting in inappropriate carbohydrate, protein, and fat metabolism, type 2 diabetes is a condition in which the pancreatic islet cells' ability to secrete insulin becomes impaired, receptor sites become insensitive to insulin, and the liver produces excess glucose.

Etiology
- There is no autoimmune destruction of the pancreatic beta cells but a defect in the secretion of insulin and decreased sensitivity in the liver, muscle, and adipose tissues to insulin, conditions that usually develop over time. Initially, hyperinsulinemia develops as the pancreas beta cells overcome insulin resistance in the tissues to create a state of normal glucose tolerance. Eventually, insulin resistance increases and beta cells cannot produce sufficient insulin to overcome it. Adipose tissues begin to break down and release free fatty acids, which increase insulin resistance in muscle and liver tissues. Liver tissues lose responsiveness to insulin's restrictive effect on glucose production, thereby increasing glucose production, causing hyperglycemia, which in turn destroys beta cells in the pancreas and reducing insulin production.
- Type 2 diabetes typically exhibits a slow and insidious onset with few symptoms.

Incidence and Demographics

- An estimated 25 million Americans have type 2 diabetes mellitus, accounting for 90% to 95% of all cases of diabetes in the United States. Approximately 30% of these have not yet been diagnosed.
- Diagnosis is typically after 45 years of age but can be diagnosed at any age and is currently increasing in the pediatric population.

Risk Factors

- Obesity, particularly central obesity or excessive weight centered around the abdomen
- Physical inactivity and sedentary lifestyle
- Age over 45 years with other risk factors present
- Ethnic/racial minority such as Black, Hispanic, Pacific Islander, or American Indian
- Family history of diabetes
- Lower socioeconomic status and educational level
- History of high blood pressure, high cholesterol, heart disease, or stroke
- Gestational diabetes or an abnormal result on a previous fasting blood sugar test will require close follow-up
- Any condition that effects how the body uses insulin, such as polycystic ovary syndrome (PCOS)

Prevention and Screening

- Weight control and exercise can help prevent development of diabetes as well as reduce the severity of the disease.
- All individuals over 45 years of age should be screened by their primary care providers and if not found to have diabetes, be rescreened every 3 years or if symptoms develop.
- Screening should begin at a younger age if any of the above risk factors are present.
- Overweight children and adolescents should be screened if they have a family history of type 2 diabetes; belong to high-risk ethnic groups such as Native Americans, Blacks, Hispanic Americans, Asians/South Pacific Islanders; or if they have conditions associated with insulin resistance such as hyperlipidemia, polycystic ovary syndrome, or dyslipidemia. This screening should begin at age 10 and continue every 2 years.
- Assess for development of gestational diabetes during pregnancy, as these women have a higher incidence of development of diabetes type 2.

Assessment

HISTORY
- Recurrent infections without resolution
- Generalized wound-healing difficulties
- Chronic obesity
- Glucosuria (glucose in urine), which causes an osmotic diuresis
- Polyuria (frequent urination), which is the result of the osmotic diuresis
- Nocturia (nighttime frequent voiding) associated with the polyuria
- Dehydration as a result of the diuresis and volume depletion
- Polydipsia (frequent thirst) resulting from the dehydration
- Polyphagia (increased hunger) as a result of the loss of calories as the glucose is excreted in the urine
- Feeling tired and fatigued due to altered metabolism of carbohydrates, proteins, and lipids

- Complaint of blurred vision or vision changes
- Complaint of numbness or tingling in hands and feet

PHYSICAL EXAM
- Dry skin and mucous membranes
- Fruity breath
- Rapid, deep respirations (Kussmaul respirations)
- Nausea and vomiting
- Signs of dehydration such as poor skin turgor, sunken eyes, low blood pressure, and tachycardia as a result of the dehydration and diuresis
- Decreased sensation and skin integrity in lower extremities

DIAGNOSTIC STUDIES
- Urinalysis to assess presence of glucose and low specific gravity. Ketones will not typically be found in the urine of patients with type 2 diabetes.
- *Fasting plasma glucose test* (FPG) involves fasting overnight before an early morning blood draw. A result of 126 mg/dL or higher suggests the presence of diabetes. Results of 100 mg/dL to 125 mg/dL may indicate prediabetes.
- *Oral glucose tolerance test* (OGTT) involves fasting overnight, having a fasting blood sugar drawn in the early morning, then ingestion of a sugary solution and a second blood specimen drawn 2 hours later. A serum blood glucose level of 200 mg/dL or greater may indicate the presence of diabetes. Blood glucose levels of 140 mg/dL to 199 mg/dL indicate the possibility of a prediabetic condition. Blood glucose levels of 139 mg/dL or lower indicate a normal OGTT.
- *Hemoglobin A1c test* (HbA1c) reflects the average blood glucose levels over the prior 6 to 8 weeks. Hemoglobin A1c, sometimes referred to as glycosylated hemoglobin or glycohemoglobin, is a component of hemoglobin to which glucose is bound. Levels of HbA1c are not influenced by daily fluctuations or the current blood glucose concentration, so HbA1c is a useful indicator of how well the blood glucose level has been controlled in the recent past and may be used to monitor the effects of diet, exercise, and drug therapy on blood glucose in people with diabetes. Testing for the HbA1c level involves no special preparations for the patient. No diet or medication changes are needed and the sample of blood can be drawn at any time. The normal HbA1c level is less than 5.7% of total hemoglobin. HbA1c levels of 6.5% or higher indicate the presence of diabetes or poor glucose control in the patient known to have diabetes. A level of 5.7% to 6.4% indicates a prediabetic state.
- Diagnosis should be based on the results of any of the above tests or any combination of the tests taken 24 hours apart.
- Other blood studies such as lipid profile, renal studies to assess kidney function, and thyroid studies may be needed to establish a baseline for follow-up as well as to assess for the presence of complications.

Nursing Management

NONPHARMACOLOGIC TREATMENT
- Goals should be focused on the prevention of long-term complications such as renal failure, cardiovascular disease, and blindness as well as short-term episodes of hypoglycemia, hyperglycemia, and hyperosmolar hyperglycemic state (HHS).

- Frequent monitoring of blood glucose levels, both self-monitoring and laboratory assessments, are used to adjust medications as needed and to monitor effectiveness of the treatment plan.
- Establish target glycemic and metabolic goals such as HbA1c < 6.0%, blood pressure < 130/80 mm Hg, low-density lipoprotein (LDL) < 100 mg/dL, high-density lipoprotein (HDL) > 40 mg/dL for men and > 50 mg/dL for women, and triglycerides < 150 mm/dL.
- Meal plans should be developed to meet individual nutritional needs, control blood glucose and lipids, and maintain or achieve appropriate weight. Caloric intake may need to be adjusted with changes in activity level. Control of timing and amount of food is essential for maintaining blood glucose control and insulin regimes.
- An exercise regimen is very important in the treatment plan of patients with diabetes. The program should be designed to fit the individual patient's fitness level and interests to enhance compliance, and adapted for any risk factors and complications present.
- Pancreatic transplantation may be considered, although donor pancreases are in short supply and patients will require immunosuppressive therapy to prevent rejection or destruction of transplanted beta cells.

PHARMACOLOGIC TREATMENT
- Oral and injectable hypoglycemic agents (see Table 15–3) are prescribed to achieve and maintain goal serum glucose levels. Patients must understand the need for oral hypoglycemic agent adjustment during times of stress, illness, or surgical interventions. Patients with type 2 diabetes may require insulin injections for a period time immediately after diagnosis until homeostasis is re-established.
- Angiotensin-converting enzyme (ACE) inhibitors, antihyperlipidemic, and other medications may be needed to treat potential cardiac, renal, and peripheral complications.

Table 15–3. Oral and Injectable Hypoglycemic Agents

Classification	Route	Generic Name	Brand Names	Action
Sulfonylureas	Oral	Glimepiride Glipizide Glyburide Tolazamide Tolbutamide	Amaryl Glucotrol Glucotrol XL DiaBeta Micronase Tolinase Orinase	Stimulate the pancreatic cells to secrete more insulin and increase sensitivity of peripheral tissues to insulin
Biguanides	Oral	Metformin	Glucophage	Decreases overproduction of glucose by the liver and increases binding of insulin to tissues
Meglitinides	Oral	Repaglinide Nateglinide	Prandin Starlix	Stimulates pancreatic islet cells to release insulin
Alpha-glucoside inhibitors	Oral	Acarbose Miglitol	Precose Glyset	Slows carbohydrate digestion and delays glucose absorption

cont.

Table 15–3. Oral and Injectable Hypoglycemic Agents (cont.)

Thiazolidinediones	Oral	Rosiglitazone Pioglitazone	Avandia Actos	Reduces glyconeogenesis and cellular insulin resistance
Incretin mimetics	Injection	Exenatide	Byetta	Enhances glucose-dependent insulin secretion
Amylin analogs	Injection	Pramlintide	Symlin	Slows gastric emptying, suppresses glucagon secretion, and regulates food intake; often requires significant reduction of injectable insulin dose
Insulin	Injection	See Table 15–2		

Special Considerations

- Because of the need for strict management of diabetes and the potential for development of complications and comorbidities, it is essential to stress compliance with the prescribed regimen of medication, diet, and activity. Weight loss and a weight maintenance program are essential for control of the morbidity conditions associated with diabetes. A consideration of the patient's needs, lifestyle, and abilities must be included in the teaching plan. The specifics of self-monitoring of blood glucose, medication administration and potential side effects, importance of foot care, and treatment of hypoglycemia and hyperglycemia also should be included.
- The older adult may have difficulties with comorbidity, chronic illnesses, memory, transportation, and ability to pay for prescribed medication regimen and diet plan as well as physical limitations for exercise and following medication regimens. Discharge planning should take into consideration dietary likes and dislikes, support services, transportation, and physical limitations to enhance compliance and increase successful compliance.
- Consideration of cultural and ethnic preferences in dietary intake must be considered. Developing meal plans that meet not only the dietary requirements for diabetes management but also the cultural food preferences and traditions of the patient will enhance compliance.

Follow-up

EXPECTED OUTCOMES

- Patient's blood glucose levels will be maintained within prescribed limits with prescribed treatment regimen.
- Patient will recognize signs and symptoms (or caregiver will recognize signs) of high or low blood glucose levels and verbalize appropriate treatment measures. Candy, fruit juices, glucose tablets, and other sugar sources should be kept available for treatment of hypoglycemia. Patient also should verbalize the effects of alcohol on blood sugar control.

- Patient or caregiver will understand and be able to plan meals with appropriate nutritional intake for an individual with diabetes. When food intake is impaired, such as with symptoms of nausea and vomiting, insulin should be administered as directed and glucose self-monitoring should be completed more frequently and treated appropriately.
- Patient will understand importance of exercise and its effects on food and medication regimen, and when changes in medication regimen will be needed.
- Patient or caregiver will understand the need for consistent follow-up with healthcare providers and to report any concerns or changes in their status.
- Patient or caregiver will verbalize understanding of potential complications to be monitored for and measures to prevent such complications.

COMPLICATIONS

- Hyperosmolar hyperglycemic state (HHS) is a life-threatening complication of diabetes, the result of a seriously elevated blood glucose level > 600 mg/dL. HHS can occur as a result of inadequate treatment; increased insulin need due to acute disease processes such as infection, burns, gangrene, MI, or stroke. Chronic illnesses such as renal and cardiac diseases, hypertension, and alcoholism as well as exercise, stress, and therapeutic procedures such as surgery, dialysis, and hyperalimentation solutions can precipitate HHS. Because of the development of a hyperosmolar and dehydration state, potassium, sodium, and chloride ions will be decreased in the circulating volume. Urinalysis will reveal the presence of glucose but no ketones (see Figure 15–2). Treatment of HHS involves the aggressive administration of IV regular insulin to decrease serum glucose by 50 to 70 mg/dL/hour, as well as 0.9% NaCl intravenous fluids to treat hypovolemic and hemoconcentration state. Electrolyte replacement to reestablish an appropriate hemodynamic state and to prevent cardiac dysrhythmias, improve skeletal and smooth muscle function, and maintain endocrine function is also essential. Because of the severe hyperglycemic state in HHS, severe neurological effects can potentially occur such as seizures, shock, coma, and death.
- Diabetic ketoacidosis (DKA; see Complications under type 1 diabetes above) is rare in type 2 diabetes.

Figure 15–2. Hyperosmolar Hyperglycemic State Etiology

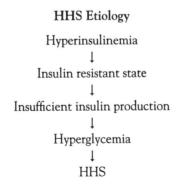

HHS Etiology

Hyperinsulinemia
↓
Insulin resistant state
↓
Insufficient insulin production
↓
Hyperglycemia
↓
HHS

- Infection is a major potential complication patients with diabetes. Hyperglycemia, altered circulatory status, alterations in the function of neutrophils, and reduced sensation due to neuropathies significantly increase the risk for development of infections.
- Blindness due to diabetic retinopathy as a result of alterations in blood flow and ischemia in the blood-retina barrier is the leading cause of blindness in persons with diabetes between the ages of 24 and 74 years.
- Kidney failure as a result of diabetic nephropathy occurs in 20% to 40% of all persons with diabetes. Diabetic nephropathy is thought to be due to the extended state of hyperglycemia and the fibrotic changes that occur in the glomerulus and tubules that allow for the excretion of albumin. Hypertension as a comorbidity also contributes to the decline in renal function.
- Hypertension, coronary artery disease, MI, and stroke are major complications of diabetes as a result of atherosclerotic changes in the blood vessels and alterations in microcirculation. Middle-age to older adults with type 2 diabetes are at high risk for the development of these complications. It is estimated that 20% to 60% of all persons with diabetes will develop hypertension, which is a major contributor to the increased mortality rate in persons with diabetes due to MI.
- Peripheral vascular insufficiency, intermittent claudication, and ulcerations are common complications of diabetes. Because of the decreased blood flow to the lower legs and resulting inadequate oxygenation, poor wound healing can lead to gangrene, the most common cause for nontraumatic amputation of toes and lower extremities in patients with diabetes.
- Diabetic neuropathies develop in the periphery and viscera. Neuropathies occur primarily in the extremities (peripheral neuropathies) but can occur anywhere. Peripheral neuropathies typically cause complaints of decreased sensation with aching, burning, or feeling of being cold, particularly in the feet and lower legs. Visceral neuropathy occurs in the autonomic nervous system. The pain and altered function of the areas depend on the location involved. Changes in sweating, constriction of the pupils, and autonomic response in the myocardium to control heart rate occur as a result of neuropathologies. Changes in gastrointestinal functioning typically include gastroparesis, constipation, and diarrhea as well as genitourinary dysfunctions such as urinary retention and decreased sexual functioning.
- Infection also is a major potential complication. Hyperglycemia, altered circulatory status, alterations in the function of neutrophils, and reduced sensation due to neuropathies significantly increase risk for development of infections.

REFERENCES

American Diabetes Association. (2010). Position statement: Diagnosis and classification of diabetes mellitus. *Diabetes Care, 33*(suppl 1), S13, 2010.

Centers for Disease Control and Prevention. (2011). *National diabetes fact sheet: National estimates and general information on diabetes and prediabetes in the United States, 2011.* Atlanta, GA: U.S. Department of Health and Human Services, Centers for Disease Control and Prevention. Retrieved from http://www.cdc.gov/diabetes/pubs/factsheet11.htm?utm_source=WWW&utm_medium=ContentPage&utm_content=CDCFactsheet&utm_campaign=CON

Ignatavicius, D. D., & Workman, M. L. (2010). *Medical-surgical nursing: Patient-centered collaborative practice.* St. Louis, MO: Saunders Elsevier.

Joslin Diabetes Center. (2010). *Joslin Diabetes Center & Joslin Clinic clinical guideline for pharmacological management of type 2 diabetes.* Boston, MA: Author. Retrieved from http://www.joslin.org/joslin_clinical_guidelines.html

Morton, P. G., & Fontaine, D. K. (2009). *Critical care nursing: A holistic approach.* Philadelphia: Wolters Kluwer/Lippincott Williams & Wilkins.

Pagana, K. D., & Pagana, T. J. (2009). *Mosby's diagnostic and laboratory test reference* (9th ed.). St. Louis, MO: Mosby Elsevier.

Wilson, B. A., Shannon, M. T., & Shields, K. M. (2009). *Prentice Hall nurse's drug guide 2009.* Upper Saddle River, NJ: Pearson Education.

16

Immune & Hematologic Systems

Deborah Jane Schwytzer, MSN, RN-BC, CEN

Immune System

GENERAL APPROACH

- The immune system is responsible for protecting the various body systems from disease-causing microorganisms and is part of the complex host defense system of the human body.
- Antigens form the basis of the immune response. All of the body's cells have antigens on their surfaces that are unique to that person. The body's immune system learns to recognize its own antigens or its "self," tolerates these cells, and destroys foreign cells.
- Immunity, commonly referred as immune response, is the body's ability to recognize its own cells and cellular structures and attempt to destroy foreign substances such as microorganisms and tumor proteins. The immune system responds in three ways:
  - Defends against the invasion of microorganisms and prevents infection by attacking foreign antigens through the development of antibodies and sensitized lymphocytes.
  - Maintains homeostasis through the removal of damaged cellular structures and maintaining the body's recognized "self" cells and structures.
  - Constantly monitors for mutations in the body's cells, recognizes them as foreign, and destroys them.
  - Only the cells of the immune system perform these functions.
- There are generally considered to be two types of immunity.

- *Innate or natural immunity* exists in the body without prior exposure to a foreign antigen. Physical barriers such as skin and mucous membranes, chemical barriers such as hydrochloric acid in the stomach and lysosomes found in bodily secretions such as tears and saliva, and the neutrophils and monocytes (white blood cells) constitute the body's innate protection against infectious agents.
- *Acquired immunity* develops either actively or passively.
    - Active acquired immunity develops in response to the invasion of a foreign substance. The body develops an antibody, sensitized lymphocytes, or both, to attack and destroy the invader on subsequent exposures. Active acquired immunity can develop as a result of exposure to a disease such as measles or chickenpox, or through inoculation with the antigen through immunization. Immunity developed this way can be long-lasting. Polio and diphtheria immunizations are examples of active acquired immunity for people who have not experienced the disease.
    - Passive acquired immunity is the result of the introduction of another person's antibodies to an antigen rather than the body's development of its own antibodies. This process can occur naturally, as with the passage of immunoglobulins in breast milk from mother to infant, or artificially via injection of human serum antibodies (gamma globulin) for an immediate but short-term effect.
- When a foreign organism invades the body, two types of immune responses can occur.
    - Cell-mediated immunity protects the body against bacterial, fungal, and viral infections as well as tumor cells and transplanted cells. Macrophages and T-lymphocytes are the primary cells involved in this form of immunity. Macrophages function to recognize, ingest, and process the foreign antigen of bacteria, fungus, or viruses for destruction by the various types of T-lymphocytes and produce interleukin-I, which serves in the inflammatory process to produce fever symptoms. T-lymphocytes, which constitute approximately 70% to 80% of the circulating lymphocytes, differentiate into five types of T-cells that each performs a specific function in cell-mediated immunity, but all identify foreign materials in the body.
        - The memory cells are sensitized cells that remain dormant until the second exposure to an antigen and then provide an immunity response.
        - The lymphokine-producing cells release a chemical substance that stimulates the activation of B-lymphocytes, cytotoxic T-cells, suppressor T-cells, and phagocytoxic macrophages to destroy foreign antigens.
        - Cytotoxic T cells directly destroy the antigen or the cells carrying the antigen.
        - Helper T cells or T4 cells facilitate the humoral as well as cell-mediated responses.
        - Suppressor T cells or T8 cells inhibit the humoral and cell-mediated responses.
    - Humoral immunity response, also called an antibody response, involves the production of immunoglobulins or antibodies created in response to the B-lymphocyte cell-bound foreign antigen. When a foreign antigen or pathogen invades, the body can respond in one of two ways. A B-lymphocyte cell may immediately bind the invader and produce the necessary immunoglobulin to destroy it, or a monocyte or macrophage can attack the foreign antigen and phagocytize the bacteria and then present the antigen to a B-lymphocyte cell. Either process ultimately destroys the bacteria or foreign matter. Table 16–1 lists the various immunoglobulins and their primary functions.

Table 16-1. Classification of Immunoglobulin

Classification	Approximate Serum Concentration	Characteristics
IgA	15%–20%	Found in body secretions such as tears, saliva, breast milk, respiratory, GI, and genitourinary. Lines mucous membranes and protects epithelial linings from antigenic attacks. Protects against viral infection.
IgD	1%	Is present on lymphocyte surfaces and is believed to control lymphocyte activation or suppression.
IgE	0.002%	Affixed to basophiles and mast cells. Causes the symptoms experienced in allergic reactions. Assists in the defense against parasites.
IgG	76%	Smallest immunoglobin; crosses cell membranes as single structure. Found in all body fluids. Major antibacterial and antiviral antibody which functions as a secondary protector.
IgM	8%	Largest immunoglobulin; cannot cross cell membrane because of size. Serves a primary antibody protection function. Usually found in the vascular system. Responsible for the classic antibody reactions such as precipitation, agglutination, and neutralization such as occurs in ABO reactions.

- Infections are the result of invasion of the body by a pathogen and the body's response to this invasion. Infections typically provoke inflammation, and if unresolved, tissue and cell injury and eventual cell death can result.
- Inflammation also can occur as a local reaction to irritation or injury, or as an allergic response to a foreign agent. The signs and symptoms of acute inflammation include:
  - Redness as a result of arteriole dilatation and increased blood circulation at the site.
  - Warmth as the area undergoes local vasodilatation, fluid leaks into the surrounding tissues, and blood flow to the area increases.
  - Edema at the site caused by local vasodilatation and leakage of fluid into the interstitial spaces. Swelling will also occur as a result of blockage of the lymphatic system in the area.
  - Pain occurs as the pain receptors are stimulated by swollen tissues, fluid leakage, and the serous chemicals released into the area of inflammation.
  - Decrease or loss of function can occur as a result of the pain and swelling in the area.
- A state of immunocompetency exists when the body's immune system is able to identify and destroy or inactivate foreign antigens. If deficiencies or unresponsiveness develops, a state of immunodeficiency occurs and malignancies, severe infections, and immunodeficiency diseases can occur.
- An immunodeficiency state results from missing or damage to one or more components of the immune system.

- Often it is the function of the B or T cells of the immune system that are compromised. These components can be missing or damaged due to a congenital factor and apparent from birth, such as lack of growth hormone or chronic granulomatous disease, a rare inherited blood disorder in which the body's phagocytes are unable to destroy bacteria and the patient suffers repeated bacterial infections. These conditions are referred to as primary immunodeficiency because they are the result of no known underlying disorder. Some immunodeficiency disorders can be acquired or the result of a secondary loss of some component of the immune system as a result of a disease, injury, or medical treatment, or they may be idiopathic (i.e., not the result of a genetic predisposition or failure of lymphoid tissue to develop appropriately). Malnutrition, exposure to radiation or chemotherapeutic agents for cancer treatment, use of immunosuppressant drugs after organ transplantation, and disease such as HIV/AIDS are classified as secondary or acquired immunodeficiency.

RED FLAGS

- Changes in the values of components of the immune system are not always a disease in themselves but rather a symptom of a disease process.
- Many conditions can indicate the presence of an immunologic deficiency and should be investigated. More frequent, severe, longer-lasting, and more difficult to cure infections than is typical in persons with normal immune systems can indicate an immune deficiency. Examples include chronic infections such as recurrent otitis media, sinusitis, and upper respiratory infections as well as inflammatory processes that do not resolve despite treatment such as chronic abscess formations. Hemolytic anemia also can be a sign of immune compromise.
- Monitoring for infection is very important for persons infected with HIV. Becoming infected with organisms that a healthy immune system would normally be able to defeat is known as contracting an opportunistic infection. Exposure to parasites such as *Toxoplasma* and *Pneumocystis carinii* normally will not produce disease in individuals with normal immune systems, but in the individual with an immunodeficiency can produce life-threatening disease.
- Having autoimmune problems (i.e., a condition in which the person's immune system attacks the body's own organs and tissues) indicates a potential immune deficiency.
- It is important to remember and to reinforce education that a person with HIV infection can transmit the virus at all stages of the disease process. Even during the asymptomatic stage, the virus is present and can be spread through body secretions.

Diseases of the Immune System

HUMAN IMMUNODEFICIENCY VIRUS (HIV) & ACQUIRED IMMUNODEFICIENCY SYNDROME (AIDS)

Description

- Human immunodeficiency virus (HIV) is a retrovirus that attacks and gradually destroys the immune system, leaving the host unprotected against infection. The Centers for Disease Control and Prevention (CDC) classifies of HIV infection in three stages, with AIDS as the third stage. The classification system is divided not only into types of clinical diseases present

(Categories A, B, or C) but also the CD4+ cell count (stage 1: CD4+ count ≥ 500 cells/mcL; stage 2: CD4+ count 200–499 cells/mcL; stage 3: CD4+ cell count < 200 cells/mcL). CDC defines AIDS as an illness characterized by the confirmed presence of HIV infection, plus CD4+ T-cell count below 200 cells/mcL (HIV stage 3) or the presence of one or more AIDS-defining conditions.

Etiology

- The human immunodeficiency virus invades the body through the blood or mucous membranes and primarily attacks the T-cells bearing the CD4+ antigen. As is common to retroviruses, HIV transcribes its RNA genetic material into the DNA of its host cells through the use of reverse transcriptase. This viral DNA enters the nucleus of the cell and is replicated with the cell's own DNA, producing numerous copies of the virus. These viral copies produce lifelong infection in the host cells and can infect other cells at any time.
  - The infected host cells can replicate immediately and cause cell death or can become latent and begin viral replication at a later time. Once replication begins, it leads to lymphocyte structural and functional changes, direct destruction of CD4+ cells, or dysfunction of the CD4+ T-cells and resultant immunosuppression.
  - The effects of this lymphopenia and the infectious process of HIV are seen as immunodeficiency, autoimmunity dysfunction, neurologic dysfunction, or any combination of these.
  - Progression of the infectious process involves several stages, the timing of which is variable. The World Health Organization (WHO) classifies HIV infection into 4 stages based upon clinical findings and does not depend on a CD4 count. These stages are as follows.
    - Typically, the individual will be exposed to HIV through contact with infected blood, blood products, or body fluids such as semen. If the individual becomes infected with the virus, seroconversion (i.e., development of detectable HIV antibodies) will occur. This is Stage 1. The ELISA (enzyme-linked immunosorbent assay) test and Western blot test will be positive for the HIV antibody. The infected individual may not experience seroconversion for 6 to 12 weeks or as long as several months depending on the extent of initial exposure. Classified as Primary HIV infection, the patient is asymptomatic.
    - Stage 2 is the period when the patient is experiencing mild symptomatology such as mild weight loss, recurrent respiratory infections, skin rash, and viral and fungal infections such as herpes zoster and fungal nail infections. The virus is present, slowly replicating and destroying normal cells. The CD4+ T-cell count gradually decreases during this stage, which may last 12 years or even longer.
    - Stage 3 occurs when the infected individual develops signs and symptoms of immunodeficiency and decline in immune system functioning such as generalized lymphadenopathy, weight loss, fatigue, fevers, night sweats, and persistent opportunistic infections. At this point, the CD4+ T-cell count has significantly declined.
    - Stage 4 is the advanced stage of the disease when severe opportunistic diseases are experienced and it is obvious that the immune system has failed. Typically, the CD4+ T-cell count has declined to less than 200 cells/mcL and several opportunistic infections are obviously present.
    - The length of time for progression from stage 3 to stage 4 depends on when antiretroviral treatment begins and the availability of treatment for opportunistic infections. Advances in diagnosis and treatment have prolonged the time from seroconversion to stage 4 in many cases.

- The CDC utilizes a classification system based on the lowest CD4 cell count and previously diagnosed HIV-related conditions. Clinical Category A are those individuals diagnosed with HIV but asymptomatic with varying CD4 counts (A1—CD4 ≥ 500 cells/mcL, A2—CD4 200–499 cells/mcL, A3—CD4 < 200 cells/mcL).
- Clinical category B are those individuals who are symptomatic or have been diagnosed with at least 1 HIV attributed infection or have a disease complicated by the presence of the HIV infection as well as varying CD4 counts (B1—CD4 ≥ 500 cells/mcL, B2—CD4 200–499 cells/mcL, B3—CD4 < 200 cells/mcL).
- Clinical category C are those individuals who are exhibiting conditions indicative of AIDS such as recurrent bacterial pneumonias, Candidiasis, Kaposi sarcoma, or wasting syndrome, as well as varying CD4 counts (C1—CD4 >/= 500 cells/mcL, C2—CD4 200–499 cells/mcL, C3—CD4 < 200 cells/mcL)

Incidence and Demographics

- HIV is common throughout the world, with a prevalence of approximately 33.4 million people living with HIV and 2.7 million people newly infected with HIV in 2008. Approximately 2 million AIDS-related deaths were recorded in 2008. In the United States in 2010, it was believed that the number of persons living with HIV was more than 1 million and 56,300 people were newly infected with the HIV virus annually. AIDS-related deaths in the United States were believed to be approximately 18,000 each year.
- HIV infection in the United States is caused by sexual transmission (male-to-male and male-to-female) and sharing injecting equipment among drug abusers. Transmission is often associated with sexually transmitted infections (STIs).

Risk Factors

- Exchange of body fluids between individuals such as during sexual intercourse and sharing of blood-contaminated drug injection equipment; a significant quantity of virus is present in blood, semen, vaginal and cervical secretions, and cerebrospinal fluid
- Unprotected sexual relations
- Presence of sexually transmitted infections
- Uncircumcised male
- Multiple sex partners
- Transfusion with unscreened blood or blood products
- Hemophilia, because of the large amount of clotting factors received
- Occupational exposures among healthcare providers, medical waste handlers, and laboratory personnel through percutaneous or mucosal exposures
- Infants of HIV-positive mothers through pregnancy or during delivery or breastfeeding

Prevention and Screening

- People with any of the risk factors should be screened frequently and regularly.
- Educating high-risk populations about the potential risks and modes of transmission can help to prevent the spread of HIV.
- Assure high-risk persons that confidentiality will be maintained to reduce fear of testing because of the stigma of the diagnosis, and educate them about the availability of counseling if diagnosis is made.
- CDC recommends including HIV testing as part of routine screening in healthcare settings for adults, adolescents, and pregnant women. Early detection and treatment can reduce the risk of prenatal HIV transmission.
- Educate people who have tested positive for HIV on how to advise their contacts to be tested.

- Although progression of HIV to AIDS is nearly inevitable, the timing of progression depends upon the extent and frequency of exposure, risk behavior changes, nutritional status, stress, and early treatment. Close monitoring of symptoms and early initiation of treatment can delay progression.

Assessment
- Chief complaints and symptoms found on history and physical assessment are based on the extent of HIV progression and opportunistic diseases.

HISTORY
- Presence of any of the risk factors
- Recent bout of mononucleosis-type illness after potential contact with the virus
- Nausea, vomiting, diarrhea
- Abdominal cramping
- Fever
- Sore throat
- Rash
- Headache
- Arthralgia
- Myalgia
- Lymphadenopathy
- History of recent flu-like symptoms, viral syndrome, or upper-respiratory infection
- Night sweats
- Weight loss
- Mouth sores
- Memory loss, confusion, lethargy, impaired thought processes
- Apathy
- Ataxia, tremor
- Incontinence

PHYSICAL EXAM
- Assess for signs and symptoms of any type of infection or cancer . Examples:
  - AIDS dementia: mental status changes, motor disturbances, neurological deficiencies
  - *Pneumocystis carinii* pneumonia: fever, cough, shortness of breath, tachypnea, tachycardia, sputum production
  - Candidiasis: oral thrush or esophagitis seen as white, friable plaques on tongue, buccal membranes, or in throat; painful or difficulty swallowing
  - Herpes virus infections such as cytomegalovirus, herpes simplex, or herpes zoster
  - Kaposi's sarcoma: vascular macules and papules; purple lesions of skin; tumors of the gastrointestinal tract, lungs, or lymphatic system
  - Hodgkin's, non-Hodgkin's, and primary lymphoma of the brain: lymphadenopathy, enlarged spleen, bone pain, mental status changes
  - Cervical dysplasia and carcinoma: cervical cell changes on Papanicolaou smears
  - *Toxoplasma gondii:* usually affects the brain as shown in the presence of changes in mental status, seizures and focal neurologic signs
  - *Cryptococcus neoformans*—exemplifies as meningitis or lung infection
  - *Cryptosporidium:* protozoan that commonly causes prolonged diarrhea
  - Bacterial salmonella: diarrhea
  - *Mycobacterium avium:* chills, fever, weakness, night sweats, abdominal pain, diarrhea, and weight loss; most common cause of "wasting syndrome" in people with AIDS

- Psychosocial assessment should include sources of support, usual coping strategies, and whether healthcare proxy or durable power of attorney has been completed.

DIAGNOSTIC STUDIES
- Standard HIV testing
  - ELISA (enzyme-linked immunosorbent assay) tests for the presence of antibodies to HIV; a positive result must be confirmed by the Western blot test.
  - A positive Western blot test will confirm the diagnosis of HIV infection.
- CD4+ T-cell count detects the depletion of CD4+ T cells in the body as an indication of the extent of HIV disease progression. The normal CD4+ T cell count is 600 to 1,500 cells/mcL. During treatment, an increase in the number of cells typically indicates successful antiviral therapy while a decrease in the cell count indicates worsening of the disease.
- Quantitative plasma HIV RNA or viral load: measures the quantity of HIV genetic material in the blood. It quantifies the amount of virus for not only diagnosis and prognosis but also the effectiveness of treatment.
- Immune-complex–dissociated p24 assay: detects the viral protein p24 in the peripheral blood. The test is sensitive as early as 2 to 6 weeks after infection, detects the presence of HIV before seroconversion, and can be used to monitor progression of the infection.
- Tuberculin skin test: diagnoses tuberculosis infection, common in some groups with HIV.
- Specific viral and bacterial cultures: diagnose specific opportunistic infections.
- Serology examinations: diagnostic for opportunistic infections and diseases.

Nursing Management
- There is no cure for HIV/AIDS at present.
- Management is focused on collaborative care in the early identification of the disease and opportunistic infections, prolonging the asymptomatic period, prevention and treatment of opportunistic infections and cancers, and provision of emotional and psychological support.
- Universal precautions are the best way for healthcare workers to prevent workplace transmission.

NONPHARMACOLOGIC TREATMENT
- Patient education
  - HIV is not spread by casual contact or biting insects such as mosquitoes.
  - Safe sex practices such the use of condoms is advisable in all cases. Oral and anal sex can increase the spread of the disease because potentially high infective seminal and vaginal fluids come in contact with mucous membranes where absorption is increased. Anal sex can also result in tears of the rectal mucous membranes, allowing increased potential for infection via direct access to the blood.
  - Abstinence and monogamous sex with noninfected individuals are the surest ways to prevent HIV infection.
  - Infected individuals must always be cautious during sex because transmission is always possible regardless of the current viral load.
  - Reduction in the transmission of HIV between injection drug users can be achieved through thorough cleaning of equipment using bleach or, preferably, a community needle exchange program that makes needle-sharing unnecessary.
  - Perinatal transmission can occur when blood passes across the placenta during pregnancy, during childbirth when the infant comes in contact with blood and vaginal secretions, and when the infant breastfeeds after birth. Prenatal testing and treatment during pregnancy or at the time of birth can decrease the likelihood of transmission to the infant.

- Sources, signs, and symptoms of opportunistic infections should be discussed. Preventive measures should be discussed with the patient and significant others.
- The importance of adequate nutritional intake must be stressed. Patient and family or caregiver should demonstrate the ability to select foods high in calories and protein and understanding of the importance of adequate fluid intake.
- Psychological support: provide support services and reassurance about confidentiality. Patients may need a list of support groups, community resources, and mental health professionals.
- Nutritional support should be provided with an emphasis on high-calorie, high-protein foods within the patient's preferences. Fluid intake should be at least 3 to 4 liters of fluid per day.
- Laboratory studies should be scheduled to monitor the effectiveness and potential side effects of antiviral medications. Basic chemistries, glucose levels, liver enzymes, CBC, lipids, CD4, viral load and urinalysis should be completed approximately 2 to 8 weeks after the initiation or modifications in antiretroviral therapy. Once clinically stable, laboratory testing may be decreased to every 3 to 12 months.

PHARMACOLOGIC TREATMENT
- The goals of drug therapy are to suppress synthesis and replication of the viral DNA, inhibit virus fusion to new host cells, and prevent and treat opportunistic infections.
- Medications are usually individualized to the patient's viral load and CD4+ T-cell counts. Due to the long-term side effects of some medications, therapies are frequently not started at diagnosis but rather when the CD4 count decreases.
- Preferred initial medication regimens are designed to optimize efficiency, be tolerable, minimize toxicity, and facilitate ease of use. Highly active antiretroviral therapies (HAART) are currently the most commonly used regimens. These suggested regimens include one of the following combinations:
  - Nonnucleoside reverse transcriptase inhibitor and 2-nucleoside reverse transcriptase inhibitor
  - Protease inhibitor and 2-nucleoside reverse transcriptase inhibitor
  - Integrase strand transfer inhibitor and 2-nucleoside reverse transcriptase inhibitor
- Nucleoside analog reverse transcriptase inhibitors suppress the production of reverse transcriptase and inhibit DNA synthesis and replication. The medications in this category include:
  - Zidovudine (Retrovir)
  - Lamivudine (Epivir)
  - Emtricitabine (Emtriva)
  - Didanosine (Videx EC)
  - Zalcitabine (ddC)
- Protease inhibitors block the effectiveness of the viral enzyme protease by binding to the enzyme's active receptor site, thereby preventing the virus from infecting new cells.
  - Saquinavir (Invirase)
  - Indinavir (Crixivan)
  - Ritonavir (Norvir)
  - Nelfinavir (Viracept)
  - Amprenavir (Agenerase)
  - Fosamprenavir (Lexiva)
- Nonnucleoside analog reverse transcriptase inhibitors attach themselves to reverse transcriptase and prevent the enzyme from converting RNA to DNA.
  - Nevirapine (Viramune)

- Efavirenz (Sustiva)
- Delavirdine (Rescriptor)
- Integrase strand transfer inhibitor: Integrase typically catalyzes the insertion of viral DNA into the host cell. Integrase strand transfer inhibitor blocks this function.
- Raltegravir (Isentress)
- Fusion inhibitors prevent the virus from fusing to the CD4 cell.
  - Enfuvirtide (Fuzeon)
- Other adjunctive therapies found to be beneficial to some persons include:
  - Immunomodulatory agents are drugs that suppress or stimulate the immune system.
  - Human granulocyte colony-stimulating agents enhance proliferation of immune cells.
  - Anti-infective agents for opportunistic infections:
    - Trimethoprim/sulfamethoxazole (Bactrim, Septra)
    - Pentamidine isethionate (Pentam)
    - Dapsone (Avlosulfon)
    - Metronidazole (Flagyl)
    - Ketoconazole (Nizoral)
    - Fluconazole (Diflucan)
    - Rifampin (Rifadin)
    - Amphotericin B (Fungizone)
    - Azithromycin (Zithromax)
    - Ciprofloxacin (Cipro)
    - Clarithromycin (Biaxin)
    - Isoniazid (Laniazid)
    - Ganciclovir (Cytovene)
    - Acyclovir (Zovirax)
  - Anti-emetics are used to manage nausea and vomiting that can be caused by many of the antiviral medications.
  - Analgesics are used for pain relief.
  - Immunizations against potential opportunistic diseases can be given when the T-cell count is adequate. Recommended immunizations include pneumococcal, annual influenza, hepatitis B, tetanus-diphtheria, inactivated polio virus, measles, mumps, and rubella vaccines.

Special Considerations

- HIV is a chronic illness, but progression of the disease can be delayed with maintenance of a healthy immune system through good nutrition, rest, routine medical care, and healthy behaviors. Close monitoring for the early symptoms of opportunistic infections and the development of adverse side effects from medications are also helpful.

Follow-up

EXPECTED OUTCOMES
- Patient and significant others will verbalize knowledge related to disease process and risk factors.
- Absence of infection.
- Reduction or elimination of fear and hopelessness.
- Adequate nutrition and hydration will be maintained.
- Patient will comply with medication regimen and make recommended lifestyle changes.
- Skin integrity will be maintained.

- Physical comfort will be maintained at a tolerable range.
- Thought processes will remain intact to maintain ability to perform activities of daily living.

COMPLICATIONS
- Repeated opportunistic diseases
- Noncompliance with medication regimen
- Low self-esteem
- Social isolation
- Diabetes mellitus as a result of protease inhibitor use
- Lipodystrophy as a side effect of nucleoside analog reverse transcriptase inhibitors
- Hyperlipidemia as a side effect of protease inhibitors and nucleoside analog reverse transcriptase inhibitors
- Lactic acidosis as a side effect of nucleoside analog reverse transcriptase inhibitors

Hematologic System

GENERAL APPROACH

- The hematologic system encompasses blood and its components, as well as its supportive structures such as the bone marrow, lymphatic system, spleen, liver, and reticuloendothelial phagocyte systems.
- Blood is a connective tissue that serves as a medium for transport of oxygen, nutrients, and hormones throughout the body as well as the transport of waste products and toxins to the liver, lungs, and kidneys for excretion. This function helps to maintain the body's pH, electrolyte balance, and body temperature as it circulates.
- The volume of blood is approximately 8% of the total body weight.
- The major components of blood are:
  - Blood cells, which originate in the bone marrow as stem cells before differentiating into red blood cells (RBCs; erythrocytes), white blood cells (WBCs; leukocytes), and platelets (thrombocytes). This process of hematopoiesis is ongoing.
  - Plasma, the straw-colored liquid portion of the blood in which all the blood cells are suspended. The plasma makes up about 50% to 55% of the blood sample and contains water, amino acids, proteins, electrolytes, hormones, carbohydrates, lipids, vitamins, and cellular waste materials.
- Serum, the liquid result of the clotting of whole blood, is the residual plasma minus fibrinogen and other clotting factors.
- The immunological products of the hematologic system, primarily white blood cells, serve as defense mechanisms against infection and other foreign materials.
- The normal red blood cell is a nonnucleated, biconcave, disc-shaped structure that composes about 99% of the total blood cells. This shape assists in the maximization of surface area for oxygen-carrying capacity. The production of RBCs (erythropoiesis) is the result of tissue hypoxia signaling kidneys to release erythropoietin, which stimulates the red bone marrow to produce reticulocytes, which mature into erythrocytes in about 24 to 48 hours. Maturation of RBCs is dependent on the availability of several vitamins and minerals such as folic acid and vitamin B12. Absence or decrease in the amounts of these substances alters the size, shape, and lifespan of the RBCs as they mature. The life span of the RBC is approximately 120 days. The normal reticulocyte count is generally 1% of the total RBC count.

- Hemoglobin is contained in the RBC and its production depends upon the amount of iron available for synthesis. As the oxygen-carrying unit of the RBC, hemoglobin is responsible for not only the transport of oxygen to the tissues and cells but also the removal and transport of the carbon dioxide to the lungs for excretion.
- White blood cells (leukocytes) defend the body against infection and on average there are about 5,000 to 10,000 WBCs per cubic milliliter of blood or about 1% of the total blood volume. WBCs are also produced in the bone marrow from stem cells and differentiate into two basic types: granular leukocytes (granulocytes) and nongranuloctyes (agranulocytes).
- The granulocytes have horseshoe-shaped nuclei and their cytoplasm contains large granules that act as phagocytes in the presence of foreign matter. There are three types of granulocytes: neutrophils, eosinophils, and basophils.
- The agranulocytes consist of two types of cells: monocytes and lymphocytes. Monocytes are large cells with a prominent nucleus that serve a phagocyte function; after being transformed into macrophages, they have a life span of months to years. The lymphocytes play a primary role in immunological, hypersensitivity, and rejection reactions.
- Thrombocytes (platelets) are produced in the bone marrow and are essential for blood clotting functions.
- Table 16–2 outlines the normal value, functions, and examples of conditions resulting in an elevation or reduction in the number of cells of the hematological system.

Table 16-2. Hematologic Cells

Cell Type	Normal Value	Function	Changes
Erythrocytes (RBCs)	Male: 4.2–5.4 million/mm³ Female: 3.6–5.0 million/mm³	Transport oxygen and carbon dioxide to and from cells	↑ polycythemia ↑ dehydration ↓ anemia ↓ fluid overload ↓ hemorrhage
Reticulocytes	1.0%–1.5% of total RBC	Synthesize hemoglobin to continue release of new RBCs into circulation	↑ recent blood loss ↑ chronic hemolysis
Hemoglobin	Male: 14–16.5 g/dL Female: 12–15 g/dL	Iron-containing protein in RBCs that transports oxygen	↑ congenital heart disease ↑ chronic obstructive pulmonary disease (COPD) ↑ congestive heart failure ↑ severe burns ↑ high altitudes ↓ anemia ↓ lymphoma ↓ hemorrhage ↓ dietary deficiency ↓ leukemia ↓ kidney disease ↓ hemolytic reaction

Hematocrit	Male: 40%–50% Female: 37%–47%	Measure of the total blood volume that the red blood cells comprise	↑ severe dehydration ↑ burns ↑ COPD ↑ polycythemia ↓ anemia ↓ cirrhosis ↓ hemorrhage ↓ dietary deficiency ↓ leukemia ↓ bone marrow failure ↓ hemolytic reaction
Leukocytes (WBCs)	5,000–10,000/mm³	Protect the body against foreign matter	↑ inflammation ↑ tissue necrosis ↑ infection ↑ hematologic malignancy ↓ bone marrow depression ↓ chronic disease
Neutrophils	3,000–7,000/ mm³	Phagocytosis of infective matter and release of enzymes to destroy bacteria	↑ inflammation ↑ surgery ↑ infection ↑ myocardial infarction ↓ aplastic anemia ↓ hepatitis
Eosinophils	50–400/mm³	Detoxification of foreign proteins and defense against parasites	↑ allergic reactions ↑ autoimmune diseases ↑ parasite infections ↑ dermatologic conditions ↓ stress reaction ↓ severe infection
Basophils	25–200/mm³	Inflammatory response; release of heparin, serotonin, and histamine in allergic reactions	↑ postsplenectomy ↑ hemolytic anemia ↑ radiation ↑ hypothyroidism ↑ leukemia ↑ chronic hypersensitivity ↓ stress reaction
Monocytes	100–600/mm³	Mature into macrophages; phagocytosis of necrotic tissue, debris, and foreign particles	↑ bacterial infections ↑ viral infections ↑ parasitic infections ↑ chronic inflammation ↓ stress reaction
Lymphocytes	1,000–4,000/mm³	Defense against microorganisms	↑ bacterial infections ↑ viral infections ↑ lymphocytic leukemia ↓ immunoglobulin deficiency

cont.

Table 16–2. Hematologic Cells (cont.)

Thrombocytes (platelets)	150,000–400,000/ mm³	Blood clotting and hemostasis	↑ polycythemia vera ↑ postsplenectomy ↑ cancer ↑ living at high altitude ↑ use of oral contraceptives ↓ leukemia ↓ bone marrow failure ↓ disseminated intravascular coagulation ↓ hemorrhage ↓ radiation exposure ↓ hypothermia ↓ hyperthermia ↓ severe infection

RED FLAGS

- Changes in the values of the components are not a disease in themselves but rather a symptom of a disease process.
- Bone marrow function must be considered whenever assessing for diseases of the hematologic system because this is the site of stem cell residence.
- Many conditions can affect the bone marrow or its ability to generate healthy blood cells or can alter the functioning of mature and maturing cells as well as the destruction of old cells. A thorough history should be taken to ensure consideration of these causative factors.
- Many conditions can lead to hematological disorders, such as:
  - Lead poisoning or exposure
  - Ionizing radiation exposure
  - Exposure to pesticides or other chemicals
  - Heredity
  - Excessive alcohol consumption
  - Allergies
  - Liver disease
  - Poor nutrition
  - Renal disease
  - Neoplasms
  - Blood clots
- The aging process can cause changes in the hematological system. Generally, the percentage of marrow space occupied by the hematopoietic tissue is decreased, reducing both cell production and the ability to promptly respond to changes in the quality of blood cells.

Diseases of the Hematologic System

ANEMIA

- Anemia is generally considered to be any process that causes a reduction in the number of circulating red blood cells or hemoglobin that leads to inadequate oxygenation of the tissues.
- Anemias are classified on the basis of red cell morphology (microcytic, normocytic, or macrocytic), quantity of pigment (hypochromic or normochromic), or etiology (nutritional or blood loss).

IRON-DEFICIENCY ANEMIA

Description
- A microcytic, hypochromic anemia caused by insufficient iron for hemoglobin synthesis

Etiology
- Inadequate iron intake in persons who are alcoholic or on vegetarian diets
- Increased demand for iron in pregnancy or adolescence
- Impaired absorption in persons with a gastrectomy or celiac disease
- Slow, persistent loss caused by menorrhagia, gastritis, polyps, aspirin ingestion, GI neoplasms, peptic ulcer disease (PUD), esophageal varices, hemorrhoids, or chronic hemorrhage

Incidence and Demographics
- Common throughout the world with a prevalence of approximately 20% among adult women, 50% among pregnant women, and 3% among adult males

Risk Factors
- Poor dietary intake of foods rich in iron, such as in a vegetarian diet because iron from grains and vegetables are not absorbed as well as iron from meats
- Blood loss with heavy menstrual bleeding
- Chronic blood loss caused by peptic ulcer disease; bladder, colon, or renal tumors; or uterine polyps
- Crohn's or celiac disease, which affect the body's ability to absorb nutrients from the small intestines

Prevention and Screening
- Routine screening in individuals with chronic blood loss or any disease process that prohibits or decreases ability to absorb iron in the intestines
- Knowledge of financial, cultural, and regional dietary restrictions decreasing iron-rich foods (e.g., vegetarians, elderly)
- Prenatal screening for all pregnant women; prenatal vitamins can decrease the potential for iron-deficiency anemia and neonatal issues

Assessment

HISTORY
- Easily fatigued or listless
- Dyspnea on exertion
- Dizziness, faintness, or weakness
- Pallor
- Headaches
- Tachycardia or heart murmurs
- Wide pulse pressure
- Cardiac hypertrophy
- Angina
- Anorexia
- Pica (unusual craving for nonnutritive substances such as ice, dirt, or starch)
- Recent infection
- GI disorders
- Family history
- Failure to respond to iron supplements

PHYSICAL EXAM
- Assess for pallor of conjunctiva, nail beds, mucous membranes
- Tachycardia and tachypnea
- Postural hypertension
- Flattened, ridged, concave, or spoon-shaped nails
- Brittle hair and nails
- Altered mental status in severe anemia

DIAGNOSTIC STUDIES
- Routine CBC will reveal:
  - Hemoglobin < 14 g/dL in males, < 12 g/dL in females
  - Hematocrit < 42% in males, < 36% in females
  - Low mean corpuscular volume (microcytic) and low mean corpuscular hemoglobin concentration (hypochromic)
  - Low RBC count
  - Increased red cell distribution width
- Iron studies
  - Total iron-binding capacity usually normal
  - Serum ferritin < 12 mcg/L
  - Serum iron generally < 50 mcg/L
  - Serum transferrin < 20%
- Bilirubin—normal
- B_{12} and folate levels within normal limits
- Bone marrow studies will show low iron stain

Management

NONPHARMACOLOGIC TREATMENT
- Nutritional support to include foods high in iron, including organ and lean meats, egg yolks, shellfish, apricots, prunes, peaches, raisins, green leafy vegetables, iron-fortified breads and cereals.

- Education that iron medications can cause GI upset, nausea, and vomiting. Even though foods and juices taken concurrently can interfere with absorption, education about alternatives to facilitate ingestion should be included. Ascorbic acid (vitamin C) can assist with absorption.
- Some over-the-counter medications can cause excessive absorption. Medications such as those used for incontinence can lead to iron overdose.
- Keep medications out of the reach of children.
- Frequent rest periods should be taken.

PHARMACOLOGIC TREATMENT
- Oral iron replacement is most effective and least expensive.
- Ferrous sulfate tablets at 300 to 325 mg. Blood levels should return to normal within 2 months but stores will take approximately 3 to 6 months. Failure to respond to treatment frequently is due to noncompliance. Iron should be taken on an empty stomach. Milk, milk products, and antacids will interfere with absorption so patients must be knowledgeable of these considerations.
- Parenteral replacement can be used for extreme cases of iron-deficiency anemia or if patient is noncompliant with oral regimen. Intramuscular (IM) or intravenous (IV) iron preparations can be costly, painful, and cause phlebitis, skin discoloration, and regional adenopathy.
- Dosage is determined by patient weight.

Special Considerations
- None

Follow-up

EXPECTED OUTCOMES
- Anemia signs and symptoms will be controlled with serum iron levels returning to normal.
- Patient or caregiver will express understanding of the need to follow treatment plan and to maintain follow-up regimen. Patient or caregiver must also understand the dietary contraindications when taking iron supplements, and that constipation caused by iron supplements can be prevented by additional oral intake of fluids and fiber.

COMPLICATIONS
- In pregnancy, iron-deficiency anemia has been associated with premature births and low birth-weight babies.
- Iron deficiency anemia has been associated with tachycardia and irregular heartbeats as well as angina due to the body's need to compensate for the decreased oxygen-carrying capacity of the blood.
- Constipation can be caused by oral iron supplements. Knowledge of dietary considerations and ways to prevent this complication should be included in the patient education provided.

VITAMIN B$_{12}$ DEFICIENCY ANEMIA (PERNICIOUS ANEMIA)

Description
- A macrocytic anemia commonly caused by insufficient gastric production of hydrochloric acid and intrinsic factor in the gastric mucosa essential for the absorption of vitamin B$_{12}$ in the ileum.

Etiology
- Because vitamin B$_{12}$ is absorbed in the ileum, patients who have gastric mucosal atrophy or surgical gastrectomy, partial gastrectomy, or gastrojejunostomy can develop a deficiency.
- A deficiency in B$_{12}$ inhibits red blood cell growth and leads to deformed and insufficient RBCs with poor oxygen-carrying capacity.
- A lack of vitamin B$_{12}$ can alter the structure and function of peripheral nerves, spinal cord, and brain, leading to permanent neurologic disability and death.
- Poor dietary intake of foods rich in vitamin B$_{12}$ also can be a cause.

Incidence and Demographics
- Inevitably occurs in patients who have undergone total gastrectomy and in about 15% of those with partial gastrectomy.
- There is also a familial incidence among people of Northern European ancestry, which may indicate a single dominant autosomal factor.
- Onset typically occurs after age 35 and incidence increases with aging.
- It is present in approximately 2% of persons over 60 years of age.

Risk Factors
- Gastric surgery
- Genetic predisposition
- Vegetarian diet

Prevention and Screening
- Screen individuals with a family history.
- Treat all individuals with total gastrectomies or altered gastric mucosa to prevent development of the effects of pernicious anemia.

Assessment

HISTORY
- Easily fatigued or listless
- Weakness
- Sore tongue
- Numbness and tingling of extremities
- Nausea, vomiting, diarrhea, constipation
- Anorexia due to sore and bleeding gums and tongue
- Balance problems
- Diplopia and blurred vision
- Complaint of frequent infections
- History of gastric surgery or chronic diseases

PHYSICAL EXAM
- Pale lips and gums
- Smooth, sore, beefy red tongue
- Jaundiced sclera
- Impaired proprioception
- Tachycardia and premature beats
- Widened pulse pressure
- Dyspnea
- Orthopnea
- Extremity weakness, numbness, reduced vibratory senses and paresthesia of hands and feet
- Altered vision
- Loss of bowel and bladder control
- Irritability, poor memory
- Frequently fair-haired or prematurely gray

DIAGNOSTIC STUDIES
- Routine CBC will reveal:
  - Decreased hemoglobin
  - Increased mean corpuscular volume (macrocytic) and increased mean corpuscular hemoglobin concentration
  - Low RBC count
  - Serum vitamin B_{12} assay level < 0.1 mcg/mL
  - Elevated serum lactate dehydrogenase level
- Gastric secretion analysis reveals absence of free hydrochloric acid with a pH of 3.5
- 24-hour urine Schilling test to measure the amount of orally administered radionuclide-labeled B_{12} excreted over time; low levels will confirm the presence of vitamin B_{12} deficiency anemia

Management

NONPHARMACOLOGIC TREATMENT
- Review dietary sources of vitamin B_{12} such as dairy products, animal proteins, and eggs.

PHARMACOLOGIC TREATMENT
- Parenteral replacement of B_{12} to increase RBC regeneration
- Oral supplementation may be used in some cases

Special Considerations
- If intrinsic factor is missing in the gastric mucosa, it may be difficult to correct the anemia despite high doses of vitamin B_{12}. Neuromuscular dysfunctions may persist.

Follow-up

EXPECTED OUTCOMES
- Resolution of neurological complications.
- Activity level returned to normal tolerance level.
- Patient and family will verbalize that replacement is a lifelong therapy even when symptoms have subsided.

COMPLICATIONS
- Rapid RBC regeneration can increase a patient's iron and folate requirements, so iron and folic acid supplementation should occur concurrently with treatment for B_{12} deficiency.
- Potential for increased susceptibility to infections should be monitored. Patient or caregiver should be advised to report signs of infection immediately to primary healthcare provider.
- Pain and irritation of the oral cavity may affect communication and cause inability to ingest appropriate foods. Dietitian consult should be obtained to facilitate appropriate oral intake. Alternative communication means should be provided until oral cavity issues have resolved.
- Neurological damage may cause behavioral problems. Safety measures should be instituted to prevent injury until symptoms resolve.

FOLIC ACID DEFICIENCY ANEMIA

Description
- Anemia caused by a deficiency of folic acid resulting in the interruption of DNA synthesis and normal maturation of red blood cells

Etiology
- Poor dietary intake of foods rich in folate, such as citrus fruits and leafy green vegetables
- Malabsorption syndromes

Incidence and Demographics
- Occurs in patients with poor dietary intake of fresh fruits and vegetables or who frequently overcook foods
- Alcohol abuse increases incidence of folic acid deficiency due to decreased absorption
- Pregnancy will increase need for folic acid for the developing fetus

Risk Factors
- Alcoholism
- Patients receiving total parenteral nutrition
- Pregnancy
- Patients requiring hemodialysis
- Some medications such as oral contraceptives, anticonvulsants, and methotrexate can impede folate absorption

Prevention and Screening
- Screening individuals with any of the risk factors listed.
- Persons with diseases of the small intestine such as Crohn's or celiac disease or surgical removal of large portions of the small intestine should be monitored for development of deficiency.
- Persons undergoing hemodialysis and pregnant females have a higher requirement for folate and should be monitored frequently or prescribed supplemental vitamins.

Assessment

HISTORY
- Easily fatigued or listless
- Shortness of breath
- Palpitations
- Sore gums and tongue
- Nausea, vomiting, diarrhea

PHYSICAL EXAM
- Pale lips and gums
- Smooth, sore, beefy red tongue
- Jaundiced sclera
- Tachycardia and premature beats
- Dyspnea

DIAGNOSTIC STUDIES
- Decreased serum folate assay level
- Routine CBC will reveal:
  - Decreased hemoglobin
  - Increased mean corpuscular volume (macrocytic)
  - Low RBC count

Management

NONPHARMACOLOGIC TREATMENT
- Dietary counseling about the need for adequate oral intake of folate-rich foods such as fish, citrus fruits, green leafy vegetables, yeast, nuts, and grains
- Patient education and referrals related to decreasing or abstaining from alcohol intake
- Social service referrals in cases of financial constraints on dietary intake; food stamps and Meals On Wheels are options frequently available.

PHARMACOLOGIC TREATMENT
- Oral folate 1 to 5 mg/day for 3 to 4 months until levels return to normal or risk factor is resolved.

Special Considerations
- The symptoms of folic acid deficiency can develop over time and remain unnoticed or attributed to co-morbidities.
- The lack of neuromuscular symptoms can be utilized to differentiate folic acid and vitamin B_{12} deficiencies.

Follow-up

EXPECTED OUTCOMES
- Resolution of symptoms of deficiency.
- Patient or caregiver verbalizes understanding of treatment regimen.
- Patient selects foods high in folic acid.

COMPLICATIONS
- Lack of folate during pregnancy can lead to birth defects of the brain and spinal cord in newborns.

APLASTIC ANEMIA

Description
- Pancytopenia resulting from decreased production of erythrocytes, leukocytes, and platelets in the bone marrow

Etiology
- The pancytopenia can be classified as congenital, resulting from a chromosomal alteration, or acquired, resulting from radiation, chemical agents, toxic drugs, viral or bacterial infections, or pregnancy effects on the bone marrow that reduce its production of cells.
- An autoimmune disorder is one possible cause: white blood cells attack the bone marrow, causing decreased production of blood cells.
- Production of red and white blood cells and platelets decreases or stops as a result of damage to the bone marrow stem cells, the bone marrow itself, or the bone marrow being replaced by fat cells.
- The condition can be classified as acute or chronic depending upon the cause; however, in many cases the original cause is unknown.

Incidence and Demographics
- Occurs in patients of all ages and both genders.
- In about 50% of all cases, the cause is unknown.
- Aplastic anemia is present in about 2% of patients with acute viral hepatitis.

Risk Factors
- Occupational or other exposure to toxic agents such as benzene chloramphenicol, alcohols, and insecticides
- Exposure to radioactive materials or radiation-producing devices
- Neoplasm, particularly those that invade the bone marrow
- Use of some antibiotics, antimicrobials, anticonvulsants, and rheumatoid arthritis medications.

Prevention and Screening
- Screen individuals whose occupation potentially exposes them to radiation or toxic materials; monitor annually unless symptoms develop.
- Monitoring of blood studies of patients receiving anemia-producing drugs should be completed every 1 to 3 months to assess status of the disease.
- Early diagnosis can substantially increase survival time from rapid death to 5 to 10 years' survival.

Assessment

HISTORY
- Easily fatigued or progressive weakness
- General malaise

- Dyspnea
- Headache
- Palpitations
- Frequent infections

PHYSICAL EXAM
- Pale lips and mucous membranes
- Petechia and ecchymotic areas
- Active hemorrhage in mucous membranes
- Retinal hemorrhage
- Palpitations
- Dyspnea
- Fever
- Skin ulcerations

DIAGNOSTIC STUDIES
- Decreased RBCs
- Very low absolute reticulocyte count
- Elevated serum iron level but total iron-binding capacity is reduced
- Low platelet, neutrophil, and WBC counts
- Increased bleeding time
- Bone marrow aspiration will show:
  - Aplastic marrow
  - Fat, fibrous tissue and gelatinous material replacement of normal marrow cells
  - Decreased erythroid elements

Management

NONPHARMACOLOGIC TREATMENT
- Eliminate cause and provide supportive care through the administration of packed red blood cells, platelets, and antigen-matched leukocytes.
- Bone marrow transplantation.
- Oxygen administration as support for low hemoglobin levels until levels return to near normal.
- Limit visitors and potential sources of infection during acute phase.
- Frequent rest periods and adequate nutritional intake.

PHARMACOLOGIC TREATMENT
- Antithymocyte globulin (ATG) or other immunosuppressant agents such as cyclosporine may be used to suppress the immune system to allow for blood-cell regeneration.
- Corticosteroids can be used to stimulate red blood cell production.
- Colony stimulating factors may be administered to encourage cell growth.

Special Considerations
- Workplace education about the dangers of toxic agent and radiation exposure should be increased, with emphasis on protective wear, decreased exposure time, and monitoring of exposure levels to prevent bone marrow depression.

Follow-up

EXPECTED OUTCOMES
- Resolution of symptoms of deficiency and regeneration of cells
- Patient or caregiver verbalizes understanding of treatment regimen.

COMPLICATIONS
- Bleeding can be a concern due to decreased platelet counts. Safety precautions should be enacted to prevent falls, cuts, or other sources of bleeding.
- Due to the increased risk for infections, hygiene and environmental precautions and frequent cultures should be taken. Good handwashing hygiene, nutrition, and oral and perianal hygiene should be encouraged to prevent infection.
- After a stem cell transplant, graft-versus-host disease may develop if the newly formed white blood cells attack the recipient's other cells.

SICKLE CELL ANEMIA

Description
- A chronic, hereditary hemolytic anemia characterized by episodes of altered, abnormally crescent-shaped cell formation (sickling).

Etiology
- The disease is transmitted as an autosomal recessive genetic defect causing the synthesis of abnormally formed hemoglobin with the red blood cells. When deoxygenated, this hemoglobin (HbS) can crystallize into rod-shaped structures that clump and can obstruct capillary blood flow. Sickle cell crisis results when obstructed areas become ischemic, resulting in severe pain and potential infarction.
- The sickled red blood cells resume their normal shape as oxygen levels return to normal but this change in shape can cause weakening and early destruction of the cells, requiring increased production of new red blood cells.

Incidence and Demographics
- Can occur in people of African, South or Central Americas (especially Panamanian), Caribbean, Mediterranean (such as Turkish, Greek, and Italian), Indian, and Saudi Arabian ancestry, but in the United States occurs most commonly in Blacks.
- Approximately 7% to 13% of Blacks are heterogeneous for the sickle cell gene and therefore are classified as having sickle cell trait.
- Approximately 1% of Blacks have sickle cell disease and are at risk for the development of sickle cell crisis.

Risk Factors
- Because the disease is caused by an autosomal recessive gene, only those who inherit two copies are at risk for severe sickling of the cells. The children of parents who are heterogeneous (carry sickle cell trait) have a one-in-four chance of having sickle cell anemia.
- Conditions likely to initiate a sickle cell crisis are hypoxia, excessive exercise, decreased body temperature, high altitudes, or deoxygenation during anesthesia. Conditions that increase blood viscosity—such as dehydration, infection, or acidosis—also can trigger a crisis.

- Individuals with sickle cell trait can develop sickle cell crisis but typically to a less severe degree because only a small percentage of their hemoglobin is affected.

Prevention and Screening
- Genetic counseling and family planning are the best way to increase awareness and decrease the occurrence of the disease.
- Screening in newborns can be used to diagnose the disease and to educate parents on methods to prevent crisis development.
- Methods to prevent sickle cell crisis include maintaining adequate hydration; avoiding stress, cold, overexertion, and areas of low oxygenation such as high altitudes; and treating infections quickly.

Assessment

HISTORY
- Genetic predisposition
- Fatigue
- Pain

PHYSICAL EXAM
- Pallor
- Jaundice
- Irritability
- Swollen and painful large joint and surrounding tissues
- Pain
- Priapism

DIAGNOSTIC STUDIES
- Presence of sickled cells on blood smear
- Elevated reticulocyte count
- Elevated serum bilirubin level
- Presence of hemoglobin S on electrophoresis

Management

NONPHARMACOLOGIC TREATMENT
- Eliminate crisis trigger and provide supportive care through administration of oxygen and adequate oral or intravenous hydration
- Blood transfusion during surgery and pregnancy as needed
- Bone marrow transplantation
- Frequent rest periods
- Psychosocial support

PHARMACOLOGIC TREATMENT
- Opioid narcotic analgesics during the acute phase at appropriate dosage to relieve pain
- Folic acid supplements
- Procardia for priapism

Special Considerations
- The severity and frequency of sickle cell crisis is variable. Increased occurrences have been related to the amount of hemoglobin S (Hb S) present in the individual.

Follow-up

EXPECTED OUTCOMES
- Resolution of symptoms of crisis, oxygen levels within normal limits, adequate hydration status, resolution of pain, and absence of signs and symptoms of vaso-obstruction such as priapism and joint swelling and tenderness.
- Care and counseling will be provided without cultural bias.
- Patient or caregiver will verbalize understanding of methods to prevent and treat acute episodes of sickling.
- Patient will be free of signs of infection.

COMPLICATIONS
- Vaso-occlusive disease such as thrombosis, stroke, renal dysfunction, splenic occlusion, priapism resulting in impotence, dyspnea, chest pain, and substance abuse.

HEMOPHILIA

Description
- There are two types of hemophilia, A and B. Both are caused by deficiencies in the amount of clotting factor in the blood (VIII or IX). When one of these clotting factors is missing or insufficient, bleeding may end very slowly or not stop at all. The two types of hemophilia are linked by their similar clinical pictures and inheritance patterns.

Etiology
- Hemophilia is a sex-linked recessive genetic disorder passed on by the X chromosome, which carries the clotting factor gene. It is generally transmitted by an unaffected mother and exhibited almost exclusively in males.
- Hemophilia A (classic hemophilia) results from deficiency in factor VIII, an alpha globulin that stabilizes fibrin clots.
- Hemophilia B (Christmas disease) results from deficiency in factor IX, a beta globulin that is essential in stage I of the intrinsic coagulation system. It affects the amount of thromboplastin present.
- The two types of hemophilia have similar clinical pictures and inheritance patterns.

Incidence and Demographics
- About 17,000 people in the United States have the disease; globally, it affects 400,000 people in 40 countries.
- Hemophilia A is more common.

Risk Factors
- The most dangerous aspect of hemophilia is internal bleeding, which if left untreated can lead to deformity, disability, or even death. If untreated, bleeding continues until the causative agent heals or the person bleeds to death.
- Hemophilia may lead to arthritis because bleeding into the joints can inflame the joint lining and destroy cartilage.
- Patients with hemophilia do not bleed any faster than others, but they bleed longer.
- Ordinary bruises are rarely serious but cuts and abrasions may bleed for days without treatment.

- Sports or other outside activities may lead to injuries and bleeding.
- Periodontal diseases can lead to bleeding of the gums.

Prevention and Screening
- Genetic counseling and family planning can be important in both education and prevention of the disease.
- Amniocentesis or chorionic villus sampling can be used to detect the presence of the genetic defect of hemophilia in utero.
- Good oral hygiene can prevent periodontal diseases that lead to bleeding of the gums.

Assessment

HISTORY
- Frequent episodes of bruising and bleeding that is slow to stop
- Excessive joint pain, swelling, and bruising following trauma
- Family history or genetic predisposition

PHYSICAL EXAM
- Assess joints for tenderness, range of motion, and evidence of bruising. The joints, particularly the knees, hips, ankles, shoulders, and elbows, are most commonly affected.
- Inspect the muscles of the upper arm, upper leg (front and back), the calf and the front of the groin for indications of bleeding. Hemarthrosis is a common occurrence.
- Easy bruising and cutaneous hematoma formation with minor trauma such as injections, bumps, and minor falls. Sometimes bleeding may be delayed.
- Spontaneous epistaxis
- Hematuria
- Gingival bleeding
- Hematemesis or blood in stool
- Pain in abdominal area following minor injury, indicating possible internal bleeding
- Altered mental status following even minor head injury, indicating potential intracranial hemorrhage
- Pain or paralysis of extremity due to possible hematoma pressure on nerve

DIAGNOSTIC STUDIES
- Amniocentesis or chorionic villus sampling can be used to detect the presence of the genetic defect of hemophilia in utero.
- Increased activated partial thromboplastin time (APPT)
- Normal prothrombin time
- Factor assays will be low depending on the type of hemophilia.
  - Factor VIII decreased in hemophilia A
  - Factor IX decreased in hemophilia B

Management

NONPHARMACOLOGIC TREATMENT
- Replace deficient clotting factors prophylactically as needed.
- Supportive treatment of arthrocentesis and physiotherapy for hemarthrosis.
- Control bleeding with topical pressure and application of ice.

PHARMACOLOGIC TREATMENT
- Cryoprecipitate of appropriate missing factor VIII or IX depending on type of hemophilia. Frequently the missing factors will be given prior to surgery or invasive procedures.
- Desmopressin acetate (DDAVP) is sometimes used preoperatively in patients with mild hemophilia A to stimulate release of factor VIII.

Special Considerations
- Because this is a chronic disease, routine medical appointments and knowledge of home management and home administration of replacement clotting factors can improve the quality of life and prevention of complications.

Follow-up

EXPECTED OUTCOMES
- Patient and family identify strategies to prevent injury, provide a safe environment, and prevent bleeding complications.
- No evidence of bleeding present.
- Patient and family will verbalize and demonstrate knowledge and ability to prepare and administer intravenous replacement blood products as needed.
- The patient should wear medical alert jewelry (such as a MedicAlert bracelet) at all times.

COMPLICATIONS
- Use of analgesics should be limited to prescriptions and over-the-counter medications that do not contain aspirin, which would further increase bleeding.
- Although most blood products are screened and tested for infectious diseases, patients should be monitored closely for infectious diseases such as hepatitis and HIV by their primary care providers.

THROMBOCYTOPENIA

Description
- A condition presenting with a decrease in the number of platelets or a platelet count of less than 100,000 per milliliter of blood, resulting in delayed hemostasis. Typically it is considered a symptom of a disease process and not a disease of itself.

Etiology
- Thrombocytopenia can result from three mechanisms.
  - Immune thrombocytopenia purpura (ITP), an immune system defect that coats the platelets with an antibody that the spleen recognizes as foreign, which results in the platelets being destroyed in 1 to 2 days rather than circulating for the normal 8 to 10 days. Systemic lupus erythematosus (SLE) and snake bites, such as from pit vipers, also can cause increased destruction of platelets.
  - Aplastic anemia, bone marrow malignancy, infection, radiation, chemotherapy, or administration of medications that destroy the stem cells in the bone marrow can decrease the production of platelets. Diseases such as vitamin B_{12} deficiency anemia, folic acid deficiency, sepsis, and leukemia also can lead to reduced platelet production. Medications

such as methotrexate, interferon, carboplatin, and valproic acid can directly cause myelosuppression.

- Disseminated intravascular coagulation (DIC) or hemorrhage injuries increase platelet consumption for the clotting process, resulting in an increased number of immature and less functional precursor cells in the bone marrow.

Incidence and Demographics

- Chronic immune thrombocytopenia purpura (ITP) is most common in women 20 to 50 years of age.
- The incidence of drug-induced thrombocytopenia is related to the use of medications which either destroy the body's ability to produce platelets or destroy the platelets themselves. The use of some chemotherapeutic agents and seizure medications such as valproic acid can decrease the body's ability to produce platelets. Heparin, an anti-coagulant, can cause an antibody reaction that destroys platelets. Approximately 8% to 15% of patients receiving heparin will develop thrombocytopenia.

Risk Factors

- The most significant risk factors are chemical and radiation myelosuppression therapies.
- Vitamin B_{12} or iron-deficiency anemia.
- Hospitalized and home-care patients on heparin therapy can develop heparin-induced thrombocytopenia (HIT).
- Viral infections can be a precursor to the development of ITP in children and young adults.

Prevention and Screening

- Patients with known myelosuppression should be monitored for the development of thrombocytopenia.
- Patients with any of the known risk factors should be followed closely.

Assessment

HISTORY
- Family history
- Frequent bleeding and bruising episodes
- Petechiae and purpura, particularly on the anterior thorax, arms, and neck
- Excessive bleeding during menses or from puncture sites
- History of drug ingestion, exposure to toxins, or radiation

PHYSICAL EXAM
- Assess joints for degree of tenderness, range of motion, and evidence of bruising following trauma.
- Easy bruising and cutaneous hematoma formation after minor trauma such as injections, bumps, and minor falls. Sometimes bleeding may be delayed.
- Spontaneous epistaxis
- Hematuria
- Gingival bleeding
- Hematemesis or blood in stool
- Pain in abdominal area following minor injury, indicating possible internal bleeding
- Altered mental status following even minor head injury, indicating potential intracranial hemorrhage

DIAGNOSTIC STUDIES
- Decreased platelet count
- Decreased hemoglobin and hematocrit if bleeding present
- Prolonged bleeding time
- Normal prothrombin time (PT) and PTT
- Bone marrow aspiration and smear will reveal decreased platelet activity and increased megakaryocytes.

Management

NONPHARMACOLOGIC TREATMENT
- Determine if cause is toxic exposures, medication, or genetic, and treat cause if possible.
- Splenectomy is the ultimate treatment for patients with chronic ITP because it removes the organ responsible for the destruction of antibody-sensitized platelets.
- Good nutrition if anemia-related.

PHARMACOLOGIC TREATMENT
- Discontinue causative medications if possible.
- Corticosteroid therapy can reduce platelet destruction.
- Replacement of blood components, including platelets.

Special Considerations
- Bleeding can be life-threatening if it occurs in the brain or other organ. Early identification of potential bleeding problems is essential.
- A pregnant woman who has antibodies to platelets produced by an immune response to a medication can pass the antibodies to the baby in the womb and cause bleeding to occur.

Follow-up

EXPECTED OUTCOMES
- The patient and family or caregivers understand the importance of observing for petechiae, ecchymoses, and other signs of recurrence. Patient will avoid aspirin, ibuprofen, and warfarin, which interfere with platelet function and blood clotting.
- Patient and family or caregiver identifies strategies to prevent injury, provide a safe environment, and prevent bleeding complications.
- No evidence of bleeding present.
- Patient and family or caregiver will verbalize the effects of medications that inhibit thrombocyte production.
- The patient should wear medical alert jewelry (such as a MedicAlert bracelet) at all times.

COMPLICATIONS
- Patients receiving immunosuppressant medications should be closely monitored by the healthcare provider because these medications cause many incidences of thrombocytopenia.

LEUKEMIA

Description
- A malignant disorder of the blood-forming tissues in the bone marrow, spleen, and lymph nodes resulting in the unregulated formation of white blood cells and their precursors.

Etiology
- The type of white blood cells affected (such as the granulocyte, lymphocyte, or monocyte) and the duration of the disease form the basis for the classification of the various types of leukemia.
  - If the majority of the leukemia cells are immature, undifferentiated, and primitive in formation, the leukemia is classified as *acute*. Acute leukemias typically have an acute onset and progress rapidly.
  - If the leukemia cells are mature, well-differentiated, but of abnormal appearance, the leukemia is classified as *chronic*. Chronic leukemias typically show a gradual onset with a prolonged disease course.
  - In *lymphocytic* or *lymphoblastic* leukemia, the immature lymphocytes and their precursors in the bone marrow invade the spleen, lymph nodes, central nervous system, and other tissues.
  - In *myelocytic or myeloblastic* leukemia, the myeloid stem cells in the bone marrow fail to mature and RBC, WBC, and platelet cell counts may all be reduced.
- In general, a single stem cell can mutate and slowly proliferate in the bone marrow as leukemia cells unable to function as normal white blood cells. These abnormal cells replace the normal, mature WBCs in inflammatory and immune responses and displace the erythrocyte-producing and platelet-producing cells causing anemia, bleeding, and splenomegaly. As the leukemia cells leave the bone marrow and infiltrate other tissues, life-threatening symptoms can develop from anemia, malignant cell expansion, and loss of the body's ability to fight infection.

Incidence and Demographics
- More than 250,000 people are living with leukemia in the United States.
- Approximately 43,000 new cases of leukemia were diagnosed in the United States in 2010.
- Chronic leukemias account for about 11% more cases of leukemia than acute forms.
- Leukemia occurs more often in adults than in children.
- The most common types of leukemia in adults in descending order are chronic lymphocytic leukemia (CLL), acute myelogenous leukemia (AML), and chronic myelogenous leukemia (CML). Acute lymphocytic leukemia occurs most commonly in children.
- Incidence is higher in males (57%) than in females and in Caucasians than in other racial groups.
- The incidence of development of any of these leukemias increases after 70 years of age.
- Classification, incidence, and survival rates are shown in Table 16–3.

Table 16–3. Summary of Leukemia Classifications

Classification	Incidence	Specific Characteristics	5-year Survival Rate With Treatment	Usual Treatment
Acute lymphoblastic leukemia (ALL)	Primarily children and young adults	Bleeding Recurrent infections Sore throat Bone pain Weight loss Fatigue and weakness Night sweats	66.4%	Chemotherapy Bone marrow transplant (BMT) Stem cell transplant (SCT)
Chronic lymphocytic leukemia (CLL)	Primarily older adults 50–70 years of age	Fatigue Lymphadenopathy Splenomegaly Recurrent infections Edema Thrombophlebitis	79.7%	Chemotherapy BMT Often no treatment is needed
Acute myelocytic leukemia (AML)	Primarily older adults with a peak at 60 years of age, but can affect children and young adults	Fatigue and weakness Anemia Fever Bone pain Bleeding and bruising Lymphadenopathy Splenomegaly Hepatomegaly	24.2%	Chemotherapy BMT
Chronic myelocytic leukemia (CML)	Primarily adults, with incidence rising with age	Three stages: *Chronic:* Asymptomatic with diagnosis on routine blood test which reveals leukocytosis, thrombocytosis, and splenomegaly *Accelerated:* Fatigue, sweating, weight loss, and heat intolerance *Acute:* Takes on characteristics of AML with the development of fatigue and weakness, anemia, fever, bone pain, bleeding and bruising, lymphadenopathy, splenomegaly and hepatomegaly	54.6% if treated prior to development of accelerated and acute phases	Chemotherapy SCT

Risk Factors

- Although almost all cases of leukemia have no identifiable etiology, several risk factors have been proposed including genetics, environmental exposures such as benzene and chloramphenicol, radiation exposure (including cancer therapy), some medications, viral infections, and immunodeficiency.
- Children and adults with Down syndrome (Trisomy 21) are 20 times more likely to develop leukemia.
- A specific genetic abnormality called the Philadelphia chromosome, a translocation between the long arms of chromosomes 22 and 9, is found in chronic myelogenous leukemia (CML).

Prevention and Screening

- Persons with known exposure to radiation, toxic chemicals, or other risk factors should be screened routinely by their primary healthcare providers.

Assessment

HISTORY

- History of exposure to toxic chemicals or radiation
- Subjective complaints of:
  - Fever
  - Night sweats
  - Easy bleeding or bruising
  - Fatigue and weakness
  - Recurrent or persistent infections
  - Bone pain
  - Anorexia and weight loss
  - Visual disturbances
  - Headache

PHYSICAL EXAM

- Lymphadenopathy
- Bruising, petechiae, purpura
- Dyspnea
- Pallor
- Splenomegaly
- Hepatomegaly
- Occult bleeding
- Palpitations and tachycardia
- Orthostatic hypotension
- Hematuria
- Weakness

DIAGNOSTIC STUDIES

- Increased WBCs in CLL and CML
- Normal, decreased, or increased WBC in ALL and AML
- Bone marrow biopsy and aspirate assessment is the definitive diagnostic test.
- The acute classification and staging of the leukemia is essential to the acute treatment and prognosis.

Management

- The overall management of leukemias is to induce remission or cure with chemotherapy or radiation therapy, relief of symptoms, and potentially bone marrow or stem cell transplant to prolong both life expectancy and quality of life.

NONPHARMACOLOGIC AND PHARMACOLOGIC TREATMENT

- Because all patients with a diagnosis of leukemia have an increased risk for infection, establish measures to minimize risk by providing a protective environment (e.g., isolation; restriction of visitors, fresh fruits, plants).
- The primary goal of treatment of patients with a diagnosis of *acute* leukemia is elimination of the malignant cells, restoration of normal hemopoiesis, and production of complete remission. Multiple courses of aggressive chemotherapy may be administered over several years depending on the patient's age, comorbidities, clinical status, and type of leukemia. Generally treatment consists of three phases:
  - *Induction phase:* Chemotherapeutic agents administered until there are no leukemic cells in the bone marrow or peripheral blood smears. During this phase, patients are hospitalized and supported with the administration of blood products and antibiotics. This period lasts about 1 month or until the patient's blood counts recover to a safe level for discharge.
  - *Consolidation phase:* The same chemotherapeutic agents administered at lower doses and over a longer duration of potentially 4 to 8 months. The goal of this phase is to eradicate any remaining leukemic cells.
  - *Maintenance phase:* If the patient stays in remission after the previous phases, monitoring and follow-up continues to assure that the goal of destroying and preventing the return of diseased cells has been accomplished. If malignant cells return, chemotherapy is reinstituted. This phase can last for several years.
- Treatment of patients diagnosed with *chronic* leukemia generally depends on the type.
  - Chronic myelogenic leukemia (CML) has chronic, accelerated, and blast phases. Although CML can remain stable and generally asymptomatic for many years, progression to the acute phase with a blast crisis is inevitable and usually occurs within 3 years of diagnosis. Treatment can be undertaken with several tyrosine kinase inhibitor agents such as imatinib mesylate (Gleevec), but allogenic bone marrow or stem cell transplantation is the only definitive curative option.
  - Chronic lymphocytic leukemia (CLL) is the most common chronic leukemia and has variable treatment options depending on the progression of leukocytosis. Because it is slow-growing, treatment is generally reserved until the patient moves into advanced stages. Treatment may include chemotherapy and radiation therapy to reduce the size of masses in the lymph nodes and spleen. A splenectomy may be considered as well.
- Preventing, monitoring, and treating infections in these patients are essential.
- Bone marrow transplant can be either autologous (patient's own bone marrow removed during remission) or allogenic (closely matched sibling or unrelated donor). After the patient has undergone high-dose irradiation or chemotherapy to destroy all leukemic cells in the marrow, the new marrow is infused through a central venous catheter. Because of the nature of allogenic bone marrow transplant cells, graft-versus-host disease may develop because the donated cells recognize the recipient's own cells as foreign, leading to a rejection reaction. Immunosuppressant drugs, steroids, and antibiotics may be used to prevent or treat this reaction.

- Stem cell transplantation can be used as an alternative to bone marrow transplantation in some cases. Stem cells are harvested from closely tissue-matched donors and infused into the patient, similar to bone marrow transplantation. The same graft-versus-host reaction can occur as well. Stem cells also may be available from umbilical cord blood for use if HLA tissue match is compatible. An advantage to stem cell transplantation is the replacement of the entire blood cell line to produce WBCs, RBCs, and platelets.
- Biologic therapies, such as cytokines, have been used to treat some leukemias along with other treatment modalities. These biologic agents modify the body's response to cancer cells by moderating immune responses and inhibiting cell proliferation and abnormal growth, as well as having some cytotoxic effects. Interferon-α and tyrosine kinase inhibitor agents are two examples of biologic therapies used currently.

Special Considerations

- Psychological support is essential in the care of the patient and family with leukemia. The availability of support systems to allow the patient and family to express feelings and concerns and to adapt to changes in the patient's condition and medical regimes are important to enhance a quality of life.

Follow-up

EXPECTED OUTCOMES

- The patient will be free of signs and symptoms of infection.
- The patient and family or caregivers will verbalize understanding of the disease process, treatment options, and plan, and know that they have support systems available to them.
- Patient and family or caregivers will verbalize, understand the need for, and provide neutropenic and bleeding precautions.
- The patient will experience adequate pain control.
- Patient will have adequate nutritional intake.
- Activities will be planned to prevent fatigue and to allow for periods of uninterrupted rest and sleep.

COMPLICATIONS

- Dependent on type of leukemia, patients may experience:
  - Neurological: Seizures, coma, subarachnoid hemorrhage
  - Respiratory: Pulmonary edema, pneumonia
  - Cardiac: Hemorrhage, thrombophlebitis
  - Gastrointestinal: GI bleeding
  - Urinary: Renal insufficiency or failure
  - Hematologic: DIC
  - Immunologic: Sepsis, abcesses
- The institution of bleeding and neutropenic precautions is imperative in these patients.

REFERENCES

Centers for Disease Control and Prevention. (2006). Revised recommendations for HIV testing for adults, adolescents, and pregnant women in health-care settings. *MMWR 55*(RR14), 1–17. Retrieved from http://www.cdc.gov/mmwr/preview/mmwrhtml/rr5514a1.htm

Centers for Disease Control and Prevention. (2008). Revised surveillance case definitions for HIV infection among adults, adolescents, and children aged <18 months and for HIV infection and AIDS among children aged 18 months to <13 years—United States, 2008. *MMWR, 57*(RR10), 1–8. Retrieved from http://www.cdc.gov/mmwr/preview/mmwrhtml/rr5710a1.htm

Centers for Disease Control and Prevention. (2010). *Cases of HIV infection and AIDS in the United States and dependent areas. HIV surveillance report: Diagnosis of HIV infection and AIDS in the United States and dependent areas 2008.* Atlanta: Author. Retrieved from www.cdc.gov/hiv/topics/surveillance/basic.htm

Centers for Disease Control and Prevention. (2011). *HIV surveillance—Epidemiology of HIV infection through 2008.* Atlanta: Author. Retrieved from www.cdc.gov/hiv/topics/surveillance/resources/slides/general/index.htm

Ignatavicius, D. D., & Workman, M. L. (2010). *Medical-surgical nursing: Patient-centered collaborative practice.* St. Louis, MO: Saunders Elsevier.

Joint United Nations Programme on HIV/AIDS (UNAIDS) and World Health Organization. (2009). *AIDS epidemic update.* Geneva, Switzerland: Author. Retrieved from www.unaids.org

Leukemia and Lymphoma Society. (2010). *Leukemia facts and statistics.* Retrieved from http://www.leukemia-lymphoma.org

Lewis, S. L., Dirksen, S. R., Heitkemper, M. M., Bucher, L., & Camera, I. M. (2011). *Medical-surgical nursing: Assessment and management of clinical problems.* St. Louis, MO: Mosby Elsevier.

Linker, C. (2008). Blood disorders. In S. McPhee, M. Papadakis, & L. Tierney (Eds.), *Current medical diagnosis and treatment* (47th ed., pp. 439–450). New York: McGraw Hill Medical.

Morton, P. G., & Fontaine, D. K. (2009). *Critical care nursing: A holistic approach.* Philadelphia: Wolters Kluwer/Lippincott Williams & Wilkins

National Heart Lung and Blood Institute. (2011). *Sickle cell anemia: Who is at risk?* Retrieved from http://www.nhlbi.nih.gov/health/dci/Diseases/Sca/SCA_WhoIsAtRisk.html

Pagana, K. D., & Pagana, T. J. (2009). *Mosby's diagnostic and laboratory test reference* (9th ed.). St. Louis, MO: Mosby Elsevier.

Wagner, K. D., Johnson, K. L., & Hardin-Pierce, M. G. (2010). *High-acuity nursing.* Upper Saddle River, NJ: Pearson Education.

Wilson, B. A., Shannon, M. T., & Shields, K. M. (2009). *Prentice Hall nurse's drug guide 2009.* Upper Saddle River, NJ: Pearson Education.

17

Shock and Multisystem Organ Failure

Deborah Jane Schwytzer, MSN, RN-BC, CEN

GENERAL APPROACH

- Shock is a life-threatening syndrome that results in a decrease in tissue and organ oxygenation and perfusion.
- Immediate intervention to reinstate oxygenation and perfusion of the tissues is required to prevent organ dysfunction and failure with a subsequent high mortality rate.
- Overall goals of management of shock:
  - Treatment of the cause if known
  - Restoration of oxygen delivery to the tissues
  - Reduce oxygen consumption
- Types of shock are categorized based on the primary physiologic cause of the decreased oxygenation of tissues
  - Hypovolemic: inadequate circulating volume or cellular oxygen-carrying capacity
  - Cardiogenic: decreased or absent pumping of the heart muscle or structural changes resulting in a mechanically reduced cardiac output
  - Obstructive: decreased circulation due to mechanical obstruction of blood flow to the lungs
  - Distributive: systemic vasodilatation resulting in a state of relative hypovolemia
    - Anaphylactic: triggered by an allergic reaction
    - Neurogenic: caused by loss of sympathetic vasoconstriction control
    - Septic: immune response to overwhelming infection

- Basic stages common to all types of shock
  - *Compensatory stage*: arterial pressure and tissue perfusion are reduced; compensatory mechanisms are activated to maintain perfusion to the brain and heart. An increase in release of epinephrine and norepinephrine will increase peripheral resistance, blood pressure, and myocardial contractility. The renin-angiotensin-aldosterone system is activated to cause vasoconstriction and increased sodium retention to increase circulating volume, resulting in maintained cardiac output and tissue perfusion.
  - *Progressive stage*: when the compensatory stage fails to maintain an adequate cardiac output for tissue perfusion, tissue hypoxia develops and cell metabolism changes from aerobic to anaerobic, resulting in a buildup of lactic acid, metabolic acidosis, and depression of cardiac function. The release of endothelial mediators causes vasodilatation, venous pooling, increased capillary permeability, and sluggish blood flow, the last of which increases the patient's risk for the development of disseminated intravascular coagulation (DIC).
  - *Irreversible stage*: further hypoxic organ and tissue damage occurs. Increasing metabolic acidosis resulting from lactic acid accumulation further increases capillary permeability, fluid loss from the vascular space contributing to hypovolemia, and decreased cardiac output. Blood flow to the coronary arteries is decreased, increasing myocardial depression. Eventually, cardiac and respiratory failure occurs and the patient dies.

RED FLAGS

- Patient with generalized debilitating disease or lack of systemic reserves is more likely to develop shock syndromes.
- Likelihood of mortality from shock syndromes depends on the underlying cause, patient age, comorbidities, and time of intervention. About 10% of young people and about 90% of elderly people who develop shock die from it.
- Clinical manifestations of shock depend on the type. Typical signs include tachycardia; tachypnea; pale, cool, clammy skin; low blood pressure; decreased urinary output; altered mental status or level of consciousness as the body attempts to conserve blood flow and oxygenation to the vital organs of brain and heart during the compensatory and progressive stages. Without adequate treatment, organ failure, a slow and thready pulse, severe hypotension, slow and shallow respirations, anuria, adult respiratory distress syndrome (ARDS), coagulopathies, and coma will occur, leading eventually to full cardiac and respiratory cessation.

Types of Shock

HYPOVOLEMIC SHOCK

Description

- Decreased intravascular circulating volume causes decreased ventricular filling pressure and decreased cardiac output, which impairs oxygen delivery to the body tissues and organs.

Etiology

- Causes can include fluid losses such as occult bleeding, internal hemorrhage, vomiting, diaphoresis, and diarrhea, or the shifting of fluids from the intravascular circulation to the interstitial space as in edema or ascites.
- Loss of as little as 20% (about 1 liter) of circulating blood volume can cause hypovolemic shock.

Incidence and Demographics

- The overall incidence of shock is unknown.
- Hypovolemic (hemorrhagic) shock is the primary cause of death in trauma patients.
- Shock occurs in all ages and populations.

Risk Factors

- Recent trauma: motor vehicle collision, burn injury, falls, elderly
- History of cardiac, respiratory or renal disease or gastrointestinal disease with bleeding
- Currently on anticoagulation therapy

Prevention and Screening

- Early identification and treatment of the cause of fluid volume loss
- Early control of bleeding
- Monitoring of fluid volume status and early replacement of fluids

Assessment

HISTORY
- Traumatic injury such as motor vehicle collision
- Falls with blunt trauma to abdomen, chest, or femur
- Lacerations, particularly of head, scalp, or extremities
- GI bleeding or disorders
- Excessive nausea, vomiting, or diarrhea
- Clotting disorders such as hemophilia or currently on anticoagulation therapy
- Strenuous exercise without adequate fluid replacement or exposure to heat extremes
- Complications of liver disease such as esophageal varices, hemorrhoids, ascites

PHYSICAL EXAM
- Rapid respirations
- Low blood pressure
- Obvious uncontrolled bleeding
- Rapid, weak, thready pulse
- Altered mental status, anxiety, agitation, confusion, unconsciousness
- Pale, diaphoretic skin
- Poor skin turgor
- Generalized weakness
- Decreased urine output

DIAGNOSTIC STUDIES
- Blood chemistries including renal, liver function, electrolytes, and serum lactate
- Complete blood count (CBC)
- Clotting studies such as prothrombin time (PT) and partial thromboplastin time (PTT)

- Urinalysis and urine output
- Pregnancy test for women of childbearing age
- Arterial blood gas
- Oxygen saturation monitoring
- X-ray, CT scan, or ultrasound of suspected site of blood loss
- Diagnostic peritoneal lavage
- Electrocardiogram (ECG)
- Endoscopy
- Type and screen for possible blood replacement

Nursing Management

NONPHARMACOLOGIC TREATMENT

- Lie patient flat with lower extremities elevated 12 inches (Modified Trendelenberg position) to facilitate venous return to central circulation.
- Keep patient warm to avoid hypothermia.
- Apply direct pressure to sites of obvious bleeding.
- Start large-bore intravenous (IV) access for fluid and blood replacement. Two large bore IVs preferred if hemorrhage is present.
- Immobilize any obvious fractures.
- Give nothing by mouth.

PHARMACOLOGIC TREATMENT

- High-flow oxygen unless contraindicated by comorbidity of respiratory disease
- Intravenous infusion of normal saline or lactated Ringer's initially
- Blood and/or blood product replacement
- Medications listed in Table 17–1

Table 17–1. Medications for Treating Hypovolemic Shock

Therapeutic Effect	Medication	Dosage Range	Comments
Vasoconstrictor	Dopamine Hydrochloride	2–50 mcg/kg/min IV	Titrate to dose to desired effect USE ONLY AFTER ADEQUATE FLUID VOLUME STATUS HAS BEEN ACHIEVED
Inotropic agent	Dobutamine Hydrochloride	2.5–15 mcg/kg/min MAX: 40 mcg/kg/min	Titrate to dose to desired effect USE ONLY AFTER ADEQUATE FLUID VOLUME STATUS HAS BEEN ACHIEVED
Vasoconstrictor	Epinephrine	1–10 mcg/min	Titrate to dose to desired effect
Vasoconstrictor	Norepinephrine	0.5–1.0 mcg/min	Titrate to dose to desired effect

Special Considerations
- Knowledge of comorbidities is necessary to avoid potential fluid overload that may exacerbate cardiac and respiratory conditions.
- Knowledge of cultural and religious attitudes about use of blood and blood products.
- Length of time of hypoperfusion can impact outcome despite appropriate interventions.

Follow-up

EXPECTED OUTCOMES
- Maintenance of adequate cardiac output and oxygen perfusion to tissues and organs
- Normalization of blood pressure (BP), pulse, and urinary output
- Reduction in potential long-term complications

COMPLICATIONS
- The decrease in delivery of oxygen and nutrients to tissues and organ systems can cause kidney damage and acute tubular necrosis, cardiac damage, liver failure, respiratory damage and ARDS, clotting abnormalities such as DIC, and brain damage such as stroke and encephalopathy.
- Lack of blood flow to extremities also may result in gangrene and loss of limb.

CARDIOGENIC SHOCK

Description
- A decrease in cardiac output and perfusion due to decrease in mechanical function of the myocardial muscle

Etiology
- The overall cause is any disease or damage to the heart muscle that decreases the heart's ability to pump enough blood to the tissues. This can include:
  - Myocardial infarctions
  - Valvular heart disease
  - Rupture of the cardiac septum
  - Cardiac arrhythmias such as ventricular tachycardia, ventricular fibrillation, supraventricular tachycardia, bradycardia, or heart conduction blocks
  - Pericarditis
  - Congestive heart failure or cardiomyopathies

Incidence and Demographics
- Most common cause is myocardial infarction (MI)
- Can occur in all age groups if risk factors area present

Risk Factors
- History of coronary artery disease, peripheral vascular disease, diabetes, hypertension, high cholesterol and triglycerides, tobacco and alcohol use
- Family history of heart or coronary artery disease
- Obesity
- Septic shock, which releases cardiac depressant factor

Prevention and Screening

- Early identification and treatment of risk factors
- Aggressive treatment of potential causes such as MI and valvular malfunctions

Assessment

HISTORY

- Complaint of chest pain or pressure
- Shortness of breath
- Restlessness or agitation

PHYSICAL EXAM

- Diaphoresis
- Pale, cool skin
- Rapid respirations
- Rapid or weak and thready pulse
- Low blood pressure: systolic blood pressure below 90 mm Hg for 30 minutes
- Confusion or loss of ability to concentrate
- Unresponsiveness

DIAGNOSTIC STUDIES

- ECG
- Chest x-ray
- Echocardiogram to diagnose mechanical and structural malformations such as mitral valve regurgitation, ventricular septal defect, cardiac tamponade, papillary wall rupture
- Arterial blood gasses
- Blood chemistries such as renal, metabolic, electrolytes, lactate
- Cardiac enzymes including creatine kinase isoenzyme MB (CK-MB), troponin I and T, brain natriuretic peptide (BNP), C-reactive protein (CRP)
- Complete blood count
- Clotting studies such as prothrombin time(PT) and activated partial thromboplastin time (aPTT)
- Cardiac catheterization

Nursing Management

NONPHARMACOLOGIC TREATMENT

- Oxygen saturation monitoring
- Fluids to assure adequate circulating volume
- Invasive hemodynamic monitoring through insertion of a central pressure monitoring device such as pulmonary artery catheter to monitor heart function and evaluate effectiveness of treatment
- Cardiac defibrillation or cardioversion to treat dysrhythmias
- Pacemaker or automated implantable cardioverter-defibrillator (AICD) placement to treat dysrhythmias
- Angioplasty and stenting of coronary artery to enhance blood flow to prevent further damage
- Coronary artery bypass surgery to improve coronary perfusion
- Heart valve replacement to improve cardiac filling

- Assist with care of implanted left ventricular assist device (LVAD) or intra-aortic balloon counterpulsation device to augment cardiac output and to rest heart muscle
- Heart transplantation

PHARMACOLOGIC TREATMENT
- Oxygen to supply tissue oxygen demands
- Thrombolytic therapy for acute MI
- Medications that may be used to increase blood pressure and improve heart function are listed in Table 17–2.

Table 17–2. Medications for Treating Cardiogenic Shock

Therapeutic Effect	Medication	Dosage Range	Comments
Vasoconstrictor	Dopamine Hydrochloride	2–50 mcg/kg/min IV	Titrate to dose to desired effect USE ONLY AFTER ADEQUATE FLUID VOLUME STATUS HAS BEEN ACHIEVED
Inotropic agent	Dobutamine Hydrochloride	2.5–15 mcg/kg/min MAX: 40 mcg/kg/min	Titrate to dose to desired effect USE ONLY AFTER ADEQUATE FLUID VOLUME STATUS HAS BEEN ACHIEVED
Vasoconstrictor	Epinephrine	1–10 mcg/min	Titrate to dose to desired effect
Vasoconstrictor	Norepinephrine	0.5–1.0 mcg/min	Titrate to dose to desired effect
Vasodilator	Sodium nitroprusside	0.3–10 mcg/kg/min	Titrate to dose to desired effect
Vasodilator	Nitroglycerine	5 mcg/min	Titrate to dose to desired effect desired
Inotropic agent	Amrinone	Loading dose 0.75–3 mg/kg Maintenance dose 2–15 mcg/kg/min	Titrate to dose to desired effect
Inotropic agent	Milirione	Loading dose 50 mcg/kg Maintenance dose 0.375–0.75 mcg/kg/min.	Titrate to dose to desired effect

Special Considerations
- Early treatment of cardiac dysrhythmias and restoration of normal heart rhythm can potentially prevent development of cardiogenic shock.

- Patient should be moved to the critical care area as soon as possible.
- Modified Trendelenburg position may not be appropriate for the treatment of cardiogenic shock due to the possibility of pulmonary edema or underlying respiratory disease.

Follow-up

EXPECTED OUTCOMES
- Goal of care is to identify and treat the cause to restore adequate mechanical heart pumping, cardiac output, and blood pressure.
- Even with treatment, the mortality rate for cardiogenic shock is 50% to 75%.

COMPLICATIONS
- Kidney damage and acute tubular necrosis, cardiac damage, liver failure, respiratory damage and ARDS, clotting abnormalities such as DIC, and brain damage such as stroke and encephalopathy may be caused by the decrease in delivery of oxygen and nutrients to tissues and organ systems.

OBSTRUCTIVE SHOCK

Description
- A condition resulting from the blockage of blood flow to the lungs

Etiology
- Conditions such as pulmonary embolism, pericardial tamponade, dissecting aortic aneurysm, and tension pneumothorax can predispose the development of shock symptoms due the underlying decrease of perfusion of oxygenated blood to the tissues and organs.
- Symptoms are caused by decreased preload rather than myocardial dysfunction.

Incidence and Demographics
- Higher incidence of aortic aneurysm in patients with history of hypertension

Risk Factors
- Blunt chest trauma can cause cardiac tamponade or tension pneumothorax
- Immobility
- Hypertension

Prevention and Screening
- Recognize disease syndromes or situations that may predispose the patient to mechanical obstruction of blood flow.

Assessment

HISTORY
- Chest or abdominal pain
- Recent trauma to chest or extremity
- Extended immobility

PHYSICAL EXAM
- Dyspnea
- Tachycardia
- Cyanosis
- Pleuritic pain
- Hemoptysis
- Pulsus paradoxus: > 10 mm Hg decrease in systolic BP on inspiration
- Distant, muffled heart sounds (pericardial tamponade)
- Pericardial friction rub
- Tracheal deviation (tension pneumothorax)
- Bradycardia

DIAGNOSTIC STUDIES
- Chest x-ray for pneumothorax
- Ultrasound to view pericardial sac or arterial structures
- Perfusion lung scans and pulmonary angiography
- CT of chest and abdomen

Nursing Management

NONPHARMACOLOGIC TREATMENT
- Removal of mechanical obstruction through surgical intervention or invasive procedure
  - Insertion of chest tube or needle decompression to remove trapped air and relieve tension pneumothorax
  - Needle pericardiocentesis to remove blood from pericardial sac to allow full cardiac pumping to resume
  - Surgical embolectomy for pulmonary embolism
  - Surgical repair of aortic aneurysm

PHARMACOLOGIC TREATMENT
- Anticoagulation therapy such as heparin for pulmonary embolism

Special Considerations
- Continuous monitoring of preload is essential to enhance survival from dissecting aortic aneurysm repair.
- Continual assessment of airway stability is necessary under conditions of tracheal deviation and increased intrathoracic pressure as seen in tension pneumothorax.

Follow-up

EXPECTED OUTCOMES
- Goal of care is to identify and treat the cause of obstruction to restore adequate cardiac output and blood pressure.
- Even with treatment, mortality from the development of dissecting and repair of aortic aneurysms is high.

COMPLICATIONS
- Kidney damage and acute tubular necrosis, cardiac damage, liver failure, respiratory damage and ARDS, clotting abnormalities such as DIC, and brain damage such as stroke and encephalopathy may be caused by the decrease in delivery of oxygen and nutrients to tissues and organ systems.

ANAPHYLACTIC SHOCK

Description
• A severe, whole-body allergic reaction that results in overwhelming vasodilatation and hypotension.

Etiology
• An antigen-antibody reaction to an allergen triggers the sudden release of histamine causing overwhelming vasodilatation of arterioles and constriction of bronchioles, resulting in hypotension and bronchospasms.

Incidence and Demographics
• Anaphylactic reactions can occur in all genders, ages, and populations.

Risk Factors
• Known allergies to insect bites, venoms, foods, medications, vaccines, environmental agents, anesthetic agents, latex, or diagnostic contrast dyes
• Family history of allergies

Prevention and Screening
• Avoidance of know allergens
• Skin-testing new medications, latex, and food or drug additives can identify the allergen to prevent future episodes of anaphylaxis

Assessment

HISTORY
• Known allergy
• Itching
• Sensation of tingling or warmth
• Shortness of breath
• Cough
• Nasal congestion
• Lightheadedness or dizziness
• Palpitations
• Difficulty breathing or swallowing
• Diarrhea, nausea, or vomiting

PHYSICAL EXAM
• Respiratory distress: wheezing or shortness of breath
• Hypotension
• Hoarseness
• Hives (urticaria)
• Generalized erythema
• Flushed appearance
• Rapid or irregular heart rate
• Altered level of consiousness
• Angioedema (swelling of face, lips, neck or throat)
• Vomiting or diarrhea

- Abdominal pain
- Anxiety or sense of impending doom

DIAGNOSTIC STUDIES
- Symptoms are usually treated first
- Skin testing for specific allergen

Nursing Management

NONPHARMACOLOGIC TREATMENT
- Identify and remove causative agent
- Assuring adequate airway
- Monitor respiratory rate, pulse rate, blood pressure, and level of anxiety as indicators of oxygenation status
- IV access
- If bee sting, remove stinger by gently scratching it out; do not squeeze or pinch to grasp the stinger, which may release additional toxin

PHARMACOLOGIC TREATMENT
- Oxygen
- If available, personal emergency allergy medication (such as EpiPen) should be administered immediately
- Antihistamine such as diphenhydramine (Benadryl)
- Epinephrine for bronchodilitation and vasodilatation
- Corticosteroids to reduce allergic response

Special Considerations
- Do not use oral medications if patient is having any difficulty swallowing or breathing.
- Patients known to have anaphylactic allergic reactions should wear medical alert jewelry (such as MedicAlert bracelet) and carry emergency allergy medications (EpiPens).

Follow-up

EXPECTED OUTCOMES
- Although anaphylaxis is a severe, life-threatening disorder, prompt treatment can be life-saving.
- Re-establishment of adequate oxygenation and cardiac output.
- Patient will name causative agent if known and verbalize proper treatment.
- Follow-up for testing and severity of reaction if allergen cause not known.

COMPLICATIONS
- Airway blockage due to bronchoconstriction
- Cardiac arrest due to anoxia
- Respiratory arrest due to anoxia

NEUROLOGIC SHOCK

Description
- A decrease in tissue perfusion despite adequate circulating volume and cardiac output as a result of increased vascular space and decreased vasoconstriction capabilities. This occurs most commonly in injuries that disrupt the vascular sympathetic response, resulting in a sudden decrease in peripheral vascular resistance, increased vascular space, and decreased blood pressure.

Etiology
- Causes include spinal cord injury, spinal anesthesia, epidural block, severe pain, and decreased vasomotor center function.

Incidence and Demographics
- Can occur in any age or gender group, but spinal trauma is more common in adolescents and young adults

Risk Factors
- Spinal trauma
- Hypoperfusion of spinal cord during surgery, leading to ischemia
- Degenerative spine changes that interfere with blood flow to the spinal cord

Prevention and Screening
- Education in trauma prevention, particularly head and spine, can help reduce the incidence of neurogenic shock.
- Early identification of spinal shock and symptoms of developing spinal shock can decrease the progression.

Assessment

HISTORY
- Spinal cord injury
- Spinal or epidural anesthesia administration
- Decrease in sweating ability
- Lightheadedness
- Loss of motor/sensory function at T6 level and below

PHYSICAL EXAM
- Skin warm and dry due to loss of sympathetic response
- Hypotension
- Severe bradycardia due to loss of sympathetic response to low cardiac output
- Loss of ability to sweat above injury

DIAGNOSTIC STUDIES
- X-ray of chest and spine to assess bony structure integrity
- CT scan to assess bony structures
- MRI for assessment of soft tissue injuries

Nursing Management

NONPHARMACOLOGIC TREATMENT
- Supine position with legs elevated approximately 12 inches to facilitate venous return to central circulation

PHARMACOLOGIC TREATMENT
- Oxygen to create high level of availability for perfusion
- Vasopressors to promote vascular constriction to increase venous return to heart and thereby increase in cardiac output
- Atropine to increase heart rate for enhanced cardiac output
- Judicious fluid resuscitation if cause of neurogenic shock symptoms is transient, such as anesthetic agent effects, which will decrease with time

Special Considerations
- Patients with spinal cord trauma are prone to the development of autonomic dysreflexia. Knowledge of causative factors such as full bladder, rectal impaction, pain below the level of injury, and temperature changes can decrease the occurrence of symptoms.
- If cause is transient, closely monitor fluid volume replacement to prevent development of pulmonary edema.

Follow-up

EXPECTED OUTCOMES
- Increased vascular tone in blood vessel walls
- Complications of lack of perfusion to tissues will be prevented

COMPLICATIONS
- Kidney damage and acute tubular necrosis, cardiac damage, liver failure, respiratory damage and ARDS, clotting abnormalities such as DIC, and brain damage such as stroke and encephalopathy may be caused by the decrease in delivery of oxygen and nutrients to tissues and organ systems.

SEPTIC SHOCK

Description
- A progressive disease that occurs when an overwhelming infection produces vasodilatation with subsequent decreased cardiac output and inadequate perfusion of oxygenated blood to essential tissues and organs

Etiology
- Sepsis causes life-threatening low blood pressure and hypoperfusion.

Incidence and Demographics
- Approximately 750,000 new episodes of sepsis occur each year. If not treated aggressively, these cases can progress to septic shock.
- Septic shock has a 40% mortality rate.
- Although all age groups can develop septic shock, it is more common in the elderly.

Risk Factors

- Extreme age
- General debilitation
- Chronic diseases such as diabetes, chronic renal failure, hepatitis
- Malnutrition
- Immunocompromised, such as from cancer, HIV, alcohol abuse
- Invasive catheters such as central venous access devices or endotracheal tubes
- Surgical and diagnostic procedures, particularly those such as cystoscopy and endoscopy with a high potential for bacterial cross-contamination
- Chemotherapy, steroid or antibiotic therapy

Prevention and Screening

- Meticulous monitoring for signs of early shock symptom development in patients with risk factors
- Meticulous handwashing before procedures and cleansing of invasive catheter sites
- Peptic ulcer prophylaxis
- Monitor for signs and symptoms of catheter-associated urinary tract infections
- Avoid excessive catheterizations, change catheter drainage system, and maintain unobstructed drainage of urine

Assessment

HISTORY
- Fever
- Chills
- Cough
- Presence of risk factors
- Nausea
- Recent or current infection

PHYSICAL EXAM
- Phase 1: warm phase (early stage)
  - Fever
  - Hyperthermia
  - Tachycardia
  - Generalized weakness
  - Nausea, vomiting, diarrhea
- Phase 2: cool phase (late stage)
  - Cold, clammy
  - Bradycardia
  - Hypotension
  - Altered level of consciousness
  - Decreased GI motility

DIAGNOSTIC STUDIES
- Culture all body fluids and potential sources of infection such as sputum, blood, urine, invasive lines such as IV and central venous access devices, and in-dwelling urinary catheters.
- Lactic acid level to monitor for acidosis.

- Renal profile to assess renal function.
- Liver profile to monitor for liver dysfunction.
- PT/PTT monitor for coagulation abnormalities.
- CBC in presence of leukocytosis and thrombocytopenia.
- C-reactive protein (CRP) level more than two standard deviations above normal. A high or increasing amount of CRP suggests acute infection.
- Glucose level; hyperglycemia occurs in the septic patient as a result of the inflammatory response. Glycemic control in all septic patients is essential to decrease mortality.

Nursing Management

NONPHARMACOLOGIC TREATMENT
- Cultures to identify source and control infection
- Modified Trendelenburg position to facilitate venous return to central circulation
- Monitor vital signs and urinary output for effectiveness of treatment

PHARMACOLOGIC TREATMENT
- Oxygen: high flow to facilitate availability
- Antibiotics: broad-spectrum until specific appropriate antibiotic is determined by culture results
- IV fluids to maintain adequate central venous pressure of 8 to 12 mm Hg, urine output > 0.5 mL/kg/h
- Medications for treating septic shock are listed in Table 17–3.

Table 17–3. Medications for Treating Septic Shock

Therapeutic Effect	Medication	Dosage Range	Comments
Vasoconstrictor	Dopamine Hydrochloride	2–50 mcg/kg/min IV	Titrate to dose to desired effect USE ONLY AFTER ADEQUATE FLUID VOLUME STATUS HAS BEEN ACHIEVED
Inotropic agent	Dobutamine Hydrochloride	2.5–15 mcg/kg/min MAX: 40 mcg/kg/min	Titrate to dose to desired effect USE ONLY AFTER ADEQUATE FLUID VOLUME STATUS HAS BEEN ACHIEVED
Vasoconstrictor	Epinephrine	1–10 mcg/min	Titrate to dose to desired effect
Vasoconstrictor	Norepinephrine	0.5–1.0 mcg/min	Titrate to dose to desired effect
Antithrombotic	Xigris	24 mcg/kg/hr infused over 96 hours	Exact action is not completely understood, but believed to act as an anti-inflammatory, antithrombotic, and profibrinolytic agent that assists in the survival of some patients

Special Considerations

- Early diagnosis of sepsis and aggressive treatment improves the septic shock survival rate. Initiation of treatment within 6 hours of onset of symptoms has been found to be the most effective.

Follow-up

EXPECTED OUTCOMES

- Find, treat, and eliminate the source of infection.
- Maintain and support hemodynamic status of adequate BP and heart rate to allow adequate oxygen perfusion of tissues.

COMPLICATIONS

- Most common complications of sepsis and septic shock are multisystem organ failure (MOF; see next section) and disseminated intravascular coagulation (DIC).

MULTISYSTEM ORGAN FAILURE (MOF)

Description

- A condition in which two or more organ systems exhibit progressive or severe failure.

Etiology

- Cause is prolonged hypoxia and hypoperfusion of organ tissues, resulting in functional failure of the organ system.

Incidence and Demographics

- Increased incidence in the elderly and patients with preexisting organ dysfunction
- Increased incidence in persons with decreased functional reserves and impaired stress response

Risk Factors

- Shock
- Sepsis
- Transfusion reactions
- Major surgical procedures

Prevention and Screening

- Identification of those patients at risk for developing multiple organ system dysfunctions can assist in the initiation of necessary treatment of underlying disease in an attempt to prevent the progression of the organ dysfunction.

Assessment

HISTORY

- Any condition that predisposes patient to tissue hypoxia

PHYSICAL EXAM

- Signs of organ failure in the following systems:
  - Respiratory: ARDS
  - Cardiac: low cardiac output, decreased myocardial function

- Hepatic: liver failure
- Renal: acute renal failure, decreased urine output, and increased creatinine
- Coagulation: DIC
- Neurologic: confusion, coma

DIAGNOSTIC STUDIES
- CBC
- Arterial blood gases (ABG)
- PT, PTT, fibrinogen levels
- Renal studies
- Liver studies
- Cardiac enzymes
- ECG

Nursing Management

- There is no specific nursing treatment for MOF.
- Management of MOF involves interventions to support the dysfunctional organ systems to allow for possible reversing of damage to organ tissues.
- Infection control measures, monitoring of hemodynamic parameters, and monitoring for response to treatment.

Special Considerations

- The nurse can be instrumental in preventing MOF through strict monitoring of patient status, early identification of the development of any shock symptoms, and interdisciplinary care of the patient.

Follow-up

EXPECTED OUTCOMES
- Re-establishment of organ system functioning is the desired goal.
- Approximately 40% of patients with septic shock will die from multisystem organ failure, despite appropriate treatment.

COMPLICATIONS
- Death due to system failures and loss of hemodynamic equilibrium.

REFERENCES

Hirasawa, H., Oda, S., & Nakamura, M. (2009). Blood glucose control in patients with severe sepsis and septic shock. *World Journal of Gastroenterology, 15*(33), 4132–4136.

Ignatavicius, D. D., & Workman, M. L. (2010). *Medical-surgical nursing: Patient-centered collaborative care.* St. Louis, MO: Saunders/Elsevier.

Morton, P. G., & Fontaine, D. K. (2009). *Critical care nursing: A holistic approach.* Philadelphia: Wolters Kluwer/Lippincott Williams & Wilkins.

Wagner, K. D., Johnson, K. L., & Hardin-Pierce, M. G. (2010). *High-acuity nursing* (5th ed.). Upper Saddle River, NJ: Pearson Education.

Wilson, B. A., Shannon, M. T., Shields, K. M., & Stang, C. L. (2009). *Prentice Hall nurse's drug guide 2009.* Upper Saddle River, NJ: Pearson/Prentice Hall.

8

Eyes, Ears, Nose, & Throat Disorders

Paula Harrison Gillman, MSN, RN, A/GNP, BC

GENERAL APPROACH

- Problems involving the eyes, ears, nose, and throat often are disregarded in a medical-surgical setting, being overshadowed by more important or life-threatening issues.
- It is important, however, for the medical-surgical nurse to have a basic understanding of these problems because recognizing and treating them can enhance patient comfort (conjunctivitis, allergic rhinitis), improve patient safety (vision impairment), and in some cases, ongoing treatment of chronic conditions may be necessary to prevent complications (glaucoma).

RED FLAGS

- Eyes
  - Sudden vision loss is a medical emergency. Such symptoms may herald a stroke (amaurosis fugax) or could lead to blindness (acute angle closure glaucoma).
  - See Table 18–1.

Table 18-1. Indicators of Vision-Threatening Disorders

Symptoms	Signs
Blurred vision that does NOT clear with blinking	Ciliary flush
Acute loss or decreased vision	Corneal damage (opacities, trauma)
Halos around sources of light	Abnormal pupils
Flashing lights	Increased intraocular pressure
Sudden floating spots or sensation of "cobwebs" across field of vision	Shallow anterior chamber
Photophobia	Proptosis (forward displacement of the eye globe within the orbit)
Periocular headache	Severe green-yellow discharge, eye erythema, chemosis, and lid edema
Ocular pain	Absent red reflex
Nystagmus	

- Ears
  - Poor hearing may be improved by examining and removing cerumen from the ear canals.
  - A perforated tympanic membrane is a contraindication to cerumen removal.
  - Pain, bloody discharge.
- Throat
  - A sore throat (pharyngitis) has multiple possible causes: dry mucous membranes; infection; postnasal drip; gastroesophageal reflux disease; mechanical irritation (from endotracheal or nasotracheal tubes); or may be referred pain from the head, neck, or chest.
  - Severe pain or swelling that causes dysphagia.

Common Disorders of the Eyes

CONJUNCTIVITIS

Description
- Acute inflammation of the conjunctival layer of the eyes
- Commonly known as "pink eye"
- May occur in one or both eyes

Etiology
- May be due to viral, bacterial, allergen, or chemical exposures.
- Also can occur as a manifestation of systemic disease such as varicella, psoriasis, or autoimmune disorders.

Incidence and Demographics
- Common eye disorder in all ages
- Increased incidence in spring and fall due to allergens and viral infections

Risk Factors
- Exposure to allergens, infectious agents, difficulty blinking

Prevention and Screening
- Frequent handwashing
- Artificial tears may be used in persons who cannot blink (such as post cerebrovascular accident [CVA])

Assessment

HISTORY
- Irritated eyes with redness, discomfort, or itching in one or both eyes
- Crusting of eyelids on awakening
- Blurry vision that clears with blinking

PHYSICAL EXAM
- Check visual acuity, pupil reaction, and extraocular movements
- Injection limited to palpebral and bulbar conjunctiva

DIAGNOSTIC STUDIES
- None routine

Nursing Management

NONPHARMACOLOGIC TREATMENT
- Eye compresses 15 minutes q.i.d.
- Discontinue contact lenses until condition resolves

PHARMACOLOGIC TREATMENT
- Eye drops that are targeted at the cause, whether allergic or bacterial
- Treatment of viral infections involves compresses and care not to spread infections

Special Considerations
- Patients with symptoms that fail to improve should be seen by an ophthalmologist.

Follow-up

EXPECTED OUTCOMES
- Patient will show signs of clearing in expected time frame and have minimal discomfort.
  - Bacterial infections usually clear in 2–4 days with treatment.
  - Viral infections last longer (2–4 weeks).
  - Allergy symptoms may persist as long as exposure to the allergen continues.

COMPLICATIONS
- Potential for spread of infection to surrounding areas

GLAUCOMA

Description
- Produces increased intraocular pressure (IOP) from obstruction of flow of aqueous humor in the anterior chamber of the eye.

Etiology

- The acute closed-angle (CAG) form is caused by sudden obstruction of flow due to occlusion of the trabecular meshwork by the iris (pupil dilation) and may result in damage to the optic nerve and permanent blindness.
- Primary open-angle glaucoma (POAG) develops slowly and is generally asymptomatic but causes progressive loss of peripheral vision.
- Altered eye structure predisposes to development.

Incidence and Demographics

- Primary open-angle glaucoma (POAG) is the second most common cause of blindness in the United States and the leading cause in Blacks.
- Five times more likely to cause blindness in Blacks than in Whites.

Risk Factors

- Family history
  - Race (Black and Native Alaskan for POAG; Asian for CAG)
  - Enlarged optic cup
  - Diabetes
  - Cardiovascular disease

Prevention and Screening

- Measurement of IOP (especially in high-risk persons).
- In severe cases, prophylactic laser procedure may be done to prevent damage to contralateral eye.

Assessment

HISTORY
- CAG: pain, tearing, blurry vision, halos around lights, nausea and vomiting
- PAOG: may be asymptomatic or cause dull ache, mild blurring that worsens when tired

PHYSICAL EXAM
- CAG: diffuse conjunctival injection; ciliary flush; fixed, mid-dilated pupil; lid and corneal edema
- PAOG: Increased cup:disc ratio on funduscopic exam; pupil may be dilated

DIAGNOSTIC STUDIES
- Measurement of IOP (tonometry)
  - CAG: 40–80 mm Hg
  - PAOG: 10–23 mm Hg

Nursing Management

PHARMACOLOGIC TREATMENT
- Multiple eye drops are used to control chronic glaucoma.
- Occasionally oral medications such as acetazolamide (Diamox) also are given.

INTERVENTIONAL TREATMENT
- Laser iridotomy and incisional iridectomy are treatments for acute glaucoma.

Special Considerations
- Medications given in the eye are rapidly absorbed into systemic circulation.
- The nurse must be alert to possible systemic side effects of beta blocker eye drops, which can cause bronchospasm in patients with asthma or chronic obstructive pulmonary disease (COPD) and bradycardia or heart failure in patients with a history of cardiac disease. Absorption of meds can be minimized by having the patient keep eyes closed for 5 minutes after drops are instilled. This action eliminates drainage down the tear duct of the eye.

Follow-up

EXPECTED OUTCOMES
- Patient will demonstrate adherence to medical plan of care to minimize vision loss from uncontrolled disease.

COMPLICATIONS
- Blindness if untreated
- Corneal damage
- Central retinal vein occlusion

AGE-RELATED MACULAR DEGENERATION (ARMD)

Description
- Age-related condition causing loss of central vision

Etiology
- Degeneration of the fovea of the macula
- Two types of disease
  - Wet MD (exudative): associated with leakage of fluid from blood vessels (10% of cases)
  - Dry MD (atrophic): associated with ischemia (90% of cases)

Incidence and Demographics
- Leading cause of severe vision loss in adults over age 75
- Affects 1.75 million people in the United States
- Affects Whites more than other racial groups

Risk Factors
- Older age
- Genetic factors
- History of smoking
- White race
- Obesity
- High intake of vegetable fat
- Others under study: phototoxicity, inflammation, diet

Prevention and Screening
- Macular screening with a new technology measures macular pigment optical density (MPOD) and, along with other risk factors, may identify at-risk persons who might benefit from supplements.

- UV protection
- Supplements and foods containing carotinoids such as lutein and zeaxanthin may slow progression or prevent MD; foods high in lutein include spinach, broccoli, orange juice, grapes, kiwi, zucchini, and corn.

Assessment

HISTORY
- Gradual loss of central vision

PHYSICAL EXAM
- No findings

DIAGNOSTIC STUDIES
- Amsler grid assessment by eye doctor

Nursing Management
- Laser photocoagulation can stabilize vision in patients with wet MD.
- No treatment for the dry type; however, education about control of ischemic risk factors is important: smoking cessation, BP and cholesterol control.

Special Considerations
- Patients with vision loss have more difficulty with self-care and learning new information and routines.

Follow-up

EXPECTED OUTCOMES
- Patient will develop compensatory activities to maintain optimal functioning despite vision loss.

COMPLICATIONS
- Central blindness
- Medication errors
- Falls or other accidents due to poor vision

Common Disorders of the Ears

HEARING LOSS

Description
- Diminished or absent sense of hearing due to mechanical obstruction of sound transmission, neurological impairment, or both

Etiology
- Conductive: impaired transmission of sound through the auditory canal, tympanic membrane (TM), or middle ear (due to ear wax or perforation of the tympanic membrane)

- Sensorineural: caused by dysfunction of the inner ear, 8th cranial nerve, brain stem, or cortical auditory pathways (age-related, noise exposure, or medications)
- Presbycusis: age-related, bilateral, symmetric loss of high-frequency tones resulting from:
  - Atrophy of sensory cells and calcification of membranes in the inner ear
  - Degeneration of 8th cranial nerve
  - Degeneration of cells in the auditory cortex

Incidence and Demographics
- Affects about one-third of persons over age 65
- Prevalence increases with age

Risk Factors
- Frequent middle ear infections
- Noise exposure
- Heredity

Prevention and Screening
- Limit noise exposure or wear hearing protection.
- Avoid ototoxic drugs.
- Hearing screening for persons with symptoms or those at risk

Assessment

HISTORY
- Cannot hear on telephone
- Television volume turned up all the way
- Patient complains that everyone is "mumbling"
- May appear to have memory impairment or lack awareness
- Cough (cerumen occlusion of the ear canals can cause a hacking cough)

PHYSICAL EXAM
- Otoscopic exam for patency of canal and appearance of TM.
- Rinne and Weber (tuning fork) tests are helpful for distinguishing conductive from sensorineural hearing loss.
  - Rinne involves striking a tuning fork and placing on the mastoid bone. The patient indicates when he or she can no longer hear the sound and that time is noted. The tuning fork is then held in front of the ear and again the patient indicates when it can no longer be heard. Under normal circumstances, the air:bone ratio will be 2:1. If sensorineural loss is present, the ratio will be less than 2:1.
  - Weber involves striking a tuning fork and placing it in the middle of the forehead. Sound will lateralize to the ear with a conductive loss, if there is no sensorineural loss. If sensorineural loss is present, sound will lateralize to the better ear.
- Pure-tone audiometry can be checked with a handheld device called The AudioScope™ (Welch-Allyn).

DIAGNOSTIC STUDIES
- Audiometric testing by a licensed audiologist

Nursing Management

NONPHARMACOLOGIC TREATMENT
- Prevention of wax accumulation by application of oil into the ear canals periodically to prevent drying and accumulation of wax
- Use of pocket amplification device (low-cost alternative to hearing aid)
- Hearing aids (cost ranges from $300 to $4,000 per ear)

PHARMACOLOGIC TREATMENT
- None available

Special Considerations
- To improve communication with older adults, the following steps are recommended:
  - Face the patient directly when speaking.
  - Use normal volume and tone and enunciate clearly without exaggerated lip movement.
  - Don't cover your mouth while speaking.
  - If asked to repeat something, try to rephrase the question or instruction using different words.
  - Ensure that hearing aids are in place and batteries are good.
  - Encourage eyeglasses when needed.

Follow-up

EXPECTED OUTCOMES
- Nurse will engage in effective communication with patient.
- Patient will be able to participate in self-care despite hearing loss.

COMPLICATIONS
- Loss of functional ability due to hearing loss
- Social isolation and depression

Common Disorders of the Nose and Mouth

RHINITIS

Description
- Hyperfunction and inflammation of the nasal mucosa

Etiology
- Allergic (AR): IgE-mediated hypersensitivity reaction to seasonal allergens (trees, grass) or perennial allergens (pet dander, mold, cockroaches)
- Vasomotor: unclear cause, possibly an autonomic response causing vascular dilation in the submucosal tissues; can be triggered by odors, eating or drinking, or changes in temperature, humidity, or body position
- Infectious (common cold): reaction to one of several viruses infecting the upper respiratory system

Incidence and Demographics

- About one-fourth of the adult population is affected by allergic rhinitis, costing several billion dollars per year in direct medical costs.
- Nine of 10 patients with asthma also have symptoms of allergic rhinitis, but most patients with AR do not have asthma.
- Infectious rhinitis is also extremely prevalent and occurs more often in persons who have contact with children.

Risk Factors

- Exposure to allergens in susceptible persons
- Exposure to infectious agents

Prevention and Screening

- AR: limit exposure to known allergens
- Vasomotor: limit exposure to known triggers
- Infectious: frequent handwashing; limit exposure to infected individuals

Assessment

HISTORY
AR
- Subjective: sneezing, nasal itching or congestion, rhinorrhea, postnasal drip, itchy or watery eyes
- Family history of atopy (genetic predisposition to develop IgE-mediated hypersensitivity)
- Social history: tobacco use
- Medication review (including herbal and natural preparations): often patients with severe allergy symptoms will be taking multiple over-the-counter (OTC) medications without realizing that they are duplicating ingredients

PHYSICAL EXAM
AR
- Nasal mucosa pale and boggy; enlarged turbinates; often nasal polyps
- Clear, watery nasal discharge
- "Allergic shiners"
- Mouth breathing

DIAGNOSTIC STUDIES
- Diagnosis is made by history and clinical exam.
- Microscopy of nasal discharge reveals eosinophils.
- Radioallergosorbent (RAST) or skin testing can be performed by a specialist to identify specific allergens.

Nursing Management

NONPHARMACOLOGIC TREATMENT
- Avoidance of allergens
- Nasal saline flushes up to 4 times per day

PHARMACOLOGIC TREATMENT
- Antihistamines (loratadine, cetirizine, diphenhydramine)
  - Nonsedating antihistamines are preferred
  - Considerable mental clouding, worsened cognition, and increased risk of falling are possible side effects of the first-generation medications such as diphenhydramine
- Oral decongestants (phenylephrine, pseudoephedrine)
  - Sympathomimetic medications that can cause elevated BP, palpitations, restlessness, insomnia, and anxiety, especially in older adults
- Intranasal anticholinergic (ipratropium bromide 0.03%)
  - Reduces production of nasal secretions
  - Can cause nasal dryness and nosebleeds
- Intranasal glucocorticoids (fluticasone, budesonide)
  - Effectively relieve nasal symptoms
  - May be used daily (most effective) or as needed
  - Side effects may include nasal irritation or bleeding
  - Patients should point spray away from the nasal septum (with chronic use); septal perforations have been reported
- Intranasal cromolyn sodium (NasalCrom®)
  - Must be used frequently (up to 4 times per day)
- Leukotriene modifiers (discussed in asthma management; see Pulmonary System)
  - Also approved to treat seasonal and perennial AR

INTERVENTIONAL TREATMENT
- Immunotherapy
  - Referral to a specialist is needed for persons who do not achieve control with medications
  - Usually reach full effectiveness in 1 year; continued for several years to maintain control of symptoms

Special Considerations
- Antihistamines and anticholinergic medications can cause urinary retention in older men with enlarged prostates.
- Older adults are more susceptible to the adverse effects of oral decongestants (elevated BP, tachycardia).

Follow-up

EXPECTED OUTCOMES
- Patient will verbalize relief of allergy symptoms after starting medications.
- Patient will demonstrate proper technique for using nasal steroids to minimize complications.

COMPLICATIONS
- Progression to sinusitis or infection of the lower respiratory tract
- Exacerbation of asthma or chronic obstructive pulmonary disease (COPD)
- Anaphylaxis can be a rare complication of immunotherapy

SINUSITIS

Description
- Inflammation or infection of the paranasal sinus cavities

Etiology
- Bacterial, viral, or fungal pathogens

Incidence and Demographics
- Affects 31 million Americans each year
- Frequently complicates asthma and cystic fibrosis

Risk Factors
- Anatomic abnormalities: enlarged tonsils and adenoids, deviated septum, nasal polyps
- Rhinitis of any type
- Dental infections or upper-respiratory infections
- Barotrauma
- Immunodeficiency

Prevention and Screening
- Treatment of allergies or other upper-respiratory symptoms
- Daily nasal irrigation with saline
- Increasing fluid intake or ambient humidity to facilitate clearance of secretions

Assessment

HISTORY
- Subjective symptoms: URI symptoms not improving after 10 days, nasal congestion, yellow or green nasal discharge, postnasal drainage and sore throat, facial or dental pain, headache, altered taste or smell, nausea or anorexia
- Social history: tobacco use

PHYSICAL EXAM
- Tenderness over involved sinuses
- Ears: dull TMs common with eustachian tube dysfunction
- Nose: mucosal redness and purulent drainage
- Mouth: red throat and purulent drainage, halitosis
- Chest: possible wheezing or chest congestion

DIAGNOSTIC STUDIES
- None needed
- Computed tomography (CT) of the sinuses may be useful with chronic or refractory symptoms

Nursing Management

NONPHARMACOLOGIC TREATMENT
- Adequate hydration
- Nasal saline spray
- Sleeping with the head of bed elevated for comfort

PHARMACOLOGIC TREATMENT
- Antibiotics
- Nasal steroids
- Oral or nasal decongestants
- Analgesics for face pain or headache

Special Considerations
- Patients should not use topical (nasal) decongestants for more than 3 days to avoid rebound congestion and dependence.

Follow-up

EXPECTED OUTCOMES
- Patient will experience relief of symptoms and clearing of nasal discharge within 2 weeks of medical therapy.
- Patient will take full course of antimicrobial medication as prescribed.

COMPLICATIONS
- Orbital or forehead pain or swelling, severe pain, or vision disturbances constitute a medical emergency.
- Patients who develop symptoms of chronic sinusitis may require intervention by an ENT (ear, nose, and throat) surgeon.

PHARYNGITIS AND TONSILLITIS

Description
- Inflammation of pharyngeal or tonsillar tissue

Etiology
- Group A beta-hemolytic streptococcus is the most concerning pathogen due to potential for complications of scarlet or rheumatic fever or glomerulonephritis.
- 90% due to viral infections.
- Also can be caused by fungal organisms or *N. gonorrhoeae*.
- Inflammation of the posterior pharynx also can be caused by uncontrolled gastroesophageal reflux, sinusitis, or allergic rhinitis.

Incidence and Demographics
- Very common: about 30 million cases/year
- Strep pharyngitis more common in persons under 18 years old during the late winter and early spring

Risk Factors
- Exposure to pathogens
- Living in group settings
- Fatigue or debilitation
- Immunosuppression or diabetes mellitus (fungal)

Prevention and Screening
- Frequent handwashing
- Avoiding ill contacts

Assessment
HISTORY
- Throat pain, pain on swallowing, fever, malaise, headache

PHYSICAL EXAM
- Fever, tachycardia
- Red, swollen tonsils, often with exudate
- Cervical lymph node swelling

DIAGNOSTIC STUDIES
- Rapid strep antigen screen: 50% to 80% sensitivity; > 95% specificity
- Throat culture
- Mono spot test if mononucleosis is suspected
- Complete blood count (CBC) with differential may be needed

Nursing Management
NONPHARMACOLOGIC TREATMENT
- Increase fluids
- Warm salt water gargles
- Throat lozenges
- Rest

PHARMACOLOGIC TREATMENT
- OTC analgesics for throat pain
- Antibiotics for strep
  - Penicillin V (Pen VK) 500 mg b.i.d. or t.i.d. is the drug of choice for streptococcus
  - If allergic to penicillin, erythromycin (E-mycin) 500 mg b.i.d.
  - Alternative treatments: first-generation cephalosporins, azithromycin (Zithromax), clarithromycin (Biaxin)
  - Fungal or other infections are treated with different medications

Special Considerations
- Afebrile persons on antibiotics for at least 24 hours are not considered contagious.
- Persons diagnosed with mono should avoid contact sports for at least 4 weeks to avoid splenic rupture.

Follow-up
EXPECTED OUTCOMES
- Patient will maintain adequate oral intake of fluids and food.
- Patient will complete course of antibiotic therapy as prescribed.

COMPLICATIONS
- Rheumatic fever is a complication of untreated group A beta-hemolytic streptococcus.
- Peritonsillar or retropharyngeal abscess may occasionally develop.
- Rarely, pharyngitis or throat edema will progress to limit the ability to breathe or swallow.
- Infectious spread leading to pneumonia, sepsis, etc.

ORAL CANDIDIASIS (THRUSH)

Description
- Fungal infection of the oral mucous membranes

Etiology
- *Candida albicans* occurs normally in the mouth.
- Reduction in competitive oral microflora leads to overgrowth of *Candida*.

Incidence and Demographics
- Most common in persons with immunosuppression, diabetes mellitus

Risk Factors
- Diabetes
- Immunosuppressive medications or conditions
- Broad-spectrum antibiotics
- Decreased host resistance (stress, malnutrition, alcoholism)
- Using inhaled corticosteroids (ICS) without rinsing mouth after use
- Dentures

Prevention and Screening
- Rinse mouth after using ICS medications
- Clean dentures frequently
- Avoid unnecessary antibiotics

Assessment

HISTORY
- Coated, sore tongue and sometimes throat
- Altered taste
- Often weight loss

PHYSICAL EXAM
- Oral mucous membranes covered with white plaques that easily rub off leaving a red, raw area on mucosa
- Angular cheilitis common

DIAGNOSTIC STUDIES
- Diagnosed by history and exam
- Potassium hydroxide (KOH) preparation for microscopy of plaque may be used
- Differential diagnoses:
  - Exudative pharyngitis

- Leukoplakia

Nursing Management

NONPHARMACOLOGIC TREATMENT
- Frequent brushing of tongue and teeth
- Control of diabetes mellitus

PHARMACOLOGIC TREATMENT
- Topical nystatin (Mycostatin) oral suspension 100,000 units per mL; 4–6 mL (1/2 dose on each side of mouth) q.i.d., keep in mouth as long as possible before swallowing; clotrimazole troches 10 mg 5 x day

Special Considerations
- People with diabetes with poor blood sugar control are more susceptible to *Candida* infections.

Follow-up

EXPECTED OUTCOMES
- Patient will have reduced pain and improved appetite with treatment.
- Patient will verbalize measures to decrease risk of recurrence.

COMPLICATIONS
- *Candida* can spread to the esophagus and cause severe esophagitis.
- Weight loss

REFERENCES

Black, J. M., Hawks, J. H., & Hogan, M. A. (2005). *Medical-surgical nursing: Clinical management for positive outcomes* (7th ed.). Philadelphia: Saunders.

Friedman, D. S., O'Colmain, B. J., Muñoz, B., Tomany, S. C., McCarty, C., de Jong, P. T., et al. (2004). Prevalence of age-related macular degeneration in the United States. *Archives of Ophthalmology, 122*(4), 564–572.

Gillman, P., Parker, P., & Tabloski, P. (2009). *Gerontological nursing review and resource manual* (2nd ed.). Silver Spring, MD: American Nurses Credentialing Center.

Ham, R. J., Sloan, P. D., Warshaw, G. A., Bernard, M. A., & Flaherty, E. (2007). *Primary care geriatrics: A case based approach* (5th ed.). Philadelphia: Mosby.

Law, A. W., Reed, S. D., Sundy, J. S., & Schulman, K. A. (2003). Direct costs of allergic rhinitis in the US: Estimates from the 1996 Medical Expenditure Panel Survey. *Journal of Allergy and Clinical Immunology, 111,* 296–300.

Martidis, A., & Tennant, M. T. S. (2004). Age-related macular degeneration. In A. Yanoff (Ed.), *Ophthalmology.* Philadelphia: Mosby.

National Eye Institute. (2001). *Facts about glaucoma.* Retrieved from http://www.nei.nih.gov/health/glaucoma/glaucoma_facts.asp

Neri, L. (2009). Eye, ear, nose, and throat disorders. In E. Blunt (Ed.), *Family nurse practitioner review and resource manual* (3rd ed., pp. 217–284). Silver Spring, MD: American Nurses Credentialing Center.

9

Integumentary System

Jeanine Goodin, MSN, RN-BC, CNRN

GENERAL APPROACH

- The integumentary system provides protection to the body by functioning as a barrier between the internal and external environments.
- The skin is the largest organ of the body and plays a significant role in maintaining homeostasis by regulating body temperature and maintaining fluid and electrolyte balance.
- The skin also contains receptors for sensation and provides clues to racial and ethnic backgrounds and one's overall health.
- Vitamin synthesis, another important role of the skin, occurs in the epidermis.
- The function, appearance, and texture of the skin can be affected by emotional stress, systemic disease, and direct injury or disease.

RED FLAGS

- Wound or bloodstream infections with methicillin-resistant *Staphylococcus aureus* (MRSA) may lead to organ damage, sepsis, and death.
- When assessing skin lesions, utilize the "ABCD" system (see Physical Exam under Skin Cancer below). A patient who has any lesion with one or more of the criteria present should be referred for further evaluation.

Common Disorders of the Integumentary System

ECZEMA

Description
- Acute lesions consisting of multiple small fluid-filled vesicles that are located on red, edematous skin. When the vesicles rupture, the fluid weeps out and produces a thin crust when it dries on the skin surface. Most common type of eczema is atopic dermatitis.

Etiology
- Individuals with eczema tend to have a variety of abnormal immunologic findings related to genetic defects (such as an elevated IgE antibody).
- May also be triggered by environmental factors, such as excessive skin dryness secondary to a lack of skin proteins.

Incidence and Demographics
- Affects 10% to 20% of children and 1% to 3% of adults
- More than 60% of people affected with eczema develop the rash within the first year of life.
- At least 80% of people affected with eczema have the condition prior to age 5.
- More than 50% of people who develop atopic dermatitis in childhood will experience hand eczema as adults.
- One-third of patients with atopic dermatitis have food allergies.

Risk Factors
- Harsh soaps and detergents
- Solvents
- Low humidity
- Rough wool clothing
- Sweating
- Rubbing
- Occlusive rubber or plastic gloves
- Staphylococcal bacteria
- Repeated wetting and drying of the skin
- Physical trauma (such as digging in the garden with bare hands or handling large amounts of paper)

Prevention and Screening
- Avoid risk factors associated with eczema.

Assessment

HISTORY
- Obtain a completed medical-surgical history that includes information on family history of hypersensitivity reactions and a personal history of food allergies.

PHYSICAL EXAM
- The initial symptom of eczema is generally intense itching.
- Rash follows the itching and is reddened and raised or bumpy.
- Rash itches and/or burns.
- If scratched, the rash oozes and becomes crusty.
- Chronic rubbing of the rash causes thickened plaques of skin to develop.
- Painful cracks may develop over time.
- Most common locations for the rash to appear include the neck and flexor surfaces of the arms and legs.

DIAGNOSTIC STUDIES
- Physical exam
- Microscopic examination of scales from the rash
- Biopsy

Nursing Management

NONPHARMACOLOGIC TREATMENT
- Remove the cause of the skin irritation.
- Prevent dry skin by taking warm (not hot) showers or baths, and using a mild soap or body cleanser.
- Before drying off, apply an effective emollient to the wet skin.
- Avoid tight-fitting, rough, or scratchy clothing.
- Avoid scratching the rash.
- Minimize sweating, which may cause a flare-up of the rash.
- Avoid physical and mental stress.
- Use moisturizing lotions.

PHARMACOLOGIC TREATMENT
- Steroid therapy—topical, systemic, or oral—may be prescribed.
- Diphenhydramine (Benadryl) may be used to treat itching. Monitor for drowsiness, confusion, insomnia, headache, vertigo, photosensitivity, diplopia, nausea and vomiting, and dry mouth.

Special Considerations
- Instruct patients not to use a topical corticosteroid anywhere if an infectious cause of the problem is suspected; the use of a topical steroid will worsen the infection by suppressing the immune response.

Follow-up

EXPECTED OUTCOMES
- Resolution of eczema without development of chronic lichenification or secondary bacterial or viral infections

COMPLICATIONS
- Development of a secondary bacterial infection as a result of scratching and excoriation
- Invasion of the skin by viruses (e.g., herpes simplex)

PSORIASIS

Description
- A chronic scaling disorder of the skin that has underlying dermal inflammation, characterized by reddened, round, and elevated circumscribed plaques covered by silvery white scales.

Etiology
- Psoriasis results from an abnormality in the rate of growth of epidermal cells in the outer layers of the skin. Cells at the basement membrane of the epidermis usually take about 28 days to reach the outermost layer of the skin before being shed. In an individual with psoriasis, the rate of cell division is accelerated and this process is shortened to 4 to 5 days. The immature cells create an abnormal keratin, which causes the formation of thick, flaky cells on the skin surface.
- Psoriasis results from an autoimmune reaction due to overstimulation of the immune system. The antigens responsible for psoriasis have not yet been identified. Langerhans cells in the skin respond to the unknown antigen, which activates the T-lymphocytes, which affect the keratinocytes. This process causes the increase in cell division and formation of plaque.

Incidence and Demographics
- Affects approximately 1% of the U.S. population.
- Occurs more frequently in Whites.
- Affects men and women equally.
- Onset usually occurs in the 20s but may occur at any age.
- Incidence is lower and improvement in patient condition occurs in warm, sunny climates.

Risk Factors
- Alcoholism
- Family history
- HIV
- History of recurrent infections, particularly strep throat
- High stress levels
- Obesity
- Smoking

Prevention and Screening
- Knowledge of risk factors and exposure to infectious processes
- Avoid psoriasis triggers

Assessment

HISTORY
- Collect routine epidemiologic data.
- Family history, including age at onset, description of disease progression, and pattern of recurrences.
- Describe current flare-up of psoriasis.
- Explore precipitating factors.
- Inquire about previous interventions and effectiveness in treatment.

PHYSICAL EXAM
- Appearance of the disease and its course varies among patients.
- During flare-ups of psoriasis, lesions thicken and extend to new areas of the body.
- Lesions become thinner with less scaling in response to treatment.
- Psoriasis vulgaris: most common type of psoriasis; presents with thick, reddened papules or plaques covered by silvery white scales with sharply defined borders. Lesions are symmetric bilaterally. Common areas affected include the scalp, elbows, trunk, knees, sacrum, and outside surfaces of the limbs.

DIAGNOSTIC STUDIES
- History and physical examination
- Skin biopsy

Nursing Management

NONPHARMACOLOGIC TREATMENT
- Ultraviolet (UV) light therapy (includes sunlight and artificial ultraviolet light)
- Daily baths
- Avoid drinking alcohol

PHARMACOLOGIC TREATMENT
- Topical treatments
  - Topical corticosteroids: most frequently prescribed medications for mild to moderate psoriasis
    - Work by slowing cell turnover and suppressing the immune system
    - Reduce inflammation and decreases itching
  - Synthetic form of vitamin D: slows down growth of skin cells
  - Anthralin (Dritho-Scalp): normalizes DNA activity in skin cells
    - Stains on contact
    - May be used in combination with UV light
  - Topical retinoids (tazarotene [Tazorac, Avage]): normalize DNA activity in skin cells and may decrease inflammation
    - Skin irritation is a common side effect
    - May increase sensitivity to light so the patient will need to use sunscreen while taking this medication
  - Calcineurin inhibitors (tacrolimus and pimecrolimus): approved for atopic dermatitis but effective in the treatment of psoriasis
    - Skin irritation is a common side effect
    - May be helpful around areas of thin skin
  - Salicylic acid: produces sloughing of dead skin scales and decreases scaling
    - May be used with other medications to improve effectiveness
  - Coal tar: oldest treatment for psoriasis
    - Used to reduce scaling, itching and inflammation
    - Stains clothing and has a strong odor
  - Moisturizers: won't heal psoriasis but aid in decreasing itching and scaling
    - Ointment-based products are more effective than creams and lotions.

- Oral medications
  - Retinoids (acitretin [Soriatane]): related to vitamin A, and may decrease the production of skin cells
    - Side effects consist of dry skin and mucous membranes, itching, and hair loss
    - May also cause severe birth defects; women must avoid pregnancy for 3 years after discontinuing the medication
  - Methotrexate: decreases the production of skin cells and suppresses inflammation
    - Side effects include upset stomach, decreased appetite, and fatigue
    - Long-term use may cause severe liver damage and decreased production of white and red blood cells and platelets
  - Cyclosporine: immune system suppressant
    - Increases risk of infection and cancer, and susceptibility to kidney disease and hypertension
  - Hydroxyurea: may be combined with UV therapy
  - Not as effective as methotrexate and cyclosporine
  - Side effects include anemia and decrease in white blood cells and platelets
  - Avoid this medication if patient is pregnant or planning to become pregnant
- Injectable medications: include immunomodulator drugs approved for moderate to severe cases of psoriasis
  - Used for patients who have not responded to traditional therapy or have psoriatic arthritis
  - Work by stopping interactions between specific immune system cells
  - Have a strong effect on the immune system; may cause serious infections
  - These medications include:
    - Alefacept (Amevive)
    - Etanercept (Enbrel)
    - Infliximab (Remicade)
    - Ustekinumab (Stelara)

Special Considerations

- There is no cure for psoriasis. Treatment goal is to manage flare-ups of psoriasis and improve patient comfort.
- Patients with psoriasis must be educated on avoiding triggers to minimize flare-ups of the disease.

Follow-up

EXPECTED OUTCOMES

- Treatment will be effective in managing flare-ups of psoriasis and the patient will remain free of side effects from the treatment.

COMPLICATIONS

- Anxiety
- Depression
- Fluid and electrolyte imbalance (severe pustular psoriasis)
- Low self-esteem
- Social isolation
- Stress
- Thickened skin and bacterial skin infections resulting from scratching to relieve itching

COMMON INFECTIONS OF THE SKIN

Description
- Skin infections occur when there is a break in the surface of the skin, an infectious agent, and/or decreased resistance resulting from a compromised immune system. See Table 19–1 below for a description of the types of common skin infections.

Table 19–1. Common Skin Infections

Classification	Type	Clinical Manifestations	Distribution
Bacterial	Folliculitis	A bacterial infection of the hair follicle, often caused by *Staphylococcus aureus*. The infection extends from the follicle opening to down into the follicle. Lesions appear as isolated erythematous pustules occurring individually or in groups.	Found most often in areas of hair-bearing skin, primarily on the scalp, buttocks, thighs, and beard area.
	Furuncle	Commonly known as a "boil" and often begins as folliculitis. Also caused by *Staphylococcus aureus*. Lesion appears as a deep, firm, red, painful nodule 1–5 cm in diameter and develops into a large, tender, cystic nodule that produces purulent drainage.	Found most often in areas of hair-bearing skin, primarily on the buttocks, thighs, abdomen, posterior neck, and axillae.
	Cellulitis	A localized area of inflammation and infection of the dermis and subcutaneous tissue. The affected area is red, warm, edematous, tender, and painful. Blisters are rarely present. Often accompanied by fever, chills, malaise, headache, and lymphadenopathy.	Commonly found on the lower legs, areas of frequent lymphedema, and areas of skin trauma.
	Impetigo	A bacterial infection of the skin, often caused by *Staphylococcus aureus* or beta-hemolytic streptococci. Infection usually begins with a vesicle or pustule that ruptures, with an open area producing a honey-colored serous drainage that forms a crust. Additional vesicles form within hours, and the pruritus that accompanies the infection causes the infection to spread. More commonly seen in children than in adults.	May be found anywhere on the skin surface.

cont.

Table 19–1. Common Skin Infections (cont.)

Bacterial	Methicillin-resistant *Staphylococcus aureus* (MRSA)	Common cause of folliculitis and furuncles. Easily spread to other body areas and other people by direct contact with infected skin and contact with personal items used by someone infected with MRSA. Does not respond to cleansing with antibacterial soaps or to most topical and many oral antibiotics. Serious complications or death may result if MRSA infects a wound or gains access to the bloodstream. Incidence of infection is highest among adults living in communal environments and in the hospital or other residential healthcare settings.	May be found anywhere on the skin surface.
Viral	*Herpes simplex*	Vesicles are present in groups with a erythematous base. Vesicles develop into pustules which rupture, weep, and form a crust. Lesions are associated with itching, stinging, or pain and immunocompromised patients may develop a secondary bacterial infection with necrosis.	Type 1 generally appears on the face and type 2 on the genitalia, but either may develop in any area where the person was exposed to the infection. Recurrent infections reappear in the same skin area.
	Herpes zoster	Also known as shingles. Lesions similar in appearance to herpes simplex. Grouped lesions present unilaterally in an area of skin along a cranial or spinal nerve pathway. Deep pain and itching precedes eruption of lesions and immunocompromised patients may develop a secondary bacterial infection with necrosis. Postherpetic neuralgia is a common complication affecting older patients.	Face, trigeminal nerve, and eye, or the anterior or posterior trunk.
	Warts	Common; benign epithelial growths resulting from human papillomavirus (HPV). Warts are flesh-colored papules or plaques with small black dots present.	May be found anywhere on the skin surface.

Fungal	Dermato-phytosis	Single or multiple annular or serpiginous patches with raised border, scaling, and area of central clearing. Often accompanied by itching. Examples: tinea pedis (athlete's foot); tinea cruris (jock itch), and tinea capitis (fungal infection of the scalp).	Tinea pedis: affects the feet. Tinea cruris: affects the groin; upper, inner thighs; and buttocks. Tinea capitis: affects the scalp. Additional variations of fungal infections may affect other areas of the body.
	Candidiasis	Isolated pustules or papules at the border with erythematous macular eruption. Associated with itching and burning. In the oral cavity, lesions (thrush) appear as creamy white plaques on an inflamed mucous membrane. Cracks may be present at the corners of the mouth.	Commonly affects skin-fold areas: perineal and perianal regions, axillae, beneath breasts, between fingers, and beneath wet or occlusive dressings. Lesions also may be present on the oral or vaginal mucous membranes.

Etiology
- See Table 19–1.

Incidence and Demographics
- Impetigo affects about 1% of children.
- 85% of the population has antibody evidence of herpes simplex virus type 1 infection.
- Herpes simplex virus type 2 infection is the source of 20% to 50% of genital ulcerations.
- Herpes zoster (shingles) affects approximately 10% to 20% of adults, often those who are immunocompromised.
- Approximately 5% of the population is affected by warts.

Risk Factors
- Immunosuppression
- Minor skin trauma
- Poor hygiene
- Preexisting skin disease
- Exposure to an individual affected by a skin infection

Prevention and Screening
- Handwashing.
- Avoid offending organisms.
- Maintain good personal hygiene to remove organisms before infection occurs.
- Avoid sharing personal items with others.

- Zostavax vaccine for older adults who have had chickenpox but do not currently have shingles.

Assessment

HISTORY
- Collect a detailed history, including recent activity indicating possible source of exposure to skin infection.

PHYSICAL EXAM
- Thorough examination of the affected skin surface and healthy skin

DIAGNOSTIC STUDIES
- Skin biopsy
- Bacterial, viral, or fungal culture
- Potassium hydroxide preparation
- Direct fluorescent antibody (DFA)
- Serology

Nursing Management

NONPHARMACOLOGIC TREATMENT
- Small furuncles and cellulitis may be treated with warm compresses 3 to 4 times a day.
- Large furuncles may require incision and drainage.
- Herpes zoster: rest, analgesics, and compresses to affected areas in addition to antiviral therapy.
- Warts: cryosurgery, electrodesiccation, curettage, or laser therapy may be used.

PHARMACOLOGIC TREATMENT
- Bacterial skin infections
  - Folliculitis: topical treatment with clindamycin 1% or erythromycin 2% and an antibiotic wash
  - Furuncles, impetigo and cellulitis: oral antibiotics
    - Cephalexin
    - Clindamycin
    - Dicloxacillin
    - Erythromycin
- Viral skin infections
  - Acyclovir
  - Famciclovir
  - Valacyclovir
- Warts
  - Trichloroacetic acid, salicylic acid, podophyllin, and cantharadin (Canthacur)
  - Imiquimod cream (Aldara) may be used for venereal warts.
- Fungal skin infections
  - For most patients, treatment with a topical preparation is adequate if applied twice daily for 6 to 8 weeks. Preparations include terbinafine (Lamisil), clotrimazole (Lotrimin, Mycelex), and econazole (Spectazole).
  - Thrush: nystatin suspension or clotrimazole troches 4 to 6 times a day

Special Considerations
- Prompt recognition of skin infections is essential to effective treatment.
- Nursing care for the patient with a skin infection is directed toward preventing the spread of infection and restoring skin integrity.
- Instruct patient to follow good handwashing practices to reduce the spread of infection.
- Isolation precautions may be implemented to prevent the spread of infection to other patients.
- Follow standard precautions when handling soiled dressings or linens and use sterile technique when changing dressings.
- Educate patients to maintain good nutrition to facilitate wound healing.

Follow-Up

EXPECTED OUTCOMES
- Complete resolution of bacterial infections, fungal infections, and warts; remission of viral infections.

COMPLICATIONS
- Assess the patient for an increase in infection, which would be evidenced systemically by fever, tachycardia, chills, and malaise. Local response would include an increase in erythema, increase in the size of the lesion, and drainage.
- MRSA does not respond to cleansing with antibacterial soaps or most topical and many oral antibiotics. Serious complications or death may result if MRSA infects a wound or gains access to the bloodstream.

PARASITIC INFECTIONS OF THE SKIN

Description
- Skin infestations occur most commonly in people who are homeless, have poor hygiene, or live in substandard housing conditions. See Table 19–2 for a description of the types of common skin infestations.

Table 19-2. Common Infestations of the Skin

Type	Description/Clinical Manifestations	Distribution
Pediculosis	This is an infestation by human lice. The three types include pediculosis capitis (head lice); pediculosis corporis (body lice) and pediculosis pubis (pubic lice or crabs). Human lice are oval in shape and 2–4 mm in length. The eggs (nits) are deposited at the hair shaft base. Pruritus is the most common symptom. In the case of pediculosis corporis, the only visible sign of infestation is the presence of excoriations on the trunk, abdomen, or extremities.	Found most often in areas of hair-bearing skin, with each type generally located in its named area. Pediculosis pubis also may be found in the axillae, eyelashes, and chest.

cont.

Table 19–2. Common Infestations of the Skin (cont.)

Scabies	A mite infestation that results in a contagious skin disease. Transmitted by close and prolonged contacted with an infested person or bedding. Mites may be carried by pets. Symptoms include curved or linear ridges in the skin, which are caused by the mite burrowing into the outer layers of the skin. Hypersensitivity reaction to the mite is evidenced by excoriated erythematous papules, pustules, and crusted lesions on the elbows, wrist, between the fingers, nipples, lower abdomen and waist, penis, buttocks, thighs, shoulder blades, and axillary folds. The itching is reported to be more intense than with pediculosis, especially at night.	Found most often between the fingers and on the palms and inner aspects of the wrists.

Etiology
• See Table 19–2.

Incidence and Demographics
• Pediculosis occurs more frequently in women than men.
• In the United States, an estimated 6 million to 12 million infestations of pediculosis capitis occur each year among children ages 3 to 11 years.
• Infestations are less common among Blacks than other races.
• All socioeconomic classes and climates are affected.

Risk Factors
• Crowded conditions
• Homelessness
• Poor hygiene
• Prolonged contact with infested persons, bedding, towels, or furniture
• Sharing personal items such as hats, scarves, hair accessories, brushes, or combs
• Substandard living conditions

Prevention and Screening
• Handwashing.
• Avoid offending organisms and persons infested with the organisms.
• Maintain good personal hygiene.
• Avoid sharing personal items with others.

Assessment

HISTORY
• Inquire about recent close contact with others who may be infested.
• Inquire about previous interventions and effectiveness in treatment.

PHYSICAL EXAM
• Pediculosis: presence of eggs (nits) on the hair shaft, close to the scalp; complaints of intense itching; presence of adult lice in the affected area
• Scabies: appearance and distribution of the rash and presence of burrows on the skin

- Scabies: microscopic examination of the mite or its eggs or fecal matter

Nursing Management

NONPHARMACOLOGIC TREATMENT
- Pediculosis
  - Wash all bed linens, pillows, stuffed animals, clothing, and hats in hot water of at least 130° Fahrenheit and dry them on high heat for 20 minutes.
  - Soak brushes and combs in hot water for at least 10 minutes.
  - Seal all bedding, clothing, and unwashable items in airtight plastic bags for 2 weeks.
  - Vacuum thoroughly.
- Scabies
  - All bed linens, clothing, and towels used 3 days before treatment should be washed in hot water and dried on high heat. Alternatively, they may be dry cleaned or sealed in an airtight plastic bag for 3 days to a week.

PHARMACOLOGIC TREATMENT
- Topical treatments: pediculosis
  - Head lice and pubic lice
    - Pyrethrins with piperonyl butoxide (A-200, Pronto, R&C, Rid, Triple X): available over-the-counter
    - Permethrin lotion 1% (Nix): available over-the-counter
    - Malathion lotion 0.5% (Ovide): available by prescription
    - Lindane shampoo 1%: available by prescription
  - Body lice
    - Medication is typically not needed if personal hygiene is maintained and personal items are laundered appropriately.
- Topical treatments: scabies
  - Permethrin cream 5% (Elimite): drug of choice for scabies treatment
  - Crotamiton lotion 10% and Crotamiton cream 10% (Eurax, Crotan)
  - Lindane lotion 1%
  - Ivermectin (Stromectol)

Special Considerations

- On initial acquisition of scabies, the patient generally has no symptoms for the first 2 to 6 weeks of infestation but may still spread scabies to others during this time.
- Patients infested with scabies may continue to itch for several weeks after treatment.
- Children who have pubic lice on the head or eyelashes need to be evaluated for sexual exposure or abuse.
- Patients infested with pubic lice should be assessed for other sexually transmitted diseases.

Follow-up

EXPECTED OUTCOMES
- With treatment, the individual will be completely free of the skin infestation.

COMPLICATIONS
- Human lice may be carriers of disease, such as typhus or recurrent fever.
- Vigorous scratching may break the skin surface, resulting in a secondary infection.

SKIN CANCER

Description
- Skin cancer develops when skin cells become damaged. See Table 19–3 for a description of the common types of skin cancer.

Table 19-3. Common Types of Skin Cancer

Type	Description/Clinical Manifestations	Distribution
Actinic keratosis (premalignant)	Small, 1–10 mm macule or papule with dry, rough, yellow or brown scales. Base may be reddened and is associated with yellow, wrinkled, weathered skin. Thick, indurated keratoses are more likely to become malignant. These may disappear spontaneously or reappear after being treated; also may progress slowly to squamous cell carcinoma.	Cheeks, temples, forehead, ears, neck, dorsal surface of hands, forearms
Basal cell carcinoma	A pearly papule with a central crater and rolled, waxy borders. Telangiectasias and pigment flecks may be present. Metastasis is rare and may cause local tissue destruction. There is a 50% recurrence rate due to inadequate treatment.	Sun-exposed areas, especially the head, neck and center of the face
Squamous cell carcinoma	A firm, nodular lesion covered with a crust or a central area of ulceration and indurated margins, adhered to underlying tissue with deep invasion. In 10% of cases, there is rapid invasion with metastasis via the lymphatic system. Larger tumors are more likely to become metastatic.	Sun-exposed areas, especially the head, neck and lower lip; may also occur at the site of chronic irritation or injury
Melanoma	An irregularly shaped, pigmented papule or plaque with variegated colors (red, blue, and white tones). Begins with horizontal growth followed by vertical growth. Rapid invasion and metastasis is associated with high morbidity and mortality. Survival is dependent on early diagnosis and treatment.	May occur anywhere on the body, especially where moles or birthmarks are present. Often found on the upper back and lower legs. In dark-skinned people, often found on the soles of the feet and palms of hands.

Etiology
- The primary cause of skin cancer is overexposure to ultraviolet (UV) light.
- Basal cell carcinomas: genetic predisposition and chronic irritation in addition to overexposure to UV light
- Squamous cell carcinomas: chronic skin damage and overexposure to UV light
- Melanomas: genetic predisposition, excessive exposure to UV light, and the presence of one or more precursor lesions

Incidence and Demographics
- The most common form of cancer in the United States.
- Incidence is highest among light-skinned races and people over age 60
- Higher incidence among people who work outdoors or live at higher altitudes and lower latitudes.
- Higher incidence among sunbathers.
- More than 2 million basal and squamous cell skin cancers are diagnosed annually in the United States.
  - Basal cell skin cancer is more common, accounting for more than 90% of all skin cancer in the United States.
- Approximately 2,000 people die annually due to basal and squamous cell skin cancers, with the death rate decreasing 30% over the past 30 years.
- Melanoma incidence has increased over the past 30 years but still accounts for less than 5% of skin cancer cases.
- Melanoma is more than 10 times more common in Whites than in Blacks.
- Melanoma is slightly more common in men than in women.

Risk Factors
- Actinic keratosis
- Age (risk increases with increased age)
- Alcohol intake (basal cell carcinoma)
- Blond or red hair
- Blue or green eyes
- Bowen's disease
- Certain types of moles, presence of multiple moles
- Chronic skin inflammation or skin ulcers
- Diseases that make the skin sensitive to the sun
- Exposure to the sun or to arsenic or other chemical carcinogens
- Family history of skin cancer
- History of sunburns at a young age
- Immune suppression
- Inadequate niacin (vitamin B_3) in the diet
- Infection with certain human papillomaviruses (nonmelanoma cancers)
- Lighter natural skin color
- Male gender (nonmelanoma cancers)
- Personal history of skin cancer
- Pigmentation irregularities
- Radiation therapy
- Scars or burns on the skin
- Skin that burns, freckles, reddens easily, or becomes painful in the sun
- Smoking (squamous cell carcinoma)

Prevention and Screening
- Avoid midday sun (midmorning to late afternoon) whenever possible.
- Avoid sunlamps and tanning beds.
- Avoid sunburns.
- Ensure diet is adequate in vitamin B_3.
- Examine skin monthly for possible cancerous or precancerous lesions.
- Have skin cancer screenings done annually by a healthcare professional.

- Protect skin from the sun and UV radiation: wear long sleeves and long pants made of tightly woven fabrics, a wide-brimmed hat, and sunglasses that absorb UV radiation.
- Use sunscreen lotions with a sun protection factor (SPF) of at least 30.

Assessment

HISTORY
- Family history of skin cancer; past surgery for removal of skin growths
- Recent changes in the size, color, or sensation of any birthmark, mole, scar, or wart
- Geographic regions where the patient has lived and current residence
- Occupational and recreational activities occurring outdoors
- Occupational exposure to chemical carcinogens
- Inquire if skin lesions are continuously irritated by rubbing

PHYSICAL EXAM
- Systematically assess the patient for unusual lesions (birthmarks, moles, scars, warts).
- Assess hair-bearing areas of the body.
- Palpate lesions to assess texture.
- Document the location, size, color, and surface details of lesions.
- Note subjective reports of itching or tenderness associated with lesions.
- Utilize the ABCD system of evaluating all lesions for possible melanoma.
  A: Asymmetry of shape
  B: Border irregularity
  C: Color variation within a single lesion
  D: Diameter greater than 6 mm
- Any lesion with one or more of the ABCD features should be evaluated by a dermatologist or surgeon.

DIAGNOSTIC STUDIES
- Skin biopsy

Nursing Management

NONPHARMACOLOGIC TREATMENT
- Surgery is the most common intervention for treating all types of skin cancer.
  - Cryosurgery: local application of liquid nitrogen to isolated lesions
  - Curettage and electrodesiccation: used for small, nonmelanoma types of skin cancer to destroy cancerous cells while minimizing damage to surrounding tissue
  - Excision: used to biopsy small lesions
    - Mohs' surgery: specialized form of excision used for squamous and basal cell skin cancers
    - Laser surgery: use of a laser beam to remove a surface lesion
    - Wide excision: used for deep melanoma or other types of skin cancers that involve removing full-thickness skin around the lesion
    - Dermabrasion: removal of the top layer of the skin using a rotating wheel or small particles

- Radiation therapy: used in older patients with deep, large, invasive basal cell carcinomas and patients who are not surgical candidates; also may be used for melanoma patients with metastatic disease who have been treated with systemic corticosteroids

PHARMACOLOGIC TREATMENT

- Topical chemotherapy
  - 5-fluorouracilcream (Efudex, Fluoroplex): used for treatment of multiple actinic keratoses and widespread superficial basal cell carcinoma
  - Photodynamic therapy: treatment using a drug that is activated when a certain type of laser light is shined on the skin; used to treat basal cell carcinoma and actinic keratoses
  - Biotherapy with interferon: accepted treatment after surgery for melanomas at Stage III or higher

SPECIAL CONSIDERATIONS

- Early detection and secondary prevention is critical to survival when melanoma is diagnosed.
- Patients need to be instructed to be aware of their skin markings.
- A total body spot map is helpful to keep track of existing lesions and to identify changes in lesions earlier.
- Patients need to be instructed to perform a thorough skin self-examination (TSSE) monthly.
- Monthly TSSE is critical for patients who have been diagnosed previously with melanoma.
- When lesions are present, they should be monitored annually by a dermatologist.

Follow-up

EXPECTED OUTCOMES

- Nonmelanoma skin cancer is generally curable with early detection.
- If detected early, most melanomas may be cured with minor surgery.

COMPLICATIONS

- Tenderness and discomfort associated with procedures used to treat various types of skin cancer
- Metastasis may occur with melanoma.

PRESSURE ULCERS

Description

- Tissue damage that occurs when the skin and underlying soft tissue are compressed for an extended period of time.
- Pressure ulcers may appear on any body surface, but are commonly found on bony prominences.
- There are 5 stages of classification for pressure ulcers. See Table 19–4 for a description of these stages.

Table 19–4. Pressure Ulcers

Stage	Description/Clinical Manifestations
Stage I	The affected area is over a bony prominence, is intact but reddened and does not blanche with pressure. In lightly pigmented skin, it is a defined area of persistent redness. In people with darker skin tones, the skin may have persistent red, blue, or purple tones.
Stage II	Skin is not intact; partial-thickness loss of skin involving the dermis or epidermis is present. The wound is superficial and may be described as an abrasion, shallow crater, or blister.
Stage III	Full thickness skin loss occurs with damage extending down to but not through the underlying fascia. Bone, tendon, and muscle are not exposed. Subcutaneous tissue may be necrotic or damaged, and the depth of the wound can vary based on anatomic location. Undermining or tunneling may or may not be present depending on the extent of the wound.
Stage IV	Full thickness skin loss occurs with exposed or palpable bone, muscle, or tendons. Undermining and tunneling are often present and sinus tracks may develop. Slough and eschar tissue are seen frequently with this level of pressure ulcer.
Unstageable	Full thickness skin loss occurs. The base is completely covered with eschar tissue or slough, so the true depth of the wound bed is unknown.

Adapted from *Updated staging system* by National Pressure Ulcer Advisory Panel, 2007, retrieved from http://www.npuap.org/pr2.htm

Etiology
- Tissue compression impedes blood flow to the skin and results in decreased tissue perfusion and oxygenation. These factors contribute to cell death.

Incidence and Demographics
- Develops in 3% to 14% of hospitalized patients.
- Hospitalizations involving patients with pressure ulcers increased by almost 80% between 1993 and 2006.
- For hospitalizations in which pressure ulcers was the primary diagnosis, 1 in 25 admissions resulted in death.
- For hospitalizations involving pressure ulcers as a secondary diagnosis, the death rate was 1 in 8.
- In 2006, the average hospital stay was 5 days and cost approximately $10,000. During the same year, the average pressure-ulcer related stay extended to between 13 and 14 days and the cost ranged from $16,755 to $20,430.

Risk Factors
- Chronic medical condition that affects blood flow
- Decreased mental awareness
- Excessive skin moisture
- Fragile skin

- Friction
- Limited mobility
- Older age
- Protein malnutrition
- Residence in a nursing home
- Sensory impairment
- Shear
- Smoking

Prevention and Screening

- Reposition patient every 2 hours to provide pressure relief.
- Use pillows, positioning devices, and sheepskin to decrease pressure.
- Eat healthy, well-balanced meals.
- Ensure patient drinks adequate amounts of water daily.
- Exercise daily. For immobile patients, provide range of motion exercises for all joints.
- Keep skin clean and dry at all times.
- Assess skin daily.

Assessment

HISTORY
- Identify the cause of skin loss.
- Assess factors that may impair wound healing.
- Inquire about history of previous pressure ulcers or delayed wound healing.
- Determine if the patient has any of the following contributing factors.
  - Altered mental status
  - Diabetes
  - Immobility
  - Inadequate nutrition
  - Incontinence
  - Peripheral vascular disease
  - Prolonged bedrest

PHYSICAL EXAM
- Inspect the entire body, including the scalp, for any areas of pressure or skin breakdown
- According to facility policy, assess the patient using the Braden Scale (as discussed in Chapter 7, Nursing Process) to determine the patient's risk for developing skin breakdown.
- Be sure to assess bony prominences and areas vulnerable to excess moisture.
- Assess the patient's overall general appearance for any problems related to skin health.
- Note body weight and proportion of weight to height for potential risk for pressure ulcer formation and malnutrition.
- Assess overall cleanliness of skin, hair, and nails.
- Assess joint mobility for limited range of motion or loss of mobility.
- When a wound is present, note the following characteristics of the wound:
  - Location
  - Size (length, width, and depth using millimeters or centimeters)
  - Color
  - Extent of tissue involvement

- Cell types in the wound base and margins
- Presence or absence of necrotic tissue
- Exudate
- Condition of surrounding tissue
- Presence of tunneling or undermining
- Presence of foreign bodies
- Frequency of wound assessment is determined by the policies and procedures of the clinical agency or facility, although it should also be done with each dressing change.

DIAGNOSTIC STUDIES
- Bacteria or fungal swab cultures
- Wound biopsy
- Chronic wounds should be checked for cancer
- Lab work: complete blood count (CBC), prealbumin, albumin, total protein levels
- Noninvasive and invasive arterial blood flow studies

Nursing Management

NONPHARMACOLOGIC TREATMENT
- Remove source of pressure to affected area.
- Reposition patient every 15 minutes while in a wheelchair and every 2 hours if in bed.
- Provide support to lower extremities and keep the knees and ankles from touching.
- Avoid raising the head of the bed more than 30 degrees.
- Use pillows, positioning devices, and sheepskin to decrease pressure.
- Use low-air-loss beds or air-fluidized (pressure-reducing) beds to decrease surface pressure to skin.
- Avoid massaging area of the ulcer because this can cause further tissue damage.
- Avoid further trauma or friction to body surface.
- Improve nutritional status to facilitate wound healing.
- Cleanse wound according to ordered guidelines.
- Wound debridement by a specially trained nurse or physician.
- Hydrotherapy.
- Wound care as ordered. Common dressing techniques for wound debridement include:
  - Wet-to-damp saline-moistened gauze
  - Continuous wet gauze
  - Topical enzyme preparations
  - Moisture-retentive dressing
- Commonly ordered dressing materials include:
  - Alginate
  - Biologic dressing
  - Cotton gauze dressing
  - Foam
  - Hydrocolloidal
  - Hydrogel dressing
  - Adhesive transparent film

PHARMACOLOGIC TREATMENT
- Oral broad-spectrum antibiotics (as determined by culture results)
- Skeletal muscle relaxants
- Topical use of human growth factors

INTERVENTIONAL TREATMENT
- Surgical debridement
- Wound reconstruction
- New technologies
  - Electrical stimulation
  - Vacuum-assisted wound closure (wound VAC)
  - Skin substitutes
  - Hyperbaric oxygen

Special Considerations
- Multiple products are available to treat pressure ulcers.
- If a pressure ulcer does not show signs of improvement after 7 to 10 days of treatment or becomes worse, the treatment plan should be reevaluated.

Follow-up

EXPECTED OUTCOMES
- The patient will remain free of wound infection or systemic sepsis.
- The patient will maintain a sufficient caloric intake to support wound healing.
- The patient and caregiver(s) will demonstrate understanding of wound care.
- Pain associated with the wound will be controlled adequately.

COMPLICATIONS
- Cancer
- Cellulitis
- Sepsis, kidney failure, infectious arthritis, and osteomyelitis are associated with chronic pressure ulcers.

REFERENCES

Agency for Healthcare Research and Quality. (2008). *Pressure ulcers increasing among hospital patients.* Retrieved from http://www.ahrq.gov/news/nn/nn120308.htm

American Academy of Dermatology. (2010). *Eczema/atopic dermatitis.* Retrieved from http://www.aad.org/public/publications/pamphlets/skin_eczema.html

Centers for Disease Control and Prevention. (2010). *Parasites—lice—head lice.* Retrieved from http://www.cdc.gov/parasites/lice/head/index.html

Centers for Disease Control and Prevention. (2010). *Parasites—lice—head lice: Treatment.* Retrieved from http://www.cdc.gov/parasites/lice/head/treatment.html

Centers for Disease Control and Prevention. (2010). *Parasites—scabies: Medications.* Retrieved from http://www.cdc.gov/parasites/scabies/health_professionals/meds.html

Centers for Disease Control and Prevention. (2010). *Parasites—lice—pubic "crab" lice: Treatment.* Retrieved from http://www.cdc.gov/parasites/lice/pubic/treatment.html

Centers for Disease Control and Prevention. (2010). *Parasites—scabies: Treatment.* Retrieved from http://www.cdc.gov/parasites/scabies/treatment.html

Cevasco, N. C., & Tomecki, K. J. (2010–20011). *Common skin infections.* Retrieved from http://www.clevelandclinicmeded.com/medicalpubs/diseasemanagement/dermatology/common-skin-infections/#cetable1

Cuzzell, J., & Workman, M. L. (2010). Assessment of the skin, hair and nails. In D. D. Ignatavicius & M. L. Workman (Eds.), *Medical-surgical nursing patient-centered collaborative care.* St. Louis, MO: Saunders.

Cuzzell, J., & Workman, M. L. (2010). Care of patients with skin problems. In D. D. Ignatavicius & M. L. Workman (Eds.), *Medical-surgical nursing patient-centered collaborative care.* St. Louis, MO: Saunders.

National Cancer Institute. (2011). *What you need to know about melanoma and other skin cancers: Risk factors.* Retrieved from http://www.cancer.gov/cancertopics/wyntk/skin/page5.

National Pressure Ulcer Advisory Panel. (2007). *Updated staging system.* Retrieved from http://www.npuap.org/pr2.htm

U.S. National Library of Medicine; National Institutes of Health. (2011). *Pressure ulcer.* Retrieved from http://www.nlm.nih.gov/medlineplus/ency/article/007071.htm

20

Neurologic System

Jeanine Goodin, MSN, RN, CNRN

GENERAL APPROACH

- The nervous system is complex; it controls mobility, sensation, and cognition. Human needs for mobility, sensation, and cognition may be impacted by trauma and diseases involving the brain.
- Neurologic changes related to aging frequently affect mobility and sensation. Slower movement, longer response time, and decreased sensation are motor changes occurring in late adulthood. Disease processes affecting the nerves, bones, muscles, or joints affect motor skills and ability to execute activities of daily living (ADLs). Sensory changes affecting older adults may impinge on their daily activities.
- The normal aging process also affects cognition, specifically the ability to perceive, register, store, and use information. Because of this, it can be difficult to distinguish between age-related changes and symptoms of dementia, depression, and delirium. Cognitive decline often results from an inadequate supply of oxygen to the brain or is due to drug interactions or toxicity. A decline in mental status also may be the result of infection, especially urinary tract infection. Intellect is not affected by aging.
- Primary role of the nurse is to support the patient in restoring these human needs or to aid the patient to adapt to deficits.
- The autonomic nervous system (ANS) innervates multiple body systems and is responsible for their function.

RED FLAGS

- The "worst headache of my life" is typically seen with a subarachnoid hemorrhage. These patients need to be evaluated immediately; this is an emergency.
- A change in a patient's level of consciousness (LOC) is the first indicator of increased intracranial pressure. Changes in the LOC should be immediately communicated to the physician.

Common Disorders of the Neurologic System

CEREBROVASCULAR ACCIDENT

Description
- Also known as a "brain attack," a stroke occurs when there is a change in the normal supply of blood to the brain. There are two types of strokes: ischemic (which includes thrombotic and embolic), and hemorrhagic. Any type of stroke is a medical emergency and should be treated immediately to prevent or reduce neurologic deficit or permanent disability.

Etiology
- Ischemic strokes are caused by the occlusion of a cerebral artery by a clot. A thrombotic stroke is caused by the rupture of plaque inside a cerebral artery, exposing foam cells inside the artery and leading to the formation of a clot at the rupture site. If the clot is large enough, blood flow to the area of the brain supplied by this vessel is interrupted and a stroke occurs.
- Embolic strokes are caused by an embolus or a group of emboli that break off from another area of the body and travel to one of the cerebral arteries. The most common sources of emboli are the heart and carotid artery.
- Hemorrhagic strokes occur when a blood vessel in the brain is damaged, causing bleeding in the brain tissue or the spaces surrounding the brain. The primary causes of a hemorrhagic stroke are ruptured aneurysm or arteriovenous malformation, severe hypertension, and trauma.

Incidence and Demographics
- In the United States, stroke is the leading cause of adult disability and the third most common cause of death.
- There are approximately 795,000 strokes, causing 150,000 deaths, in the United States each year.
- It is estimated that one-fourth of all strokes occur in people younger than 65 years.
- Annually, approximately 55,000 more women than men experience a stroke.
- Men have a higher incidence of stroke through age 84, but women have a higher incidence beginning at age 85.
- Blacks have almost double the risk of a first stroke compared to Whites. Mexican-Americans have a higher incidence of ischemic and hemorrhagic stroke than non-Hispanic Whites.
- The stroke incidence is higher in the "stroke belt," which is located in the southern and southeastern United States.
- 87% of all strokes are ischemic and 13% are hemorrhagic.

Risk Factors

- Atrial fibrillation or heart murmur
- Arteriosclerosis or atherosclerosis
- Brain trauma
- Diabetes mellitus
- Family history of stroke
- Heart surgery
- Heavy alcohol use
- Sudden discontinuation of antihypertensive medications (increases risk of hemorrhagic stroke)
- Male gender
- Migraine headaches
- Obesity
- Older age
- Oral contraceptives
- Use of phenylpropanolamine (PPA), found in antihistamine medications
- Previous stroke or transient ischemic attack (TIA)
- Race (Black, Hispanic, or Native American)
- Sedentary lifestyle
- Elevated serum cholesterol, lipoprotein, triglyceride, low-density lipoprotein
- Sickle cell anemia
- Smoking
- Substance abuse (primarily cocaine)
- Valvular heart disease

Prevention and Screening

- Most strokes can be prevented. The biggest challenge is to educate the public on stroke prevention, the signs and symptoms of stroke, importance of calling 911 with the onset of symptoms, and the 3-hour treatment time for tissue plasminogen activator (tPA).
- Patient education should focus on lifestyle changes to reduce the risk of stroke, especially in patients with predisposing health conditions.
- Management of predisposing health conditions (hypertension, diabetes, obesity, etc.) is essential in the prevention of a stroke.

Assessment

HISTORY

- Obtain a completed medical-surgical history that includes information on risk factors for stroke as well as a complete list of prescription and over-the-counter medications, as well as recreational drug use.
- Obtain information about the patient's social history, including personal habits (e.g., smoking, exercise pattern, diet, use of alcohol and drugs), education, employment, leisure activities, and travel history.
- Obtain a history of what the patient was doing when the stroke symptoms began and determine how the symptoms progressed. Document the history of the stroke's onset, noting time symptoms began.
- Note if the symptoms changed in severity or resolved.

- During the interview, note the patient's level of consciousness and any signs of intellectual or memory difficulties. Also note character of speech and ability to process information.
- Ask the patient or family member about any changes in the patient's ability to read or write, motor or sensory changes, or problems with vision, balance, or gait.

PHYSICAL EXAM
- The patient presenting with acute symptoms of stroke must be evaluated within 10 minutes of arriving at the emergency department. This standard also applies to patients who are hospitalized already for other medical conditions and experience new-onset stroke symptoms.
- Approximately 5% of patients with an acute stroke present with a seizure and up to 30% have a headache. The symptoms of an acute stroke vary and are based on the location of the stroke and the collateral blood supply to the brain.
- The initial assessment includes airway, breathing, and circulation (ABC), assessing gag reflex, and the patient's ability to control secretions.
- Begin with a neurologic assessment. The specialized stroke scale recognized throughout the United States is the National Institutes of Health Stroke Scale (NIHSS). The completed examination measures neurologic function and aids in determining the severity of the stroke.
  - NIHSS score interpretation:
    - 0–1 is normal
    - 1–4 indicates a minor stroke
    - 5–15 indicates a moderate stroke
    - 15–20 indicates a moderately severe stroke
    - > 20 indicates a severe stroke
  - When administering the stroke scare, follow the scale in the order listed. Be sure the score reflects what the patient actually does, not what the examiner thinks the patient can do. (See Table 20–1.)

Table 20–1. NIH Stroke Scale

Category	Description	Score
1a. Level of consciousness (LOC)	Alert	0
	Drowsy	1
	Stuporous	2
	Coma	3
1b. LOC questions	Answers both correctly	0
	Answers one correctly	1
	Both incorrect	2
1c. LOC commands	Obeys both correctly	0
	Obeys one correctly	1
	Both incorrect	2
2. Best gaze	Normal	0
	Partial gaze palsy	1
	Forced deviation	2

3. Visual	No visual loss	0
	Partial hemianopia	1
	Complete hemianopia	2
	Bilateral hemianopia	3
4. Facial palsy	Normal	0
	Minor	1
	Partial	2
	Complete	3
5a. Motor arm left	No drift	0
	Drift	1
	Can't resist gravity	2
	No effort against gravity	3
	No movement	4
	Amputation, joint fusion	UN
5b. Motor arm right	No drift	0
	Drift	1
	Can't resist gravity	2
	No effort against gravity	3
	No movement	4
	Amputation, joint fusion	UN
6a. Motor leg left	No drift	0
	Drift	1
	Can't resist gravity	2
	No effort against gravity	3
	No movement	4
	Amputation, joint fusion	UN
6b. Motor leg right	No drift	0
	Drift	1
	Can't resist gravity	2
	No effort against gravity	3
	No movement	4
	Amputation, joint fusion	UN
7. Limb ataxia	Absent	0
	Present in one limb	1
	Present in two limbs	2
8. Sensory	Normal	0
	Partial loss	1
	Severe loss	2

cont.

Table 20–1. NIH Stroke Scale (cont.)

9. Best language	No aphasia	0
	Mild to moderate aphasia	1
	Severe aphasia	2
	Mute	3
10. Dysarthria	Normal articulation	0
	Mild to moderate dysarthria	1
	Near to unintelligible	2
	Intubated or other barrier	UN
11. Extinction and inattention	No neglect	0
	Partial neglect	1
	Complete neglect	2

Reprinted from *Stroke scales & clinical assessment tools*, 2010, The Internet Stroke Center. Retrieved from http://www.strokecenter.org/trials/scales/nihss.html

- Assess for cognitive problems in addition to changes in the LOC. The LOC may vary depending on the extent of increased intracranial pressure and location of the stroke. Specifically assess for denial of the illness; spatial and proprioceptive dysfunction; and impairment of memory, judgment; and ability to concentrate, problem-solve, and make decisions.
- Note the presence of motor weakness, paralysis, or sensory loss involving one extremity or side of the body. Also assess for neglect, which is common for strokes involving the right cerebral hemisphere.
- The patient's visual ability may be affected by a stroke. Assess for ptosis, homonymous hemianopsia, nystagmus, or complete blindness.
- Assess cranial nerves (CN) V, IX, and X, which affect the patient's ability to chew and swallow as well as the gag reflex. CN VII should be tested to note the presence of facial weakness and CN XII is tested to assess tongue strength.
- A cardiovascular assessment also should be completed because patients with embolic strokes often have a heart murmur, atrial fibrillation or another dysrhythmia, or hypertension.
- Perform a psychosocial assessment: assess the patient's ability to perform activities of daily living (ADLs), reaction to illness, and emotional lability.

DIAGNOSTIC STUDIES
- Computed tomography (CT) and CT angiography (CTA) are the first-line tests when a stroke is suspected. These are ordered to determine the presence of a cerebral hemorrhage. For the patient with an ischemic stroke, these tests will be negative for the first 24 hours, but after this the head CT will show ischemia, infarction, and cerebral edema.
- Magnetic resonance imaging (MRI) may be ordered. This will show the presence of cerebral edema, ischemia, and tissue necrosis sooner than a CT scan.
- MR angiography (MRA) may be ordered to identify the location of aneurysm, vessel rupture, or vasospasm.

- Electrocardiogram (ECG), along with a Holter monitor and an echocardiogram, may be ordered to assist in determining any cardiac causes of a stroke.
- Blood tests: cardiac enzymes, complete blood count (CBC), coagulation studies (PT, PTT, INR), blood glucose.
- Additional studies: single-photon emission tomography (SPECT), transesophageal echocardiogram, carotid artery ultrasound (duplex testing), and transcranial Dopplers (TCDs).

Nursing Management

NONPHARMACOLOGIC TREATMENT
- Monitor for changes in the neurologic assessment or complications associated with stroke.
- Monitor vital signs, including respiratory status every 2 to 4 hours.
- Monitor serum glucose levels and keep within normal range.
- Place patient in the optimal head-of-bed position (e.g., 0, 15, or 30 degrees) and note the patient's response to head positioning. Keep the neck in midline position to facilitate venous drainage.
- Avoid neck flexion and extreme hip and knee flexion to enhance venous drainage. Maintain proper body alignment.
- Orient the patient as needed.
- Keep items in the same place and maintain an environment free of clutter. Place frequently used objects within reach.
- Avoid sensory overload and permit frequent rest periods as needed.
- Encourage the patient to use previously learned skills and to actively participate in his or her care.
- Encourage the patient to increase activity levels as tolerated and to participate in therapy as ordered (e.g., physical therapy, occupational therapy, speech therapy). Instruct the patient to use assistive devices as needed.
- Assess the patient's ability to swallow safely using a dysphagia screen. If the patient does not meet the criteria to swallow safely, obtain an order for a formal evaluation by a speech–language pathologist.
- Ensure that the patient is receiving the correct diet and is seated in a chair or a high Fowler's position during meals and for 30 minutes afterward to reduce the risk of aspiration.
- Keep suction equipment at the bedside at all times.
- Assess for communication difficulties and facilitate clear communication with the patient (e.g., use a communication board, face the patient and speak slowly and clearly).
- A carotid endarterectomy may be performed to remove atherosclerotic plaque from inside the carotid artery. This often is done in patients with 70%–90% occlusion of the carotid artery.
- An extracranial-intracranial bypass may be performed to re-establish blood flow to part of the brain that is affected by a blocked artery. The most common techniques are the superficial middle temporal artery to middle cerebral artery (STA-MCA) graft and the occipital to posterior inferior cerebellar artery (PICA) bypass.
- Cerebral aneurysms may be repaired by either a craniotomy in which the aneurysm is clipped or secured so that it does not rerupture, or a coiling procedure in which the aneurysm is filled with a platinum microcoil and a clot is formed within the aneurysm.

Table 20–2. Pharmacologic Treatment of Stroke

Classification	Name	Route & Dosage	Action	Comments/Nursing Implications
Thrombolytic therapy	Tissue plasminogen activator (tPA)	IV: 0.9 mg/kg over 60 minutes with 10% of dose as an initial bolus over 1 minute. Max dose: 90 mg.	This medication activates plasminogen, which disintegrates the thrombus by breaking down fibrin.	May be administered intravenously or intra-arterially. This is the only drug approved for the treatment of acute ischemic stroke. tPA must be administered within the first three hours following the onset of stroke symptoms.
Anti-coagulants	Warfarin sodium (Coumadin)	p.o.: usual dose 2–10 mg daily with dose adjusted to maintain a PT of 1.2–2 times the control or an INR of 2–3.	Interferes with blood clotting by depressing the synthesis of vitamin K-dependent coagulation factors (II, VII, IX, and X); prevents the growth of existing clots and prevents new clots from developing.	Now considered controversial although widely used in the past. Determine PT and INR prior to administration and monitor daily until the maintenance dose is determined. Ensure that a thorough medication history has been obtained prior to beginning this medication; many drugs interfere with the action of warfarin. A high-fat diet or foods rich in vitamin K will shorten the PT/INR. Fever, extended hot weather, malnutrition, and diarrhea will prolong the PT/INR. The risk of bleeding is increased for up to 1 month following the influenza vaccine. Instruct the patient to take the medication at the same time each day and not to alter the dose or brand of medication.
Antiplatelet agents	Aspirin (Ecotrin)	p.o.: 81–325 mg daily or 650 mg b.i.d.	Antiplatelet action: Inhibits platelet aggregation and may impair hepatic synthesis of coagulation factors VII, IX, and X.	May be used alone or in conjunction with other acute drugs. Give with milk, food, an antacid, or use enteric-coated tablets to decrease gastric irritation. Monitor for salicylate toxicity and discontinue use if the patient shows signs or symptoms of salicylate toxicity.

Clopidogrel (Plavix)	p.o.: 75 mg daily.	Platelet aggregation inhibitor; prevents the binding of adenosine diphosphate to its platelet receptor; prolongs bleeding time.	2007 American Stroke Association best practice guidelines recommend against using Plavix or Ticlopidine alone or in combination with aspirin because these antiplatelet drugs have not been studied on their effectiveness after a stroke. Monitor platelet count and lipid profile periodically. Monitor for and report any signs or symptoms of bleeding, especially when administered in conjunction with another anticoagulant or antiplatelet agent.
Aspirin/ dipyridamole (Aggrenox)	p.o.: 25 mg/200 mg capsule b.i.d.	Antiplatelet action: inhibits platelet aggregation.	Used to reduce the risk of a subsequent stroke following a stroke or TIA. Causes coronary vasodilation and should be used carefully in people with heart disease.
Ticlopidine hydrochloride (Ticlid)	p.o.: 250 mg b.i.d. with food.	Inhibits platelet aggregation and interferes with platelet membrane functioning; bleeding time is prolonged.	Primarily used to decrease the risk of a thrombotic stroke in patients who are unable to tolerate aspirin.
Benzo-diazepine	Lorazepam (Ativan)	IV: 4 mg pushed slowly at 2 mg/min; may repeat dose once if inadequate response after 10 min.	Has antianxiety, sedative, and skeletal muscle relaxant effects mediated by GABA.	Used to manage status epilepticus. Patients > 50 years may have more significant and prolonged sedation with IV lorazepam.

cont.

Table 20–2. Pharmacologic Treatment of Stroke (cont.)

Anti-epileptic drugs (AEDs)	Phenytoin (Dilantin)	p.o.: 15–20 mg/kg loading dose, then 300 mg/day in 1–3 divided doses; may be slowly increased by 100 mg/week until seizures are controlled. IV: 10–15 mg/kg, then 300 mg/day in divided doses.	Inhibits seizure activity by elevating the seizure threshold and/or decreasing the voltage, frequency, and spread of electrical discharges in the motor cortex of the brain.	Oral: Ensure that the sustained release form is swallowed whole; do not administer within 2–3 hours of antacid ingestion. IV: Inspect solution prior to use and give only when clear and without precipitate in solution; inspect the injection site frequently during administration because soft tissue irritation may be very serious. Many other drugs are incompatible with this medication.
	Gabapentin (Neurontin)	Slowly increase dose amount to usual dose of 900–1,800 mg/day in 3 divided doses.	Mechanism of action is unknown; it is a GABA neurotransmitter analog but does not interact with GABA receptors and does not inhibit GABA uptake or degradation.	Separate doses from antacids by 2 hours. Discontinue drug gradually over 1 week because abrupt discontinuation may cause status epilepticus.
	Topiramate (Topamax)	p.o.: Begin with 25 mg b.i.d., increase by 50 mg/week to a maintenance dose of 200–400 mg/day divided b.i.d.	Effectively controls partial onset seizures in adults and children by blocking sodium channels.	Discontinue drug slowly to minimize seizures. Drink at least 6–8 full glasses of water daily to reduce risk of kidney stones. Add additional contraceptives if using hormonal contraceptives. Psychomotor slowing and speech or language problems may develop while taking this medication.

	Levetiracetam (Keppra)	Partial onset seizures: p.o.: 500 mg b.i.d. and may increase by 500 mg b.i.d. every 2 weeks to a max dose of 3000 mg/day. Tonic-clonic seizures: p.o.: 500 mg b.i.d., increase by 1000 mg every 2 weeks to max dose of 3000 mg/day.	Mechanism of action is unknown; a broad-spectrum antiepileptic agent that does not involve GABA inhibition; prevents seizure activity by preventing epileptiform burst firing.	Monitor for difficulty with gait or coordination. Assess for changes in phenytoin blood levels when both medications are ordered. Assess individuals with a history of psychosis or depression for signs and symptoms of suicidal tendencies, suicidal ideation, and suicidality.
Calcium channel blockers	Nimodipine (Nimotop)	p.o.: 60 mg every four hours for 21 days, beginning within 96 hours following a subarachnoid hemorrhage (SAH).	Used to reduce the occurrence of vasospasms in cerebral arteries following a SAH; this calcium channel blocker is relatively selective for cerebral arteries.	If patient is unable to swallow when administering, poke holes in the ends of the capsule and extract the contents into a syringe. Mix the extracted medication with NS and flush down the enteral tube with 30 mL NS. Do not administer IV. Hold if the apical pulse is < 60 and notify the MD.

PHARMACOLOGIC TREATMENT
  • Anticoagulation with heparinoids or low-molecular weight heparin is not effective in acute stroke. It is used to prevent the progression of TIAs or an evolving stroke.

Special Considerations
• The increased longevity of the United States population influences the number and needs of older adult stroke survivors. This population of stroke survivors may have greater needs based on multiple factors (multiple concurrent diseases, multiple medications, limitations in ADLs, and financial situation). Patients who are 80 years old or older with an acute stroke should be carefully evaluated and a treatment plan designed to address each of their needs.

Follow-up
EXPECTED OUTCOMES
  • A patient with a stroke may be discharged within 2 to 3 days to home, a rehabilitation center, or a skilled nursing facility depending on the degree of the disability and the availability of caregiver support. Palliative care is available for patients who have suffered severe brain damage and have no rehabilitative potential.
  • Physical therapy, occupational therapy, and speech therapy may be provided at home or on an outpatient basis.
  • Maximizing the patient's abilities in all aspects of life is the goal of rehabilitation.

COMPLICATIONS
  • Aspiration pneumonia due to dysphagia
  • Pulmonary embolism (PE) and/or deep vein thrombosis (DVT) secondary to immobility
  • Skin breakdown secondary to immobility
  • Recurrent stroke
  • Falls due to unilateral weakness or a loss of balance

PARKINSON'S DISEASE (PD)

Description
• A progressive neurodegenerative disease that affects one's motor ability and coordination. The four cardinal symptoms of Parkinson's disease (PD) are tremor, rigidity, bradykinesia or akinesia (slow or no movement), and postural instability.

Etiology
• PD occurs when the substantia nigra, which is responsible for producing dopamine, degenerates. When dopamine levels are diminished, a person is unable to refine voluntary movements.
• Most people have the primary (idiopathic) form of PD, in which the cause is unknown but thought to be related to environmental and genetic factors.
• A small percentage of people have secondary parkinsonian symptoms from brain tumors, infections, trauma, and certain antipsychotic medications.

Incidence and Demographics
• Affects more than 1.5 million people in the United States.
• Men more often affected than women.

- Symptoms of idiopathic PD generally begin between the ages of 40 and 70; peak onset is in the 60s.
- Young-onset PD occurs between 21 and 40 years.
- Disease progresses faster in people who are older when diagnosed.
- More common in industrialized nations.

Risk Factors
- Exposure to pesticides, herbicides, industrial chemicals and metals
- Drinking well water
- Age > 40
- Reduced estrogen levels

Prevention and Screening
- Knowledge of risk factors and avoidance of exposure to toxins in the environment

Assessment

HISTORY
- Collect data regarding the time and progression of symptoms

PHYSICAL EXAM
- Diagnosis of PD is based on the presence of one or more of the four clinical features on one side of the body (see Table 20–3).
- Symptoms may progress at a variable and unpredictable rate.

Table 20–3. Clinical Features of Parkinson's Disease

Four Primary Clinical Features	Other Clinical Features of PD
Tremor (resting or with movement) Rigidity Bradykinesia/akinesia Postural instability	Altered sensation: pain, burning, coldness Masklike face with decreased blinking Difficulty chewing and swallowing Drooling Dysarthria, slow speech, and voice tremors Depression in 20%–50% of patients Changes in behavior (apathy, mood swings, hallucinations, paranoia, dementia) Slow, shuffling gait with short steps Urinary incontinence Gastrointestinal symptoms: constipation, decreased peristalsis Change in handwriting or micrographia Orthostatic hypotension Skin and hair changes: increased perspiration, oily skin, seborrhea, flushing, changes in skin texture Sleep disturbances with frequent awakenings Sexual dysfunction: male impotence; decreased libido for both genders

DIAGNOSTIC STUDIES
- No specific diagnostic tests for PD.
- Diagnosis of PD is made based on the physical assessment and after other neurologic disease processes are eliminated.
- Responsiveness to levodopa administration.
- CT or MRI may be done to rule out secondary causes of PD.

Nursing Management

NONPHARMACOLOGIC TREATMENT

Table 20–4. Nonpharmacologic Management of PD

Lifestyle Changes	Surgical Management
Good general nutrition Rest periods when needed Exercising—adjust the activity level to meet energy level Avoid stress Physical, occupational, and speech therapy Safety equipment throughout the home to minimize fall risk (railings and banisters throughout the commonly used areas of the home, remove throw rugs and cords on the floor) Adaptive equipment (special grips on utensils) Community assistance as needed (counseling services, Meals-on-Wheels)	Deep brain stimulation Thalamotomy Pallidotomy Subthalamotomy Fetal tissue transplantation

PHARMACOLOGIC TREATMENT

Table 20–5. Pharmacologic Management of PD

Classification	Name	Route & Dosage	Action	Comments/Nursing Implications
	Carbidopa-levodopa (Sinemet)	p.o.: 10 mg/100 mg or 25mg/100mg t.i.d., increased by 1 tablet daily or q.o.d. up to 6 tablets/day.	Carbidopa prevents levodopa from premature conversion to dopamine outside of the brain.	Monitor patient carefully for behavior changes. Assess for off and on phenomenon—may indicate need for adjustments in the dose.

Dopamine agonists	Pramipexole (Mirapex)	p.o.: Begin with 0.125 mg t.i.d. for 1 week then 0.25 mg t.i.d. for 1 week; continue to increase by 0.25 mg/dose t.i.d. every week to a goal dose of 1.5 mg t.i.d.	Dopamine receptor agonist	Monitor for signs and symptoms of orthostatic hypotension, especially when increasing the dose.
	Ropinirole (Requip)	p.o.: Begin with 0.25 mg t.i.d. and increase dose by 0.25 mg t.i.d. each week to goal dose of 1 mg t.i.d.	Dopamine receptor agonist	Give with food to decrease nausea. Monitor for signs and symptoms of ortho-static hypotension, especially when increasing the dose.
Monoamine oxidase B (MAO B) inhibitors	Selegiline (Eldepryl)	p.o.: 5 mg b.i.d. with doses at breakfast and lunch.	Increases dopaminergic activity; interferes with dopamine reuptake at the synapse and inhibits MAO B dopaminergic activity in the brain.	Do not give daily doses exceeding 10 mg/day. Monitor for changes in behavior and for orthostatic hypotension.
	Rasagiline (Azilect)	p.o.: 1 mg/day as monotherapy and 0.5–1 mg/day as adjunctive therapy.	MAO B inhibitor that prevents the enzyme MAO B from breaking down dopamine in the brain; interferes with dopamine reuptake in the brain.	Assess for signs and symptoms of dopaminergic side effects when also taking levodopa. Assess for skin changes that may be indicative of skin cancer.
Catechol O-methyl-transferase (COMT) inhibitors	Entacapone (Comtan)	p.o.: 200 mg with each dose of Sinemet, up to 8 times/day.	COMT inhibitor increases the availability of levodopa in the CNS.	Give simultaneously with each dose of Sinemet. Assess for orthostatic hypotension or wors-ening of dyskinesia or hyperkinesias. Urine may assume a brownish-orange color with medication.

cont.

Table 20–5. Pharmacologic Management of PD (cont.)

Anti-cholinergics	Benztropine (Cogentin)	p.o.: 0.5–1 mg/day and may gradually increase as needed up to 6 mg/day.	IV/IM: 1–2 mg/day.	Diminishes excess cholinergic effect with a decreased level of dopamine. Give with food or immediately after meals to decrease gastric irritation. Improvement in symptoms may occur 2–3 days after initiating medication. Monitor I&Os, especially urinary output and voiding patterns.
Glutamate (NMDA) blocking drugs	Amantadine (Symmetrel)	p.o.: 100 mg 1–2 times/day; begin with 100 mg/day if taking other antiparkinsonism medications.	This antiviral medication has anti-Parkinson properties; mechanism of action may be related to releasing dopamine and other catecholamines from neurons.	Often prescribed with Sinemet to decrease dyskinesias. Maximum response occurs within 2 weeks to 3 months, and may wane after 6–8 weeks of treatment. Assess for changes in symptoms of PD that may develop within 2 days of beginning therapy.

INTERVENTIONAL TREATMENT
- Surgical management (see Table 20–4) may be an option for patients with PD who no longer respond to medications. These surgeries do not cure PD but may help some patients.

Special Considerations
- The progressive, debilitating nature of PD is challenging for many patients, their families, caregivers, and healthcare providers. During the early stages of the disease, many patients are able to live at home with family providing for many of their needs. With disease progression, the patient may require a higher level of care and need placement in a long-term-care facility.
- Health promotion activities are important for patients with PD to incorporate into their daily life. Education on the topics of preventing malnutrition, safety needs, constipation, skin breakdown, and contractures must be given to the patient and caregivers. Information on preventing orthostatic hypotension and proper medication administration is also essential.

Follow-up

EXPECTED OUTCOMES
- Prognosis is poor due to the continual degeneration that affects multiple physiologic systems and their ability to function. The caregiver needs increased support as the patient becomes progressively debilitated. Complete disability generally occurs 10 to 20 years after diagnosis.

COMPLICATIONS
- Pneumonia may result from aspiration, dysphagia, or impaired physical mobility
- Joint contractures
- Physical injuries due to falls
- Malnutrition
- Constipation
- Impaired verbal communication
- Sleep pattern disturbances

SEIZURE DISORDERS

Description
- An abnormal, sudden, and excessive uncontrolled electrical discharge in the brain. Seizure activity may result in a change in the level of consciousness (LOC), motor or sensory functioning, perception, and/or behavior. A seizure may consist of a staring spell lasting as briefly as a second or may be a generalized tonic-clonic seizure that lasts for several minutes. The International Classification of Epileptic Seizures identifies three broad categories of seizure disorders: generalized (involves both cerebral hemispheres from the onset), partial, and unclassified seizures. (See Table 20–6.)
- Epilepsy is defined as two or more seizures experienced by a person, and is a chronic disorder in which a person has repeated unprovoked seizures.

Table 20–6. Classification of Seizures

Category	Seizure Type	Description
Partial	Simple partial seizures	An epileptic seizure that begins in part of one side of the brain. With this type of seizure, the patient may have motor, sensory, autonomic, or psychic symptoms while maintaining consciousness. These seizures may occur as isolated events or may precede complex partial or tonic-clonic seizures.
	Complex partial seizures	These seizures may cause a loss of consciousness for 1–3 minutes. This type of seizure begins in one hemisphere and may spread to both. During these seizures, the person is unaware of the environment and may wander and display oral, hand, or gestural automatic behaviors including lip smacking, chewing, or picking at clothes; eye movements; and changes in speech.

cont.

Table 20–6. Classification of Seizures (cont.)

Generalized	Absence seizures	These seizures are more common in children and are characterized by a brief loss of consciousness lasting 10–15 seconds and may be accompanied by blinking spells or eye fluttering, facial clonus, automatic movements, and/or other features.
	Myoclonic seizures	May involve a single or multiple muscle groups, and may involve one or both sides of the body. These seizures consist of rapid muscular contractions, causing a brief jerking or stiffening of the extremities, lasting for just a few seconds. These often occur early in the morning.
	Atonic seizures	Also known as "drop attacks," these seizures last 1–2 seconds and involve a loss of muscle tone. They may be mild and involve a brief head nod or may be more severe and the patient will fall to the ground. Patients who have this type of seizure should wear helmets. Medication is the only treatment available.
	Tonic seizures	Characterized by a loss of consciousness, an abrupt increase in muscle tone, and autonomic changes lasting from less than 10 seconds to a minute. Commonly occur in clusters when a person is drowsy and during non–rapid eye movement (REM) sleep, occurring multiple times a day.
	Clonic seizures	This seizure type is rare and may be seen in children with a high fever. This type of seizure lasts several minutes and causes muscle contraction and relaxation.
	Tonic-clonic seizures	This is the most common type of seizure, lasts about 2–5 minutes and has two phases. The first is the tonic phase that causes stiffening of the muscles (generally arms and legs) and an immediate loss of consciousness. The second phase is the clonic phase which consists of jerking of all extremities. During this seizure, the patient may be incontinent of urine or stool and bite his or her tongue. The patient may be confused, lethargic, or fatigued for a while after the seizure.
Unclassified		Includes neonatal and nonepileptic seizures

Etiology

- Seizures are classified as being either primary/idiopathic or secondary/symptomatic.
- Idiopathic seizures are not associated with any specific cause or identifiable brain lesion.

- Secondary seizures occur due to an underlying brain lesion. Examples of causes of secondary seizures include:
  - Brain tumor
  - Trauma/head injury
  - Metabolic disorders
  - Acute alcohol or drug withdrawal; substance abuse
  - Electrolyte disturbances: hypoglycemia, hyperkalemia, or water intoxication
  - High fever
  - Stroke
  - Heart disease
- Epilepsy may be caused by abnormal electrical activity in the brain, an imbalance of neurotransmitters (especially gamma aminobutyric acid [GABA]), or both.

Incidence and Demographics

- Epilepsy and seizures affect almost 3 million people in the United States.
- The estimated annual cost is $15.5 billion in direct and indirect costs.
- There are approximately 200,000 new cases of seizures and epilepsy annually.
- Ten percent of the population in the United States will experience a seizure during their lifetime.
- People under the age of 20 have the highest incidence rates of having a seizure, and the incidence of seizures/epilepsy declines until the age of 65.
- Three percent of the population in the United States will develop epilepsy by age 75.

Risk Factors

- History of:
  - Mental retardation
  - Cerebral palsy
  - Perinatal problems (including toxemia, difficulty during the birth process, low birth weight, hypoxia, neonatal seizure)
  - Congenital malformations of the central nervous system (CNS)
  - Toxic and metabolic disturbance
  - Alcohol and/or drug abuse
  - Degenerative diseases: Alzheimer's disease and multiple sclerosis (MS)
  - Stroke, cerebrovascular disease, aneurysm, arteriovenous malformation (AVM)
  - Parent or family member with epilepsy and/or febrile convulsions
  - Head trauma
  - CNS infections
  - Brain tumors
  - Anoxic brain injury
  - Lead poisoning

Prevention and Screening

- Knowledge of risk factors and avoidance of exposure to toxins in the environment

Assessment

HISTORY
- Collect a complete medical history and history of seizure activity, noting if the patient has a history of epilepsy.

- A precise description of the seizure is important because the treatment differs for different types of seizures. Friends and family who witnessed the seizure activity are often better able to provide an accurate description of the event.
- When describing the seizure, be sure to note specific details and any feelings the patient experienced. Also note how the seizure progressed and the duration.

PHYSICAL EXAM
- Assess specific focal findings or any other neurologic abnormalities.

DIAGNOSTIC STUDIES
- Electroencephalogram (EEG)
- Continuous video and EEG monitoring
- Computed tomography (CT)
- Magnetic resonance imaging (MRI)
- Single-photon emission tomography (SPECT)
- Positron emission tomography (PET)
- Laboratory studies: electrolytes, blood urea nitrogen (BUN), arterial blood gas (ABG), toxicology screen, lactic acid level, antiepileptic drug (AED) levels
- Neuropsychologic evaluation and testing

Nursing Management

NONPHARMACOLOGIC TREATMENT
- Seizure precautions are taken to minimize the risk of injury if a seizure occurs.
- Seizure precautions include the following:
  - Oxygen and suction equipment are available.
  - The patient has an IV saline lock available.
  - Side rails in the up position and padded according to hospital policy.
- Seizure first aid needs to be provided to the patient during a tonic-clonic seizure and includes the following:
  - Protect the patient from injury.
  - Position the patient on the floor with the head turned to one side.
  - Remove sharp objects, eyeglasses, and other hard items from the patient and the nearby vicinity.
  - Loosen tight clothing, including the collar or belt.
  - Never apply physical or mechanical restraints.
  - Never place anything into the mouth, including a tongue depressor.
  - Stay with the patient and remain calm.
  - Maintain the patient's airway and suction as needed.
  - After the seizure has ended and the patient regains consciousness, explain to the patient in a calm manner that she/he had a seizure.
  - Record and note the type, duration, and characteristics of the seizure and the postseizure activity of the patient.

PHARMACOLOGIC TREATMENT

Table 20-7. Pharmacologic Treatment of Seizure Disorders

Name	Route & Dosage	Action	Comments / Nursing Implications
Phenytoin (Dilantin)	p.o.: 15–20 mg/kg loading dose then 300 mg/day in 1–3 divided doses; may be slowly increased by 100 mg/week until seizures are controlled. IV: 10–15 mg/kg then 300 mg/day in divided doses.	Inhibits seizure activity by elevating the seizure threshold and/or decreasing the voltage, frequency, and spread of electrical discharges in the motor cortex of the brain.	Oral: Ensure that the sustained release form is swallowed whole; do not administer within 2–3 hours of antacid ingestion. IV: Inspect solution prior to use and give only when clear and without precipitate in solution; inspect the injection site frequently during administration because soft tissue irritation may be very serious. Many other drugs are incompatible with this medication.
Gabapentin (Neurontin)	Slowly increase dose amount to usual dose of 900–1800 mg/day in 3 divided doses.	Mechanism of action is unknown; it is a GABA neurotransmitter analog but does not interact with GABA receptors and does not inhibit GABA uptake or degradation.	Separate doses from antacids by 2 hours. Discontinue drug gradually over 1 week because abrupt discontinuation may cause status epilepticus.
Topiramate (Topamax)	p.o.: Begin with 25 mg b.i.d., increase by 50 mg/week to a maintenance dose of 200–400 mg/day divided b.i.d.	Effectively controls partial onset seizures in adults and children by blocking sodium channels.	Discontinue drug slowly to minimize seizures. Drink at least 6–8 full glasses of water daily to reduce risk of kidney stones. Add additional contraceptives if using hormonal contraceptives. Psychomotor slowing and speech or language problems may develop while taking this medication.
Levetiracetam (Keppra)	Partial onset seizures: p.o.: 500 mg b.i.d. and may increase by 500 mg b.i.d. every 2 weeks to a max dose of 3,000 mg/day. Tonic-clonic seizures: p.o.: 500 mg b.i.d., increase by 1,000 mg every 2 weeks to max dose of 3,000 mg/day.	Mechanism of action is unknown; a broad spectrum antiepileptic agent that does not involve GABA inhibition; prevents seizure activity by preventing epileptiform burst firing.	Monitor for difficulty with gait or coordination. Assess for changes in phenytoin blood levels when both medications are ordered. Assess individuals with a history of psychosis or depression for signs and symptoms of suicidal tendencies, suicidal ideation, and suicidality.

INTERVENTIONAL TREATMENT
- Vagal nerve stimulator
- Corpus callosotomy
- Temporal lobectomy
- Hemispherectomy

REFERENCES

American Heart Association. (2010). *Heart disease & stroke statistics—2010 update.* Retrieved from http://www.americanheart.org/presenter.jhtm?identifier=3000090

Epilepsy Foundation. (n.d.). *About epilepsy & seizures: Epilepsy and seizure statistics.* Retrieved from http://www.epilepsyfoundation.org/about/statistics.cfm

Hausman, K. A., & Ignatavicius, D. D. (2010). Care of patients with problems of the central nervous system: The brain. In D. D. Ignatavicius & M. L. Workman, *Medical-surgical nursing: Patient-centered collaborative care.* St. Louis, MO: Saunders.

Ignatavicius, D. D., & Hausman, K. A. (2010). Care of critically ill patients with neurologic problems. In D. D. Ignatavicius & M. L. Workman, *Medical-surgical nursing: Patient-centered collaborative care.* St. Louis, MO: Saunders.

The Internet Stroke Center. (2010). *Stroke scales & clinical assessment tools.* Retrieved from http://www.strokecenter.org/trials/scales/nihss.html

Wilson, B. A., Shannon, M. T., & Shields, K. M. (2009). *Prentice Hall nurse's drug guide 2009.* Upper Saddle River, NJ: Pearson Prentice Hall.

Review Questions

1. A client is admitted to the hospital with a diagnosis of cholecystitis from cholelithiasis. The client is complaining of severe abdominal pain and extreme nausea and has vomited several times. Based on these data, which nursing diagnosis would have the highest priority for intervention at this time?

    a. Imbalanced nutrition: Less than body requirements related to vomiting.
    b. Anxiety related to sever abdominal discomfort.
    c. Pain related to gallbladder inflammation.
    d. Deficient fluid volume related to vomiting.

2. The nurse plans care for the client with hepatitis A with the understanding that the causative virus will be excreted from the client's body primarily through the:

    a. blood.
    b. urine.
    c. feces.
    d. skin.

3. The nurse teaches the patient with a hiatal hernia or GERD to control symptoms by:

    a. performing daily exercises of toe-touching, sit-ups, and weight-lifting.
    b. spacing six small meals a day between breakfast and bedtime.
    c. drinking 10–12 ounces of water with each meal.
    d. sleeping with the head of the bed elevated on 4- to 6-inch blocks.

4. The nurse determines that further dietary teaching is needed when a patient with dumping syndrome says, "I should . . .

   a. eat smaller meals about six times a day."
   b. lie down for 30–60 minutes after each meal."
   c. avoid drinking fluids with my meals."
   d. eat bread with every meal."

5. A client was hospitalized and treated for acute diverticulitis. The nurse has provided discharge teaching. Which statement by the client indicates that he understands his discharge instructions?

   a. "I'll decrease my fluid intake."
   b. "I'll decrease the fiber in my diet."
   c. "I'll take all of my antibiotics.
   d. "I'll exercise to increase my intraabdominal pressure."

6. Which of the following nurse statements would be therapeutic and likely to promote therapeutic communications?

   a. "Tell me what it is like to live with arthritis."
   b. "Why are you so restless?"
   c. "Here's what I'd do, I'd eat more fruits and whole grains."
   d. "I'm sure the test results will be positive."

7. A patient newly diagnosed with hypertension has been given a prescription to start a hydrochlorothiazide medication. The patient tells the nurse she would rather control her blood pressure with herbal therapy. Which action should the nurse take? Advise the patient to:

   a. discuss using herbal therapy with her physician.
   b. consider herbal therapies as unsafe and not to be used.
   c. give the prescribed medication time to work before using herbal therapy.
   d. monitor her blood pressure more often if she takes herbal therapy.

8. The census is 17 with 5 RNs scheduled. The assignment is posted and you are assigned to provide care to 5 patients, leaving the remaining 4 RNs with 3 patients apiece. This is the third time your assignment has been considerably heavier than the rest of the nurses. What is the best method to handle the situation?

   a. Contact the nursing supervisor and make a formal complaint.
   b. State your dissatisfaction with your assignment to everyone.
   c. Confront the charge nurse regarding your dissatisfaction with your assignment in a professional manner.
   d. Refuse to provide care to your assigned patients, stating that this assignment is putting the patients at risk.

9. A student nurse makes a medication error. Which of the following statements is accurate?

    a. Because the patient was assigned to the faculty by the charge nurse, the charge nurse has sole responsibility.

    b. Because the RN has ultimate responsibility for the patient, the error rests entirely with the RN.

    c. Because the care was assigned by the faculty member, the faculty member has sole responsibility.

    d. Because the care was assigned to the student who completed the medication administration module, the error rests with the student.

10. The nurse and an unlicensed assistive personnel (UAP) are caring for clients on a medical unit. Of the following, which task would be best for the nurse to delegate to the UAP?

    a. Transport a patient to the intensive care unit
    b. Provide a patient with discharge teaching on wound care
    c. Assist a patient to go to the smoking area
    d. Meet with a family member who has concerns about care

11. A patient with a history of myocardial infarction (MI) complains of chest pain while walking to the restroom. Which action should the nurse perform first?

    a. Assess patient's vital signs
    b. Instruct patient to sit down
    c. Obtain a STAT EKG
    d. Call the physician

12. Which assessment finding would the nurse expect to auscultate in a patient with mitral valve insufficiency?

    a. Harsh systolic murmur heard best at the right upper sternal border
    b. Rumbling diastolic murmur heard best at the left lower sternal border
    c. Holosystolic murmur heard best at the cardiac apex
    d. Mid-systolic click and soft diastolic murmur at the cardiac apex

13. A patient with asthma has been prescribed an inhaled corticosteroid for control of her disease. Which patient teaching is most important for this patient?

    a. Use 2 puffs when an attack of wheezing occurs
    b. Do not mix this medication with other inhalers
    c. Rinse mouth and spit immediately after use
    d. Use of this medication should be minimized to prevent side effects

14. Which of the following puts a patient at risk for "pre-renal" acute renal failure?

    a. Hypovolemia
    b. Hypertension
    c. Benign prostatic hypertrophy (BPH)
    d. Intravenous (IV) contrast dye

15. The nurse is discharging a patient with a urinary tract infection (UTI). Which of the following should be included in the discharge teaching?

    a. Limit fluid to decrease irritation to the urethra
    b. Practice postponing voiding to recondition the urinary tract
    c. Take all of the antibiotics as prescribed
    d. Expect continued burning on urination

16. Which of the following would be the most important to discuss with the osteoarthritis patient taking NSAIDs?

    a. Changes in mood
    b. Photosensitivity
    c. Symptoms of GI bleed
    d. Symptoms of immune suppression

17. The nurse is speaking about musculoskeletal trauma to a group of young adults at a health fair. The focus should be on:

    a. bone health.
    b. ergonomic principles.
    c. nutrition.
    d. trauma prevention.

18. The nurse is caring for a patient who has recently been told he has a prognosis of 6 months. The patient tells the nurse "I will do anything to live to see the birth of my granddaughter." The patient is in which stage of grieving?

    a. Acceptance
    b. Anger
    c. Bargaining
    d. Denial

19. A 32-year-old patient is recuperating after a motor vehicle accident resulting in a lower extremity amputation. During physical therapy, he is obviously angry when attempting to place his prosthesis. The nurse should allow him to verbalize his feelings and:

    a. assist him to deal with his anger.
    b. emphasize the importance of cooperating and engaging in therapy.
    c. make a referral to the staff psychiatrist.
    d. reschedule therapy until he is able to control his anger.

20. The nurse is caring for an 82-year-old patient who recently was widowed. The patient frequently uses the call light for a variety of requests, including a total bed bath, assistance with feeding, and having someone dial her telephone. The best intervention to employ would be to:

    a. Comply with the patient's requests in order to get the work done in a timely manner.
    b. delegate the patient's requests to a technician and have a sitter remain at the bedside.
    c. encourage the patient to do as much as possible to maintain her independence and promote her recuperation.
    d. request a referral to a geriatric specialist for an assessment to evaluate cognitive and physical abilities.

21. A post-op patient states that he would prefer to limit the amount of pain medication he takes and asks if there is some other kind of therapy that would help him to control his pain as he recuperates. The nurse suggests:

    a. acupressure.
    b. craniosacral therapy.
    c. imagery.
    d. herbal therapy.

22. When planning an educational program for a group of middle-age adults, the nurse should discuss a topic that:

    a. the nurse feels is important.
    b. is of interest to the group.
    c. is important to the families.
    d. is listed in the Healthy People 2010 report.

23. What type of education does the nurse provide when she shows a video on monthly self-examination of the breast and encourages a group of college-age women to begin monthly self-examination?

    a. Primary prevention
    b. Early detection
    c. Initial screening
    d. Tertiary prevention

24. A dopamine drip may not be helpful in the early treatment of which type of shock?

    a. Hypovolemia
    b. Cardiogenic
    c. Anaphylactic
    d. Septic

25. A 22-year old patient is admitted o the ICU after a motorcycle collision. He is intubated and has a splint on his left lower leg to immobilize a femur fracture. You notice a change in his heart rate from 100 beats/minute to 132 beats/minute and his BP has dropped by 30 mm Hg over the last 20 minutes. His pulse is thready and weak when palpated and his skin is cool to touch. You also notice significant swelling of his left thigh. What type of shock symptoms is the patient exhibiting?

    a. Neurogenic shock
    b. Cardiogenic shock
    c. Obstructive shock
    d. Hypovolemic shock

26. A client presents to the emergency unit after a fall complaining of right leg pain. Which of the following physical assessment techniques would the nurse utilize initially?

    a. Palpate to assess for tenderness
    b. Palpate for dorsalis pedis pulse
    c. Inspection for any obvious deformities or hemorrhage
    d. Interview to assess for date of last tetanus toxoid injection

27. A patient is admitted to the unit from the OR after having a sub-total thyroidectomy completed. The nurse asks the patient whether he is experiencing any numbness of tingling of the face, mouth, or extremities. The rationale for this assessment is for what purpose?

    a. Detection of facial nerve damage
    b. Early identification of hypocalcemia
    c. Early identification of hypothyroidism
    d. Effects of post-op medications

28. A client with type 1 diabetes mellitus presents to the hospital with a blood sugar of 550 mg/dL and complaints of polydipsia, polyuria, ketones in their urine, and weakness. The physician orders insulin to be administered by IV drip and to monitor serum blood sugar levels every 30 minutes. The nurse would expect that the client is experiencing an episode of which of the following?

    a. Diabetic ketoacidosis (DKA)
    b. Hyperglycemic hyperosmolar syndrome (HHS)
    c. Hypoglycemia
    d. Hypothyroidism

29. The nurse is caring for a client who has recently undergone a surgical procedure for thyroid cancer requiring a partial thyroidectomy. The patient is experiencing numbness and tingling in their extremities and a twitch in the face. The nurse would suspect the patient is experiencing which of the following?

    a. Hyperthyroidism
    b. Hyperparathyroidism
    c. Hypoparathyroidism
    d. Hypothyroidism

30. A client is being tested for the presence of pernicious anemia. Which of the following tests would the nurse expect the client to have scheduled?

    a. Schilling test
    b. Serum foliate level
    c. Bone marrow aspiration
    d. Serum total iron-bind capacity

31. While caring for a client with sickle cell crisis, the nurse would identify which of the following as the priority nursing diagnosis?

    a. Altered cardiac output
    b. Alteration in comfort
    c. Fluid volume deficit
    d. Ineffective coping

32. Which of the following activities would be a high-risk activity for contracting HIV?

    a. Drinking from public water fountains
    b. Participating in contact sports
    c. Sharing water glasses at a restaurant
    d. Contracting recurrent sexually transmitted infections

33. When taking the blood pressure of a client with AIDS, the nurse must:

    a. wear clean gloves.
    b. use barrier techniques.
    c. wear a gown and mask.
    d. wear sterile gloves and a face mask.

34. A client has recently been diagnosed with Addison's disease. The nurse is preparing discharge instructions related to diet therapy for the client. Which of the following diets would be the most appropriate diet plan to include in these instructions?

    a. High-fat meal plan
    b. Low-carbohydrate meal plan
    c. Low-protein meal plan
    d. Normal sodium plan

35. A nurse is instructing a patient taking diuretics for heart failure about foods that are high in potassium to include in her daily diet. The nurse concludes that additional education is needed when the client states that the food highest in potassium is:

    a. spinach.
    b. apples.
    c. avocado.
    d. carrots.

36. The nurse is caring for a client with severe vomiting and diarrhea for the last 24 hours. The nurse knows that this client is at risk for which of the following primary acid–base imbalance?

    a. Metabolic acidosis
    b. Metabolic alkalosis
    c. Respiratory acidosis
    d. Respiratory alkalosis

37. A couple is seeking genetic counseling for hemophilia. The wife is known to be a carrier of the hemophilia B trait. The nurse understands that the chance of the couple producing a male offspring with hemophilia B is which of the following?

    a. All of the children will have hemophilia type B.
    b. There is a 50% chance that this offspring will have hemophilia type B.
    c. None of their children will have hemophilia type B.
    d. There is a 25% chance that this offspring will have hemophilia type B.

38. Which of the following statements by a client who has recently seroconverted to a state of being HIV positive but is asymptomatic at the present time will indicate to the nurse a need for further education?

    a. Although I am HIV positive, I do not have to practice safe sex because I do not have any symptoms yet.
    b. I must remember that I can pass on the virus even though I am asymptomatic.
    c. I should not share my disposable razor with my roommate.
    d. I should contact my primary care provider if I develop any rash on my body.

39. Which finding in the client with HIV who is receiving highly affective antiretroviral therapy (HAART) indicates that the treatment is effective?

    a. Increased viral load
    b. Increased CD4 T-cells
    c. Decreased CD4 T-cells
    d. Decreased total WBC count

40. The patient has been prescribed propylthiouracil (PTU) for treatment of hyperthyroidism. When developing a discharge teaching plan, the nurse would include which of the follow information regarding this medication?

    a. Signs and symptoms of diabetes insipidus
    b. Signs and symptoms of hyperglycemia
    c. Signs and symptoms of hypothyroidism
    d. Signs and symptoms of renal toxicity

41. Arterial blood gas results for the client recently admitted to your unit reveals the following: pH 7.30, $PaCO_2$ 43 mm Hg, HCO_3 24 mEq/L, PaO_2 74 mm Hg. Based on these results, the patient would be exhibiting which of the following?

    a. Respiratory acidosis; mild hypoxia; compensated
    b. Respiratory alkalosis; normal oxygenation status, uncompensated
    c. Respiratory acidosis; mild hypoxia; uncompensated
    d. Metabolic alkalosis; mild hypoxia; uncompensated

42. While assessing a patient newly admitted to the nursing unit, the nurse finds distended neck veins, skeletal muscle weakness and pitting edema in the lower extremities. Which of the following physician orders wo,uld the nurse question?

    a. Administration of an osmotic diuretic
    b. Intravenous infusion of normal saline solution at 250 ml/hr
    c. Monitor intake and output each shift
    d. Sodium-restricted diet

43. Which of the following populations would be at higher risk for development of folic acid deficiency?

    a. Young adults
    b. Athletes
    c. Alcoholics
    d. Obese men

44. The nurse has just completed teaching about the disease processes of leukemia. Which of the following statements by the patient indicates an understanding of the disease process?

    a. Leukemia is infectious in nature and characterized by fever and chills.
    b. Leukemia is an inflammatory response and is characterized by the formation of enlarged and solid lymph node tumors.
    c. Leukemia is a disease that is the result of an allergic reaction to an exposure and is characterized by increased circulating antibodies in the blood.
    d. Leukemia is a neoplasm that is characterized by the proliferation of immature white blood cells in my blood and tissues.

45. A hospital employee had an occupational exposure to HIV via an accidently needle stick from a HIV-positive patient. The initial ELISA test was negative. The employee is back in the employee health department for the 6-week follow-up ELISA; those results were also negative. The employee asks the nurse what these findings mean. Which of the following responses represents the best response from the nurse to the employee?

    a. You have not been infected by HIV.
    b. We really still do not know your HIV status; you need to be retested again in 6 weeks.
    c. You probably do not have HIV but should still to return for more follow-up testing.
    d. You probably do not have HIV. We will know for sure when you are retested in 3 months.

Answers to the Review Questions

1. **Correct Answer: C.** Pain is a priority and may be one reason for the nausea and vomiting. Relief of pain may relieve the nausea and vomiting and thus decrease risk for fluid volume deficit.

2. **Correct Answer: C.** Hepatitis is transmitted primarily though feces. Viral hepatitis is not transmitted via the skin or urine. Hepatitis B, C, and D are transmitted through exposure to blood, but hepatitis A is not.

3. **Correct Answer: D.** Keeping the patient's head elevated assists to prevent GERD associated with a hiatal hernia and when the patient is lying supine. Small meals may assist to prevent GERD, but is a difficult regimen to follow and the patient is likely to be non-compliant. Drinking this amount of water could overfill the stomach and increase the symptoms of GERD.

4. **Correct Answer: D.** Dumping syndrome occurs in response to rapid emptying of the stomach into the small intestine. Options a, b, and c discourage the rapid emptying and thus lessen the risk for dumping syndrome. Eating bread with every meal indicates need for more instruction because bread increases the carbohydrate intake of the patient and this increases the (hyper) tonicity of the food bolus and risk of dumping syndrome.

5. **Correct Answer: C.** Continuation of antibiotics is important to promote full healing of the inflamed bowel and minimize risk of perforation. After acute care, the patient should drink a lot of fluids to replace fluids absorbed by the recommended high-fiber diet, but avoid exercise that increases intraabdominal pressure.

6. **Correct Answer: A.** This is an open-ended statement that promotes patient sharing of information. "Why" questions can put the patient on the defensive and stifle conversation. Offering opinions inhibits patient sharing and focuses on the nurse. The final option does not promote patient sharing of feelings, but instead offers possible false reassurance.

7. **Correct Answer: A.** Nurses should encourage patients to report use of herbal therapy so physicians can assist the patient to learn of safety and efficacy issues with non-prescribed therapies. Other options by the nurse bypass the priority first step of supporting the patient to communicate use of herbal therapies to the physician.

8. **Correct Answer: C.** If a nurse has a problem with the assignment, the first rule in confronting management is to talk to the individual you have the conflict with, explaining the problem and listening to the other side. Answer B will not help the nurse, but will cause trouble within the team. Answer A is not resolved.

9. **Correct Answer: D.** Because the student had completed the education module, the error rests with the student. Keep in mind that the student is held accountable to the RN scope of practice when providing care as a student. Also, the faculty has some accountability in this situation. The faculty will need to be able to state that the assignment given to the student was not above the ability of the student.

10. **Correct Answer: C.** The other three patients require skills of the registered nurse. Accompanying the patient to the smoking area is the most appropriate task for a UAP.

11. **Correct Answer: B.** Having the patient sit down reduces myocardial oxygen demand to help relieve pain and take stress off of the heart. The other actions are important, but would come after having the patient sit down.

12. **Correct Answer: C.** Mitral insufficiency or regurgitation is characterized by a holosystolic murmur at the apex.

13. **Correct Answer: C.** Rinsing the mouth after use of inhaled steroids prevents oral candidiasis (thrush). Inhaled corticosteroids are maintenance medications to be used on a regular basis (not for rescue) and can be given with other inhalers.

14. **Correct Answer: A.** Hypovolemia leads to reduced cardiac output and thus pre-renal azotemia. BPH causes post-renal obstruction and HTN and IV contrast lead to intrinsic renal damage.

15. **Correct Answer: C.** Patients with UTI should be advised to finish all antibiotics, as most people stop medication once their symptoms disappear. Dysuria will cease after the first few doses. Recommendations would include increasing fluid intake and voiding immediately when the urge occurs.

16. **Correct Answer: C.** A side effect of NSAIDs is GI irritation, and chronic use of NSAIDs can result in gastritis, ulceration, perforation, and GI bleeding. NSAIDs should be used with caution in patients older than 60, or who have preexisting renal, liver, or blood dysfunction.

17. **Correct Answer: D.** Trauma is the leading cause of death for those ages 1 to 37 in the United States. Young adults are at particular risk for injury, and education should focus on awareness of safety measures to prevent injuries at home, work, or during leisure activities. Ergonomic principles, bone health, and nutrition are all important in maintaining musculoskeletal health across the life span.

18. **Correct Answer: C.** Acceptance, the last stage, involves facing death/loss peacefully; anger, the second stage, involves blaming others and asking why; bargaining, the third stage, involves asking for additional time; denial, the first stage of grieving, allows the individual to gather coping resources.

19. **Correct Answer: A.** In order to progress and adapt to the change in body image, the nurse assists the patient to resolve angry feelings. Cooperating and engaging in therapy can be achieved after anger is resolved. Rescheduling would prevent the patient from moving forward with recuperation.

20. **Correct Answer: C.** Cumulative and interacting effects of risk factors (illness, decreased activity) most significantly affect function and quality of life. By promoting independence and care, the nurse can assist the patient to maintain or return to baseline musculoskeletal strength and function.

21. **Correct Answer: C.** For acute self-limiting pain, imagery, a cognitive-behavioral intervention, allows the patient to visualize pleasant experience. It relieves pain through distraction, increases pain tolerance, produces a relaxation response, and possibly diminishes the source of pain. Craniosacral therapy and acupressure are alternative therapies used for chronic or stress-related pain, not acute pain. Herbal therapies are not FDA-regulated, lack standardization, and may cause interactions with other medications.

22. **Correct Answer: B.** Adult learning theory concepts identify that adult learners are independent, autonomous, self-directed, and goal-oriented. They need to know that what they are learning is relevant and practical. They also build on previous life events.

23. **Correct Answer: B.** Early detection involves education of breast self-exams beginning at the age of 20. Primary prevention involves an action to prevent disease; tertiary prevention involves actions to manage a disease and prevent complications; and initial screening includes actions to identify disease prior to manifestation of symptoms occurs.

24. **Correct Answer: A.** Dopamine (Intropin) is an inotropic drug that will increase heart contractility and cardiac output when an adequate fluid volume is present. In hypovolemic shock, the underlying cause is a decreased circulating volume. Once the circulating volume has been increased, dopamine may be utilized in the later stages of the management of shock to enhance cardiac contractility to increase cardiac output.

25. **Correct Answer: D.** Tachycardia; weak, thready pulse; hypotension; and cool, clammy skin are all signs of the development of hypovolemic shock in the patient. The mechanism of injury for this patient is significant for the potential for significant blood loss into the left femoral region as seen in the swelling of the left thigh, the site of traumatic injury.

26. **Correct Answer: C.** The nurse should inspect the area initially to assess for any obvious bleeding or deformities. Palpation would follow the initial physical assessment of the extremity. Interview is not a physical assessment technique.

27. **Correct Answer: B.** Due to the location of the parathyroid gland in relationship to the thyroid gland, there is a possibility of damage to the parathyroid and a developing decrease in serum calcium levels due to the decrease of release of parathyroid hormone. Indications of hypothyroidism can include numbness and tingling in the face and extremities. The thyroidectomy procedure typically does not cause facial nerve damage and post-op medication side effect of numbness and tingling. The loss or decrease of thyroid hormone does not cause numbness or tingling.

28. **Correct Answer: A.** In a client with type 1 diabetes, an elevated glucose level and ketones in the urine is indicative of diabetic ketoacidosis (DKA). Clients experiencing HHS will not experience the presence of ketones in their urine. Elevated serum glucose levels will not be present in clients with hypoglycemia or hypothyroidism.

29. **Correct Answer: C.** The patient is demonstrating signs of low serum calcium. Numbness, tingling, and positive Chvostek's and Trousseau's signs are indications of hypoparathyroidism. A complication of thyroidectomy surgery can be the destruction or removal of the parathyroid gland and resulting decrease in serum calcium levels.

30. **Correct Answer: A.** Pernicious anemia is the result of inadequate absorption of vitamin B_{12} in the ileum. When undergoing a Schilling test, radioactive vitamin B_{12} is ingested and a dose of non-radioactive vitamin B_{12} is injected several hours later. Urine is collected for 24 hours to determine the presence of absorbed vitamin B_{12}.

31. **Correct Answer: B.** Promoting comfort and a decrease in pain level is a priority in the nursing care of a client with sickle cell crisis. Fluids are administered, either orally or through intravenous means, to prevent vascular occlusion. Altered cardiac output is typically not a problem with a vaso-occlusive process.

32. **Correct Answer: D.** One of the most frequently activities associated with the contracting of HIV is the participation in unprotected sexual activity and contracting multiple cases of sexually transmitted infections. There is a very low incidence of contracting HIV through drinking from public water fountains or sharing drinks. The possibility of contracting HIV through contact sports would only occur with the transfer of significant blood and body fluid exchange through open skin sites or mucous membranes, which does not typically occur.

33. **Correct Answer: A.** The spread of HIV is through direct contact with body secretions. Because this procedure does not involve direct contact with body secretions, additional protection is not necessary. Handwashing should be completed before and after all contact with patients as well.

34. **Correct Answer: D.** The dietary intake for a client with Addison's disease is typically high protein and high carbohydrate due to weight loss and altered metabolism. Due to the need to prevent further fluid and sodium loss, the client is typically advised to maintain normal sodium intake and increase sodium and fluid intake during times of increased hydration needs such as exercise, vomiting, diarrhea, and fever. A high-fat diet would not be appropriate for this client.

35. **Correct Answer: B.** Of the foods listed, the avocado has the highest amount of potassium, followed by spinach and carrots. Apples have the lowest potassium content of those foods listed.

36. **Correct Answer: B.** The loss of hydrogen ions in the form of acids from the body through the gastrointestinal tract will result in a state of metabolic alkalosis.

37. **Correct Answer: D.** Hemophilia is a sex-linked recessive genetic disorder and is passed on by the X chromosome. It is transmitted by the female carrier and exhibited almost exclusively in males. There is a 50% probability that the offspring will be male and a 25% chance that the offspring will be a male and have hemophilia type B.

38. **Correct Answer: A.** Although the client is asymptomatic at the present time, transmission of the virus is possible due to the presence of the virus in body secretions. The client is correct in not sharing any devices that may contain any blood or in being aware of the chance of contracting infections and viruses as a result of his immunocompromised state.

39. **Correct Answer: B.** Effectiveness of the medication therapy can be measured in the increased production of viable and functional CD4-T-cells. An increase in the viral load, decrease in CD4 T-cells, or decreased total WBC count would be an indication of a decline in the client's condition and ineffective treatment measures at the present.

40. **Correct Answer: C.** The use of PTU for the treatment of hyperthyroidism can convert the client to a hypothyroid state if dosage and effectiveness is not closely monitored. PTU does not cause hyperglycemia, diabetes insipidus, or renal toxicity.

41. **Correct Answer: C.** The pH of 7.30 is an indication of an acidotic state. The elevation of the $PaCO_2$ is indicative of a respiratory condition. The bicarbonate level is within normal limits, indicating no compensation has occurred at the present time. The PaO_2 is below normal value, indicating a hypoxic state.

42. **Correct Answer: B.** The patient is exhibiting signs of fluid overload. High volume infusion of normal saline would typically be contraindicated for this patient. The use of diuretics, a sodium-restricted diet to decrease fluid retention, and the monitoring of the patient's intake and output are appropriate interventions.

43. **Correct Answer: C.** Alcohol ingestion impairs foliate metabolism. Additionally, alcoholic individuals are typically undernourished, with a diet lacking in the adequate fresh fruits, vegetables, and fish.

44. **Correct Answer: D.** Leukemia is a neoplasmic condition resulting in the invasion of the blood-forming tissues of the body and proliferation of abnormal white blood cells. This condition is not an infectious, inflammatory, or allergic disease process; rather, it prevents the body from appropriately responding to infectious agents and clotting appropriately.

45. **Correct Answer: B.** Seroconversion can take up to 3 months to occur, depending upon the degree and type of exposure. Initial testing can remain negative for 12 weeks. It is important to remember to not give false reassurance at the 6-week testing.

Index

About the Authors

Nancy Batchelor, MSN, RN-BC, CNS, has been employed in a variety of settings in nursing since 1972. She has a broad base of medical-surgical experience, is certified in medical-surgical nursing, and has a focus in gerontology and palliative care. She has published several articles, book chapters, and continuing education modules in education, gerontology, and palliative care.

Mrs. Batchelor is currently employed as an associate professor of clinical nursing at the University of Cincinnati College of Nursing and maintains clinical practice for Hospice of Cincinnati. She received her MSN and has her CNS in adult health and is currently working toward her Doctorate of Nursing Practice at the University of Cincinnati.

She is an active member of Sigma Theta Tau International, Beta Iota Chapter; the National Gerontological Nurses Association, OKI Regional chapter; and the Hospice and Palliative Nurses Association.

Paula Harrison Gillman, MSN, RN-C, ANP-BC, GNP-BC, currently works as a gerontologic nurse practitioner in an outpatient clinic in Dallas, TX. Prior to her outpatient experience, Paula was a medical-surgical clinical specialist and ICU educator. Throughout her career spanning nearly 3 decades, Paula has worked in a variety of care settings including acute care, sub-acute, rehab, and long-term care. She has also worked in many specialty areas, including critical care, transplant, and post-anesthesia recovery. In addition, she conducted research for a start-up company developing new technology for critical care patients.

Paula loves teaching other nurses and spent 10 years as a clinical instructor at the University of Texas at Arlington (UTA) School of Nursing, where she promoted expertise among the many nurse practitioner students who she helped prepare for practice. In addition, Paula has precepted hundreds of nursing studenmts over her career. She graduated from Baylor University with a BSN in 1984, from UTA with her MSN in 1992, and then completed a post-Master's program as a gerontological and adult nurse practitioner in 1996.

Since 2004, Paula has worked with ANCC to develop and present review programs in medical-surgical and gerontological nursing. She is a co-author of ANCC's *Gerontological Nursing Review and Resource Manual* and holds four ANCC certifications.

Jeanine Goodin, MSN, RN-BC, CNRN, has been a registered nurse for over 18 years, with experiences in general medical-surgical care, critical care, long-term acute care, and rehabilitation. Her primary area of interest is neuroscience, and she remains active as a staff nurse in a large, urban Level 1 trauma center in the Neuroscience Intensive Care Unit. Prior to this experience, she was a Neuroscience Clinical Nurse Specialist and a staff nurse. She received her BSN from the University of Cincinnati in 1992 and her MSN in Adult Health from the Medical University of South Carolina in 1996.

Mrs. Goodin is an Associate Professor of Clinical Nursing at the University of Cincinnati College of Nursing and primarily teaches undergraduate students in the BSN and Accelerated Nursing Programs.

She has served as a contributor and a reviewer for several medical-surgical and critical care nursing textbooks.

Mrs. Goodin is the Vice-President of the Beta Iota Chapter of Sigma Theta Tau International, and is an active member of the Southwestern Ohio Nurses Association. She is also an active member of the American Association of Neuroscience Nurses and has served on several committees at the local and national levels.

Deborah Schwytzer, MSN, RN-BC, CEN, has been a registered nurse for more than 35 years, with experiences in general medical-surgical care as well as emergency, critical care, and peri-operative. She remains active as a staff nurse in a large, urban, Level 1 trauma center both in the Center for Emergency Care and the Post-Operative Care Unit. She holds a Master's of Nursing in Nursing Administration.

Ms. Schwytzer is a faculty member at the University of the Cincinnati College of Nursing, serving as a clinical faculty member primarily in the BSN and Accelerated Nursing Program, as well as presenting didactic content in areas of expertise. She is also the Director of the University of Cincinnati Co-Op Program, which has placed students both at the Cincinnati Children's Hospital Medical Center and the University Hospital. She has been active in the contribution and review of numerous medical-surgical and critical care nursing textbooks.

Ms. Schwytzer has remained active in many professional organizations, such as the Beta Iota Chapter of Sigma Theta Tau International, serving as President of the Southwestern Ohio Nurses Association, and as an officer and on numerous committees at the local, state, and national level of the Emergency Nurses Association.

Jo Nell Wells, PhD, RN-BC, OCN, has been a registered nurse more than 35 years, with consistent work experience in medical-surgical settings.

She received her PhD from Texas Woman's University in Denton, TX. Since 1998, she has taught at Texas Christian University in Fort Worth, TX. She teaches nursing students in the BSN program in pharmacology and medical-surgical content. She is certified in medical-surgical nursing and oncology nursing. She has received awards for teaching and scholarship excellence.

Eileen M. Werdman, MSN, RN-BC, CNS, is an Associate Professor of Clinical Nursing at the University of Cincinnati College of Nursing, where she teaches undergraduate and accelerated pathway adult health (medical-surgical nursing). Ms. Werdman received her diploma from the Good Samaritan Hospital School of Nursing, her BSN from the College of Mount St. Joseph, and her MSN from the University of Cincinnati.

Currently, she is finishing coursework toward her Doctorate of Nursing Practice from the University of Cincinnati. She is also certified by ANCC in medical-surgical nursing. In addition to teaching, she continues to practice as a staff nurse on a medical-surgical unit. In March of 2011, she was elected President Elect to the Ohio League for Nursing, continuing her service on the OLN Board of Directors. She has developed online continuing education modules and has written several hundred NCLEX-style test questions to accompany a textbook.